Healthy Canada

▌◆▌ Health and Welfare Canada   Santé et Bien-être social Canada

CANADA'S
Food Guide
TO HEALTHY EATING

Enjoy a variety of foods from each group every day.

Choose lower-fat foods more often.

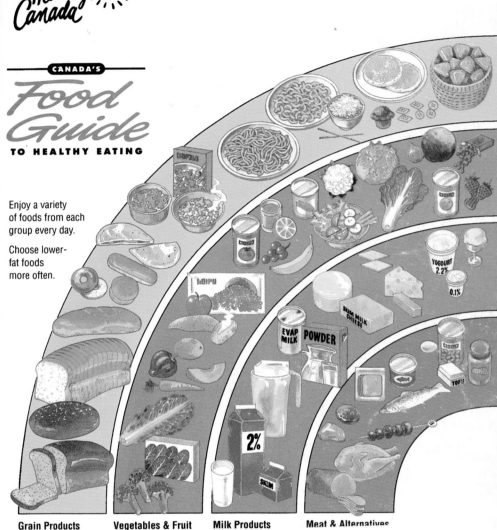

Grain Products
Choose whole grain and enriched products more often.

Vegetables & Fruit
Choose dark green and orange vegetables and orange fruit more often.

Milk Products
Choose lower milk products often.

Meat & Alternatives

Canadä

D1411583

PUTTING BREAD FIRST

Bread is front and centre in the Grain Products Group. Recommended servings per day from this group are now 5 to 12. That's good news you can sink your teeth into!

PREPARATION TIPS

■ Frozen bread toasts just as fast as fresh bread.
■ Busy day? Make a hot sandwich for dinner. Try a quick'n easy tuna melt, or use leftovers for a hot turkey or beef sandwich.
■ Allow frozen bread to thaw at room temperature *inside* its plastic bag. The moisture will then be re-absorbed into the bread.

■ For a complete protein *without* cholesterol, have bread with beans, peanut butter, lentils or peas.
■ French toast can be made ahead and stored in your freezer. Just pop it into the toaster for a great start to a weekday morning.
■ For bread crumbs and croutons, use fresh or leftover bread.

Bakery Council of Canada

tear here

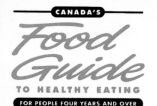
Different People Need Different Amounts of Food

The amount of food you need every day from the 4 food groups and other foods depends on your age, body size, activity level, whether you are male or female and if you are pregnant or breast-feeding. That's why the Food Guide gives a lower and higher number of servings for each food group. For example, young children can choose the lower number of servings, while male teenagers can go to the higher number. Most other people can choose servings somewhere in between.

Grain Products

5–12

SERVINGS PER DAY

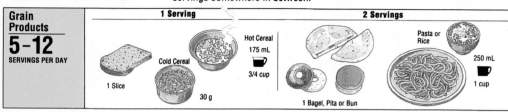

1 Serving

1 Slice — Cold Cereal 30 g — Hot Cereal 175 mL 3/4 cup

2 Servings

1 Bagel, Pita or Bun — Pasta or Rice 250 mL 1 cup

Vegetables & Fruit

5–10

SERVINGS PER DAY

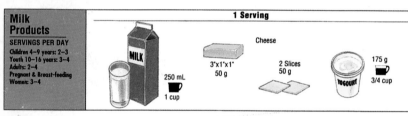

1 Serving

1 Medium Size Vegetable or Fruit — Fresh, Frozen or Canned Vegetables or Fruit 125 mL 1/2 cup — Salad 250 mL 1 cup — Juice 125 mL 1/2 cup

Milk Products

SERVINGS PER DAY

Children 4–9 years: 2–3
Youth 10–16 years: 3–4
Adults: 2–4
Pregnant & Breast-feeding
Women: 3–4

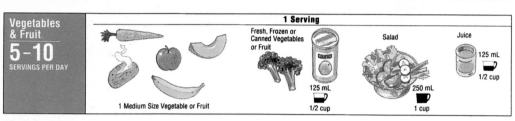

1 Serving

MILK 250 mL 1 cup — Cheese 3"x1"x1" 50 g — 2 Slices 50 g — Yogurt 175 g 3/4 cup

Other Foods

Taste and enjoyment can also come from other foods and beverages that are not part of the 4 food groups. Some of these foods are higher in fat or Calories, so use these foods in moderation.

Meat & Alternatives

2–3

SERVINGS PER DAY

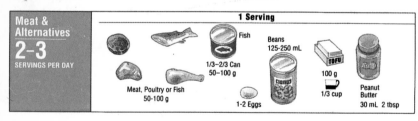

1 Serving

Meat, Poultry or Fish 50–100 g — 1–2 Eggs — Fish — Beans 125–250 mL — 1/3–2/3 Can 50–100 g — TOFU 100 g 1/3 cup — Peanut Butter 30 mL 2 tbsp

Enjoy eating well, being active and feeling good about yourself. That's VITALIT*É*

© Minister of Supply and Services Canada 1992   Cat. No. H39-252/1992E   No changes permitted. Reprint permission not required.
ISBN 0-662-19648-1

GOOD NEWS

Now more than ever, you can enjoy a lot more bread in all its different shapes and textures each and every day.

NUTRITION TIPS

■ All bread is low in fat. One slice (one serving from the Grain Products group) averages just 75 calories.
■ Fibre is great for people who want to eat less. Bread's fibre helps satisfy your hunger without adding many extra calories.

■ When you have a sandwich, the bread provides you with 9 essential nutrients: thiamin, riboflavin, niacin, folacin, pantothenic acid, phosphorus, magnesium, iron and zinc.
■ All white flour in Canada is enriched. So *all* bread contains B vitamins and iron.

Bakery Council of Canada

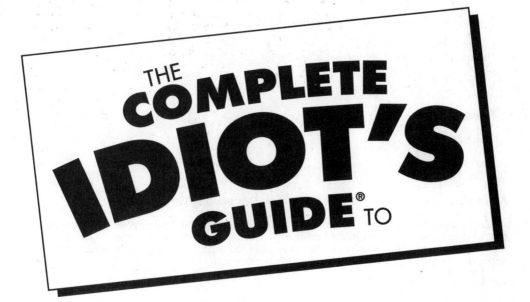

THE
COMPLETE
IDIOT'S
GUIDE® TO

Total Nutrition
for Canadians

by Leslie Beck RD and Joy Bauer MS RD

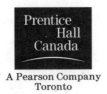

Prentice
Hall
Canada

A Pearson Company
Toronto

alpha
books

Canadian Cataloguing in Publication Data

Beck, Leslie (Leslie C.)
  The complete idiot's guide to total nutrition for Canadians

Includes index.
ISBN 0-13-086722-5

1. Nutrition. I. Bauer, Joy. II. Title.

RA784.B42 2000   613.2   C00-930174-7

ISBN 0-13-086722-5

Editorial Director, Trade Division: Andrea Crozier
Acquisitions Editor: Andrea Crozier
Copy Editor: Sarah Weber
Production Editor: Lori McLellan
Art Direction: Mary Opper
Cover Image: Tom Gates
Interior Design: Scott Cook and Amy Adams of DesignLab
Production Manager: Kathrine Pummell
Page Layout: Quadratone
Illustrator: Jody P. Schaeffer

1 2 3 4 5 WC 04 03 02 01 00

Printed and bound in Canada.

Visit the Prentice Hall Canada Web site! Send us your comments, browse our catalogues, and more.
www.phcanada.com.

A Pearson Company
Toronto

Contents at a Glance

Part 1: Time for a Nutrition Tune-Up   **1**

1   Guidelines for Healthy Eating   3
*Decoding Canada's Food Guide and learning to
incorporate the four food groups into your diet.*

2   A Close-Up on Carbohydrates   15
*Examining the "real deal" on carbohydrates: from
simple to complex.*

3   The Profile on Protein   25
*How much protein you should be eating and the best
sources.*

4   Chewing the Fat   35
*Everything you never understood about fat, including
the various types, the link to heart disease, interpreting
your cholesterol numbers, and inside tips to reduce the
amount of fat in your diet.*

5   Don't As-*salt* Your Body   47
*The reasons why you should give up the salt shaker,
and plenty of "saltless solutions."*

6   The Facts on Fibre   57
*All the specs on fabulous fibre, both insoluble and
soluble.*

7   Vitamins and Minerals: the Micronutrients   65
*Investigating the water-soluble and fat-soluble
vitamins: what they do and where they are found.*

8   Mighty Minerals: Calcium and Iron   81
*A closer look at the vital roles of two powerhouse
minerals, calcium and iron.*

Part 2: Making Savvy Food Choices   **91**

9   Decoding a Nutrition Label   93
*At last, understanding how to read all of the
information on a nutrition label.*

10   Shopping Smart   103
*Hitting the grocery store aisle by aisle and choosing the
best bets in vegetables, fruits, dairy, breads, grains,
beef, poultry, fish, eggs, legumes, frozen and canned
items, snacks, condiments, fats, and oils.*

11 Now You're Cooking   117
Learning to give your favourite personal recipes a nutrition makeover. Plus 13 mouth-watering new creations to try.

12 Restaurant Survival Guide   131
Become a dining detective while learning to select healthy meals in all types of ethnic cuisine.

13 Trimming Down the Holidays   143
Cutting fat and calories out of your holiday menus— without giving up taste or tradition.

Part 3: The ABCs of Exercise   151

14 Getting Physical   153
Learning how to start an appropriate exercise program.

15 The Gym Scene   165
Everything you'll need to know for a trip to the gym, from the lingo to the equipment.

16 Sports Nutrition   173
Fuelling your body for optimal performance in sport and other activity.

17 Going That Extra Mile: Fluids and Supplements   183
Comprehensive information on proper hydration, sports bars, and ergogenic aids.

Part 4: Beyond the Basics: Nutrition for Special Needs   193

18 Diet and Cancer   195
All about the foods that might help the fight against cancer.

19 Going Vegetarian   203
A guide to vegetarianism and a couple of dynamite meatless recipes.

20 Food Allergies and Other Ailments   217
Examining food allergies, lactose intolerance, and celiac disease.

21 Herbal Remedies   227
Alleviating bothersome ailments with an alternative approach.

Part 5: Pregnancy and Parenting   **241**

22 Eating Your Way Through Pregnancy   243
    Eating the right foods for you and your growing baby.

23 Exercising Your Way Through Pregnancy   261
    Exercising safely and effectively during pregnancy.

24 Feeding the Younger Folks   271
    Tips for getting your kids to eat healthy snacks and meals.

Part 6: Weight Management 101   **283**

25 Come On, Knock It Off   285
    The facts on fad diets and how to painlessly lose weight on a well-balanced food plan.

26 Adding Some Padding   309
    Tips to pack in the calories and increase your weight.

27 Understanding Eating Disorders   313
    When food and exercise get out of control: anorexia nervosa, bulimia nervosa, and compulsive overeating.

Appendices

A Recipes for Your Health   323

B Glossary   333

C Food Values   339

Index   **369**

v

Contents

Part 1: Time for a Nutrition Tune-Up   **1**

1 Guidelines for Healthy Eating   **3**

A Look at Canada's Food Guide 3
Where Do Calories Fit In? 7
How Many Calories Are Right for You? 7
The Keys to Successful Eating: Variety, Moderation, and Balance . . 10
Eating a Variety of Healthy Foods 11
All Foods in Moderation 11
Balancing Your Meals with Various Food Groups 12
Scheduling Time for Breakfast, Lunch, and Dinner 12
Breakfast with a Bang 12
Fuelling Your Body All Day 13

2 A Close-Up on Carbohydrates   **15**

What Exactly Is a Carbohydrate? 16
Sweet Satisfaction: the Lowdown on Simple Sugars 16
Where Do Fruits and Fruit Juices Fit In? 17
All About Complex Carbohydrates 18
Carbohydrates and the Glycemic Index 18
How Much Carbohydrate Should You Eat? 20
Do Pasta and Other Carbohydrates Make You Fat? 21
Adding Variety to Your Grain Foods 22
To Artificially Sweeten or Not 22

3 The Profile on Protein   **25**

What's So Important About Protein? 25
A Brief Return to Chemistry 101 26
Amino Acids: the Building Blocks of Protein 26
Your Body: the Amino-Acid Recycling Bin 27
Animal Protein Versus Vegetable Protein 27
Your Personal Protein Requirements 29
Protein for the Day in a Blink of an Eye 30
Should You Worry About Overeating Protein? 32
Does Excessive Protein Build Larger Muscles? 33
The Scoop on Amino-Acid Supplements 33
Should You Worry About Undereating Protein 34

4 Chewing the Fat   **35**

Why You Need a Little Fat...in Your Food and in Your Body . . . 36
Are All Fats Created Equal? 36

The Cholesterol Connection and Heart Disease 39
   Don't Be Fooled by Misleading Labels 40
   Your Cholesterol Report Card 41
Getting Fat from Eating Fat 42
   How Much Fat and Cholesterol Should We Eat? 43
   Some Fats Are Easier to Spot Than Others 43
   Slicing Off the Fat Without a Knife 44
The "Fat-Phobic" Generation 44

5 Don't As-*salt* Your Body   **47**

All About Salt 48
Feeling a Bit Waterlogged? 48
Can't Take the Pressure! 49
   What Exactly Is High Blood Pressure? 49
   What Causes High Blood Pressure? 49
   Investigating Your Blood Pressure Numbers 50
   How to Lower High Blood Pressure 51
How Much Sodium Is Recommended? 52
Salt-Less Solutions 53

6 The Facts on Fibre   **57**

Fibre Facts: What Is Fibre Anyway? 57
   Soluble Fibre 58
   Insoluble Fibre 58
   Reducing Your Risk of Colon Cancer 59
   Lowering Your Cholesterol Level 59
   Feeling Fuller with Less Food 59
How Much Fibre Do You Need? 60
   Tips to Increase the Fibre in Your Diet 60
   Don't Overdo It! 63

7 Vitamins and Minerals: the Micronutrients   **65**

What Are Vitamins and Minerals? 66
   The RNIs: Recommended Nutrient Intakes 66
   The DRIs: Dietary Reference Intakes 67
Fat-Soluble Vitamins 67
   Vitamin A (Retinol) 70
   Vitamin D: the Sunshine Vitamin 71
   Vitamin E (Tocopherols) 71
   Vitamin K 72
Water-Soluble Vitamins 72
   Thiamin (B-1) 72
   Riboflavin (B-2) 73
   Niacin (B-3) 73

Pyridoxine (B-6) 74
Cobalamin (B-12) 74
Folate (Folacin, Folic Acid) 74
Pantothenic Acid and Biotin 75
Vitamin C (Ascorbic Acid) 75
A Day in the Life of an Antioxidant 76
What Can Antioxidants Do? 77
How Much Should You Take? 78
The Scoop on Minerals 78

8 Mighty Minerals: Calcium and Iron   **81**

Calcium and Healthy Bones 81
How Much Calcium Is Recommended? 82
Are You Getting Enough Calcium? The Foods to Choose 83
Iron Out Your Body 85
Tips to Boost Your Dietary Iron Intake 86
Are You a Candidate for a Vitamin or Mineral Supplement? . . . 87
Are Your Vitamin and Mineral Supplements Absorbable? 89
Home Testing 89
Look for "GMP" on the Label 89

Part 2: Making Savvy Food Choices   **91**

9 Decoding a Nutrition Label   **93**

Serving Size 95
Energy 95
Protein 95
Carbohydrate 96
Fat 96
Saturated Fat 97
Cholesterol 97
Sodium 97
Percentage of Recommended Daily Intake 98
Take the Nutrition Label Challenge 99
Ingredient Lists 100
Buyer Beware! 101

10 Shopping Smart   **103**

The Shopping List 103
Aisle One: Starting with the Produce Section 104
Voluptuous Veggies 104
Getting to Know Vegetables 105
Fabulous Fruits 107
Aisle Two: Down Dairy Lane 110
Aisle Three: Shopping for the Whole Grains 111

Pasta, Rice, and More 112
Aisle Four: Best Bets for Protein 112
Meat 112
Poultry 113
Fish and Seafood 113
Eggs 114
Legumes (Dried Beans, Peas, and Lentils) 114
Aisle Five: Frozen Meals, Canned Soups, and Sauces 115
Aisle Six: Savvy Snacks 115
Aisle Seven: Condiments for the Health Conscious 115
Aisle Eight: Heart-Smart Fats, Spreads, and Dressings 116

11 Now You're Cooking   **117**
The Recipe Makeover: Remodelling Family Favourites 117
Top-10 List for Substitutions 120
Breakfast: Two Creative Morning Recipes 120
Lunch: Not the Same Old Sandwich Again! 121
Dinner: Recipes to "Wow" Your Taste Buds 123
Sensational Side Dishes 125
Decadent Desserts 126
Start a Cookbook Library 129

12 Restaurant Survival Guide   **131**
Common Restaurant Faux Pas 131
Become a Dining Detective 132
Ethnic Cuisine: the Good, the Not-So-Great, and the
Downright Bad 133
Chinese Food 133
French Food 134
Indian Food 135
Italian Food 136
Japanese Food 137
Mexican Food 138
North American Food 138
Fast Food 140
Going Out for Breakfast or Brunch? 141

13 Trimming Down the Holidays   **143**
Staying on Track During the Holidays 143
Easter 144
Passover 144
Summer Long Weekends 145
Thanksgiving 146
Hanukkah 147
Christmas 148

Part 3: The ABCs of Exercise — 151

14 Getting Physical — 153

Why Bother Exercising? 154
What's an Appropriate Exercise Program? 155
  Warming Up 155
  The Cardiovascular Workout: Challenge Your Heart and Lungs . . 155
  How Long, How Much, How Hard? 156
  Cooling Down 156
  Stretching 157
Are You Working Hard Enough? 157
  Test Your Heart Rate and Your Math Skills 158
  Try the "Talk" Test 158
Hit the Weights and "Pump Some Iron" 158
  Your Weekly Weight-Training Routine 159
  Cardio and Weight Training: the Perfect Combination 160
Top-Five Exercise Myths 160
How to Get Started: Your Personal Plan of Attack 161
  A Million Things You Can Do to Stay in Shape 162
When Formal Exercise Is Just Not Your Thing! 163

15 The Gym Scene — 165

Gym Jargon 101 165
A Tour of the Equipment 166
  Get to Know the Aerobic Contraptions 166
  Become Familiar with the Weight-Training Tools 168
Learn Your Muscles and "Buff That Bod" 168
Do You Need a Personal Trainer? 171

16 Sports Nutrition — 173

Carbohydrates: Fuel of Choice 173
Develop Your Own High-Carb Diet 175
  The Starchy Carbs 175
  Fruits 175
  Milk Products 175
  Vegetables 175
All About Muscle Glycogen 176
What's Carbo-Loading About? 177
Personal Protein Requirements 178
Food Before, During, and After Exercise 179
  Pre-Event Meals 179
  Fuelling Your Body During Prolonged Endurance Activity 181
  Recovery Foods 181

17 Going That Extra Mile: Fluids and Supplements   183

Guidelines for Proper Hydration 183
Sports Drinks Versus Water 184
The Bar Exam 184
What's the Story on Ergogenic Aids? 186
  Thumbs Up 186
  Thumbs Down 187

Part 4: Beyond the Basics: Nutrition for Special Needs 193

18 Diet and Cancer   195

Which Fats Can Help 196
  The Fatty Fish 196
  Flaxseed and Flaxseed Oil 196
Fight Back with Antioxidants 196
  Vitamins C and E, and Beta-Carotene 197
  Green and Black Tea 198
  Tomatoes 198
Can't Get Enough of Those Fruits and Veggies 198
Phytochemicals, Phytonutrients, and Phytoestrogens 199
The Story on Soy Products 200

19 Going Vegetarian   203

A Food Guide for Vegetarians 203
The Various Types of Vegetarians 205
How to Ensure an Adequate Protein Intake 205
  The Many Faces of Soy Protein 206
  Ironing Out the Plant Foods 207
  Searching for Nondairy Calcium 207
  Have You Had Enough B-12 Today? 208
  Don't Forget the Kitchen Zinc 208
  Tips for the Vegetarian Dining Out 209
Remarkably Meatless Recipes 210

20 Food Allergies and Other Ailments   217

Understanding Food Allergies 217
Diagnosing a True Food Allergy 218
  Treating a True Food Allergy 220
What's the Difference Between Allergy and Intolerance? 221
  What's Lactose Intolerance All About? 221
  Living with a Lactose Intolerance 222
Celiac Disease: Life Without Wheat, Rye, Barley,
  Triticale, and Oats 224
Irritable Bowel Syndrome 225
For the Caffeine Sensitive 225

21 Herbal Remedies   **227**

Judging the Quality of Herbal Products. 227

For Female Health. 228

Valerian Root 228

Black Cohosh 229

Evening Primrose Oil 229

For Male Health 230

Saw Palmetto 230

Pygeum Africanum and Stinging Nettle 230

Yohimbe 231

For Depression, Sleeping, and Aging 231

Gingko Biloba 231

St. John's Wort 232

Kava-Kava 232

Asian Ginseng (a.k.a. Panax, Korean or Chinese) 232

Chamomile 233

Heart Disease 233

Garlic 233

Hawthorn 233

Liver Disease 234

Milk Thistle 234

Respiratory Ailments. 234

Echinacea 234

Arthritis 235

Boswella 235

Glucosamine Sulphate with Chondroiten 235

Migraines 236

Feverfew 236

Cancer 236

Chinese Green Tea 236

More Herbal Remedies Worth Mentioning 236

Ginger 237

Bilberry 237

Rosemary 237

Peppermint 237

Aloe 238

...And Stay Away from These! 238

Ephedra/Ma Huang 238

Dong Quai 238

Part 5: Pregnancy and Parenting   **241**

22 Eating Your Way Through Pregnancy   **243**

Are You Really Eating for Two? 243

Increased Calories and Protein 243

A Weighty Issue: How Much Weight Should You Gain? 244
Adjusting Your Eating Plan 245
Why All the Hype About Calcium? 246
Hiking Up the Iron 247
Blast Your Baby with Vitamins! 248
Keep on Guzzlin' Those Fluids! 249
Foods to Forget! 249
The Many Trials and Tribulations of Having a Baby 250
   The "Uh-Oh, Better Get Drano" Feeling 251
   Ugh! That Nagging Nausea 251
   What's All the Swelling About? 252
   Oh, My Aching Heart 252
Five-Day Pregnancy Meal Plan 253

23 Exercising Your Way Through Pregnancy   **261**
Most Doctors Give the Green Light to Exercise 261
   What Do the Experts Say? 262
Warming Up, Cooling Down, and All the Stuff in the Middle . . 264
   Stretch Your Body...Carefully 264
   Keep a Check on the Intensity 264
"Energize" Without the Slamming and Jamming! 265
   Take a Walk with Your Baby 265
Sign Up for a Prenatal Exercise Class 266
Yes, Moms-to-Be Can Lift Weights 267
Bouncing Back After the Baby Arrives 269

24 Feeding the Younger Folks   **271**
Your Very First Food Decision: Breast Milk or Formula? 271
When and How to Start Solid Foods 272
The Wrong Stuff 273
The Right Stuff for Growing Kids 274
   Be a Healthy Role Model 275
   Cook with Your Kids, Not for Them! 275
   Fun and Easy Recipes 276
What About Sweets? 278
The Sneaky Gourmet: 15 Ways to Disguise Vegetables 279
Turn Off That Tube! 280

Part 6: Weight Management 101   **283**

25 Come On, Knock It Off   **285**
The Scoop on Some Popular Fad Diets 286
What's the Best Diet, Anyway? 287
What Should You Weigh? 287
Testing Your Body Fat: Getting Pinched, Dunked, and Zapped 289

Skin-Fold Calipers 290
Underwater Weighing 290
Bio-Electrical Impedance 290
How Many Calories Should You Eat for Weight Loss
  and Weight Maintenance? 291
Your Personal Weight Loss Plan 291
  Understanding the Food Plans 292
  Tracking Your Food on the Daily Plans 295
No More "I've Blown It" Syndrome; All Foods Are Allowed . . 304
Setting Realistic Goals 305
  Get Moving and Keep Moving 306
  Maintaining Your New Weight After You've Lost Weight 306

26 Adding Some Padding   **309**

Is Being Underweight a Health Concern? 309
Six Tips to Help You Pack in the Calories 310
Adding More of the Good Stuff 310
  Shake It Up Baby 311

27 Understanding Eating Disorders   **313**

Anorexia Nervosa: The Relentless Pursuit of Thinness 314
Bulimia Nervosa 316
Compulsive Overeating 318
How to Help a Friend or Relative with an Eating Disorder . . . 319
  Where to Go for Help 320

Appendices

A Recipes for Your Health 323

B Glossary 333

C Food Values 339

Index   **369**

Foreword

There doesn't seem to be a day that goes by where we're not bombarded by the media with some new piece of information regarding our nutritional health. There are so many books on nutrition available, many stating different ideas and philosophies. If we're not either registered dietitians or doctors, we can be left confused and no further ahead in our pursuit of good health.

For instance, one day we're told we can eat as much protein as we like, as long as we eliminate carbohydrates (breads and pastas). But once you go off the diet, watch out, weight gain comes quickly once you begin consuming carbs again. Next day comes the Mediterranean diet, where we don't have to worry about the amount of fat we have as long as it's in the form of olive oil! The authorities say, "put it on everything!" Remember one tablespoon of fat is still 120 calories and 14 grams of fat, no matter whether it's oil, butter or lard. Then we're told as long as we stay in the "zone", we'll never have to worry about our weight again. "The zone" is a complicated diet to follow. You'll need your calculator and measuring cups at all times to succeed. What about "food combining", and the promise theat you'll stay slim forever! Just don't dare mix your carbohydrates and proteins at the same meal. In other words say good bye to meat and potatoes forever!

You get the picture! I'm sure you may have tried a fad diet at some point. How many of you can say it worked for good? I bet not too many hands went up when I asked that.

So, what's the problem? With all the nutrition information out there, why do we continually obsess ourselves about food and diet? I believe it's because we want immediate satisfaction; in other words, "I want it all or nothing". We have lost our patience with proper health. We want to be "svelte" (thin) tomorrow. We can't wait 6 months to reach an ideal body weight, learn better eating behaviours and educate ourselves and families about some basic and easy to follow nutrition facts.

But admit it. None of those "fads" diets or trendy nutritional gimmicks work for long. You get bored with the restricted diet and inflexible scheduling. Within 6 months you've gained back all the weight you lost and probably a few more pounds for good measure.

Well don't despair. I've got great news. It is possible to feel passionate about food and enjoy everything you put in your mouth, and still eat healthy. You'll be able to learn everything you ever needed to know about nutrition, food and dieting without going back to school to become a nutritionist.

Leslie Beck, one of Canada's leading registered dietitians and nutrition consultants has written the only book you'll ever have to read on nutrition. For over 12 years Leslie has counselled more than 1500 people regarding their individual eating habits. She's helped them achieve their personal nutrition and fitness goals, and now she's made this possible for you.

In my career as a cookbook author and TV food personality, I have focused on delicious, low fat recipes. I was thrilled to have Leslie Beck author all the nutrition chapters of my latest book, *Sensationally Light Pasta and Grains*, I found reading her information exciting and informative. Leslie gives you the important information in a direct and easy to understand manner. You walk away feeling enlightened and in more control of your choices. Her writing is down to earth, reader friendly, and most of all, useful.

After reading *The Complete Idiot's Guide® to Total Nutrition for Canadians*, you'll have your questions answered. You'll be able to decode "Canada's Guidelines to Healthy Eating" and apply it to your life; you'll find out why you must have both carbohydrates and proteins in your diet to stay healthy, and you'll realize why "fad" diets fail. You'll learn what vitamins and minerals are essential to your individual health; you'll finally be able to interpret food labels and what you should watch out for; you'll learn how to eat in restaurants and fast food outlets without feeling deprived, and you'll understand the relationship between certain diseases and the foods we consume.

You may choose to use this book as a guide or enjoy reading it from cover to cover, as I have. No matter what you do, you'll finally be further ahead in your pursuit and understanding of good health. Remember, basic dietary education empowers you to make the proper choices so you can lead a healthier, more active and fulfilling life. A big thanks to Leslie Beck for aiming us able to understand and enjoy the world of nutrition.

—Rose Reisman, author of several low-fat cookbooks including *Sensationally Light Pasta & Grains*

Introduction

If you're confused by the enormous amount of nutrition information that bombards us on a daily basis, this book is for you! It is a comprehensive guide to eating smart and becoming fit that's up to date, trustworthy, and, most importantly, reader friendly. It was written with both my personal and professional experiences in mind for people who want to slim down, bulk up, maintain good health, or just plain look and feel great.

How to Use This Book

To make reading this book easier for you, I've divided it into six areas of interest:

Part 1, "Time for a Nutrition Tune-Up," clears up the confusion about the fundamentals of food. This section dissects the dietary guidelines and offers simple strategies to incorporate the four food groups into your life. You'll also get the inside scoop on simple to complex carbohydrates, the power of protein, and the relationship between excessive fat intake and heart disease. In addition, you'll examine the facts on fibre and salt, and become well versed in the vital vitamins and minerals that your body requires.

Part 2, "Making Savvy Food Choices," shows you that dining healthily does not mean giving up the pleasure of eating. In this section, you'll learn to become Sherlock Holmes in your grocery store—able to decode the nutrition information on product labels and make more informed food purchases. We'll take a trial run through the supermarket and load your cart with healthy food items for your kitchen. You'll also find many easy-to-make creative recipes, and learn to master the art of low-fat cooking. Furthermore, I provide the best bets in most ethnic cuisines so you'll be ready to tackle any type of restaurant, and you'll learn strategies for trimming down your holiday menus without losing taste or tradition.

Part 3, "The ABCs of Exercise," provides you with the tools and inspiration to get moving and keep moving. That's right—a crash course on becoming physically fit. You'll hear the lowdown on strengthening your heart and lungs through aerobic exercise, and get tips to buff your bodacious physique through appropriate weight training and conditioning. You'll learn the importance of properly warming up, cooling down, and stretching your body, and get the education you need to enter a gym with confidence. I also take a comprehensive look at sports nutrition and provide the skills you'll need to fuel your body for both casual exercise and competitive sport.

Part 4, "Beyond the Basics: Nutrition for Special Needs," discusses a variety of hot topics within the world of nutrition. First, I discuss how diet can potentially reduce your risk of cancer, and zoom in on the common culprits that trigger food allergies and other food sensitivities. I also present the latest scoop on herbal remedies and how they can help conquer a bunch of bothersome ailments, and offer sound information on vegetarian eating plans.

Part 5, "Pregnancy and Parenting," provides essential information that will help you manage your and your growing baby's health. I discuss the importance of sound nutrition and offer specific food guidelines for a healthy pregnancy. You'll learn how much weight you should gain, the right foods to eat, and which foods to avoid. I also give you surefire tips to help get your kids to eat healthily. This section includes ideas for lower fat after-school snacks, strategic ways to disguise vegetables, and tips to encourage more physical activity.

Part 6, "Weight Management 101," provides you with a sensible plan of attack. Whether you want to lose weight, gain weight, or, most importantly, stop obsessing, this final section covers it all. I provide weight loss programs to help knock off (and keep off) those unwanted extra pounds, along with calorie-cramming strategies to help you skinny folks beef up your bods. I also take a look at life-threatening eating disorders, and tell you where to find help when food and exercise go beyond health and get way out of control.

Extras

To help you get the most out of this book, I've sprinkled it with the following helpful information boxes.

Q & A
These are the questions we all want to ask, and their answers.

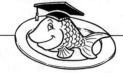

Food for Thought
Follow these tips on eating and exercising to make everyday nutrition and fitness fun.

Overrated-Undercooked
You should keep these warnings in mind when eating or exercising.

Nutri-Speak
These boxes provide definitions of food and exercise jargon.

Acknowledgments

Many thanks to the tremendous number of people who helped pull this book together. First, let me extend my eternal gratitude to my extraordinary associate Lisa Mandelbaum, who provided her expertise and long hard work!

A special thanks to my great literary agent, Mitch Douglas, and to senior editor Nancy Mikhail for making this book happen. Tremendous thanks to Jessica Faust for wrapping up the entire project and, of course, Phil Kitchel, Kris Simmons, and Donna Wright for their intense dedication on the editing and production end.

Thanks to Tom Gates and Ina for the great cover photo, and to Meredith Gunsberg for such delicious vegetarian recipes.

Sincere thanks (as usual) to Geralyn Coopersmith and Evan Spinks, two outstanding fitness consultants who shared their sense of humour and invaluable information. Thanks to Suki Hertz, a talented chef who provided great ideas and creative recipes in the holiday chapter. And a million thanks to Karen Robinowitz, a great writer and an exceptional person.

I am also grateful to many others who contributed to portions of this book, including Frances Aaron, Michael Simon, Elyse Sosin, MA, RD, Grace Leder, Meg Fein, Dany Levy, Candy Gulko, Jane Stern, Dr. Catharine Fedeli, and Dr. Susan Wagner.

On a personal note, I would like to extend a sincere thanks to these people: my incredible parents, Ellen and Artie Schloss, who have always taught me that *anything and everything* is possible; my Grandma Martha, for sticking around to see my second edition published; "The Gang"—Debra, Steve, Ben, Glenn, Pam, Dan, Nancy, Jon, Camrin, Harley, Karen, Lisi, Lisa, and Jason; my saviours on the fourth floor—Vivian, Mary, Cece, and Kiki; Andrea Mendonca for being the wonderful person she is; my super in-laws, Carol and Vic, along with Grandma Mary and Grandpa Nat for their support and encouragement; and, most of all, my partners in crime, Ian, Jesse, and Cole!

—Joy Bauer

Part 1

Time for a Nutrition Tune-Up

After they read and listen to conflicting food advice from friends, relatives, and diet gurus, it's no wonder people are more confused than ever about what they should be eating.

This first part of the book proves that eating healthy does not need to be complicated or restrictive. In fact, it is quite the contrary. This section unravels the colourful Canada's Food Guide rainbow and provides the inside scoop on carbohydrates, protein, fat, fibre, and salt. Once you've grasped these fundamentals of food, you'll be ready to read on and learn the specifics about everything you never understood or realized.

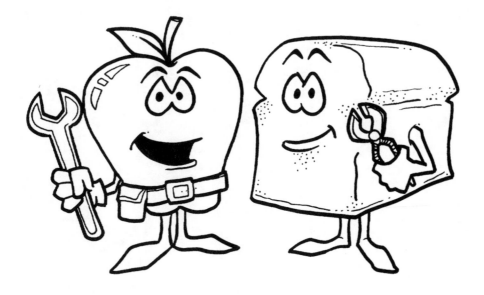

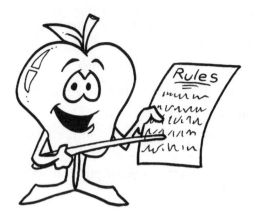

Chapter 1

Guidelines for Healthy Eating

In This Chapter

➤ Unravelling *Canada's Food Guide to Healthy Eating*

➤ Balancing your food groups

➤ Where do calories fit in?

➤ The keys to successful eating

➤ Scheduling time to fuel your body

After thumbing through hundreds of complicated nutrition articles and magazine ads, receiving random food advice from friends and relatives, and listening warily to endless infomercials promising a lean, fit body, you're probably more confused than ever about what you should be eating.

So what exactly should you be eating? Believe it or not, healthy eating doesn't mean driving miles to some obscure health food store in search of organic produce. It also doesn't mean eating bean sprouts sprinkled with wheat germ for dinner (mm, mm). In fact, according to nutrition experts, healthy eating is more basic than you think.

A Look at Canada's Food Guide

In 1992, Health Canada created *Canada's Food Guide to Healthy Eating*, an updated version of the familiar basic four food groups that have been drilled into your head since the first grade. I'm sure you've seen this colourful rainbow in books and magazines (see the reference card at the front of this book). Perhaps you even have a copy taped to your fridge. This visual approach to nutrition, a general outline of what you should eat each day, makes healthy eating a lot less complicated. Although individuals vary in their specific requirements, Canada's Food Guide provides solid information on do's and don'ts for people over age four.

Canada's Food Guide is based on the following guidelines to healthy eating:

1. Enjoy a variety of foods from and within each of the four main food groups.

2. Emphasize cereals, breads, other grain foods, vegetables, and fruit.

3. Choose lower fat dairy products, leaner meats, and foods prepared with little or no fat.

4. Achieve and maintain a healthy body weight by enjoying regular physical activity and healthy eating.

5. Limit salt, alcohol, and caffeine.

Based on these fundamentals of healthy eating, Canada's Food Guide focuses on choices that are lower in fat, higher in fibre, and rich in vitamins and minerals. It also limits the amount of fats, oils, and sweets in your diet. Here's a look at the famous four food groups:

Group 1: Grain products—breads, cereal, rice, and pasta

Group 2: Vegetables and fruit

Group 3: Milk products—milk, yogurt, and cheese

Group 4: Meat and alternatives—meat, poultry, fish, dry beans, eggs, and nuts

Let's take a look at how this model works:

1. **Grain products group:** Foods that come from grains are at the top of the rainbow, creating a foundation for building a healthy diet. This foundation provides carbohydrates (also called carbs or carbos) for energy, dietary fibre, and important vitamins and minerals. To get a good supply of fibre, B vitamins, and iron, Canada's Food Guide recommends that we choose whole-grain and enriched grain products more often. Enjoy multigrain breads, brown rice, whole-wheat pasta, ready-to-eat bran cereals, and oatmeal. Of course, you can be more adventurous and try less common grains such as quinoa, kasha, barley, or millet! Health Canada's guidelines recommend **5–12** servings of grain products per day. That might sound like a lot, but serving sizes are deceptively small, so they add up quickly!

   One serving =
   1 slice of bread, or
   $1/2$ English muffin, or
   $1/2$ small bagel, or
   $1/2$ large pita bread, or
   1 small roll, or

$^3/_4$ cup (175 mL) ready-to-eat cereal, or

$^1/_2$ cup (125 mL) cooked cereal, rice, or pasta

2. **Vegetables and fruit group:** Depending on which ones you choose, foods from this group are loaded with vitamins and minerals, including vitamins A and C, folate, iron, calcium, magnesium, and several others. Vegetables are naturally low in calories and fat, and are packed with fibre. Fruits and unsweetened fruit juices are terrific sources of vitamins A and C and potassium. Canada's Food Guide advises you to eat dark green and orange vegetables and fruit more often. These foods are higher in certain key nutrients such as vitamin A, vitamin C, beta-carotene, and folate. Go for green salads, broccoli, spinach, sweet potato, carrots, oranges, and cantaloupe. To boost your fibre intake, eat whole fruits most often.

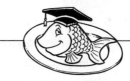

Food for Thought

Look how quickly grain portions can add up! Did you know that...

A common pasta entrée = 4–5 servings

A large bagel = 4–5 servings

A large hot pretzel = 3 servings

Health Canada's guidelines recommend **5–10** servings of vegetables and fruit per day, but there's no need to stop there. When it comes to vegetables and fruit, you can never get enough.

Vegetables:

One serving =

1 cup (250 mL) raw, leafy green vegetables, or

$^1/_2$ cup (125 mL) cooked or chopped vegetables, or

$^3/_4$ cup (175 mL) vegetable juice

Fruits:

One serving =

1 medium fruit (apple, banana, orange), or

$^1/_2$ mango, or

1 cup (250 mL) strawberries, blueberries, or raspberries, or

$^3/_4$ cup (175 mL) fruit juice, or

$^1/_2$ cup (125 mL) chopped, canned, or cooked fruit, or

$^1/_4$ cup (50 mL) dried fruit, or

1 wedge of melon

Overrated-Undercooked

When buying fruit juice, pay close attention to the wording on the juice containers; the contents might not be as healthy as they sound. For instance, "fruit drinks" and "fruit cocktails" generally contain a lot of added sugar with small amounts of real fruit juice. To get more nutrients and less sugar into your diet, examine the label and choose fruit beverages that contain only "100% fruit juice."

Food for Thought

Stock your fridge with low-fat dairy products. You'll still get all the good stuff (calcium, vitamin D, protein, and so on), but you'll get a lot less fat. Smart choices include 1% or skim milk, low-fat cheese and yogurts, reduced-fat or fat-free ice cream, or low-fat frozen yogurt.

3. **Milk products group:** The hands-down winners of the calcium contest, these foods also provide protein and other vitamins and minerals. To help you consume less fat and fewer calories, Canada's Food Guide encourages you to choose lower fat milk products. Look at labels and choose products with a lower percentage of milkfat (MF) or butterfat (BF). Health Canada's guidelines recommend **2–4** servings per day—two to three for most people and four for teenagers, and men and women who are over age 50.

One serving =

1 cup (250 mL) milk, or
3/4 cup (175 mL) yogurt, or
1 1/2 ounces (45 g) cheese, or
2 slices (45 g) cheese

4. **Meat and alternatives group:** The bottom of the rainbow contains foods that are good sources of protein, B-vitamins, iron, and zinc. Choose leaner meats, poultry breast, fish, and seafood to reduce your fat intake without losing important nutrients. Use dried beans or soy foods more often in place of meat to get less fat and more fibre. Health Canada's guidelines recommend **2–3** servings per day, the equivalent of 4–9 ounces.

One serving =

2–3 ounces (60–90 g) of cooked lean meat, or
2–3 ounces (60–90 g) of cooked fish or
  skinless poultry, or
1/2 to 1 cup (125–250 mL) cooked beans,
  or eggs

5. **Other foods:** Although the rainbow doesn't display this group, if you look at Canada's Food Guide you'll see foods and beverages that are not a part of any group. These include spreads, oils, jams, honey, snack foods, tea, coffee, water, soft drinks, and condiments. While some are often

referred to as "empty calories" because they don't give you nutrients, others can be used as part of a healthy meal. Health Canada's guidelines recommend limiting your intake of other foods that are higher in fat and calories—salad dressings, butter, margarine, sugars, soft drinks, candies, rich desserts, and snack foods.

Where Do Calories Fit In?

Practically everyone over the age of 10 has heard the word "calorie"—but few actually understand how calories work in regard to their diets. For some reason, the word calorie has a bad reputation, even though a calorie is simply the measurement of food as energy. The more calories you eat, the more energy you supply your body.

All the foods we eat contain calories, some more than others. Here's the ideal situation: *Take in the amount of food energy—calories—that your body needs. No more, no less.*

Although this is easier said than done, this tightrope walk will help maintain a normal body weight. Unfortunately, it is quite easy to eat more calories than your body actually needs or burns, resulting in weight gain. On the other hand, taking in fewer calories than your body needs can result in weight loss.

How Many Calories Are Right for You?

How can you find the perfect balance between calories in and calories out? Not by nit-picking over calorie counting, that's for sure! You *should* pay attention to what and how much you eat, but not to the point that you carry around a calculator and use it to determine your next bite of food.

Food for Thought

Although eggs are a good source of protein, the yolks contain a large amount of cholesterol. But that doesn't mean you have to give up eggs! Most experts agree that eating five or six eggs a week won't affect the risk of heart disease in healthy men and women. If you enjoy eggs more often, try using the egg substitutes (no cholesterol) or mix one whole egg with two or three whites.

Nutri-Speak

A **calorie** is the amount of energy food provides. The number of calories is determined by burning it in a device called a **calorimeter** and measuring the amount of heat produced. One calorie is equal to the amount of energy needed to raise the temperature of 1 litre of water 1°C. Carbohydrates and protein contain 4 calories per gram, fat contains 9 calories per gram, and alcohol has 7 calories per gram.

To get a *rough* idea of how many calories you should be taking in, look at the following chart. This chart offers only three general caloric ranges, so keep in mind that your personal daily requirements might fall somewhere between two that are listed. Remember, everyone is different. The amount of food (or number of calories) you need every day from Canada's Food Guide depends on your age, body size, activity level, whether you are male or female, and whether you are pregnant or breast-feeding. After you select the caloric amount that seems right for you, simply experiment with the various numbers of servings in each food group (listed underneath your caloric level) until you find what feels most comfortable. You may even keep a food diary for a week or so; that way, you can keep track of the groups from which you need to increase your intake and those from which you might be overeating.

General Daily Calorie Requirements

1,600–1,800 calories	Number of calories needed for many sedentary women and some older adults.
1,800–2,100 calories	Number of calories needed for most children, teenage girls, active women, and many sedentary men. Women who are pregnant and breast-feeding may need somewhat more.
2,700–3,000 calories	Number of calories needed for teenage boys, many active men, and some very active women.

Source: Nutrition Recommendations for Canadians, Health Canada 1990

Food for Thought

Not all calories are created equal! Although the following foods contain the same number of calories, notice the difference in nutrition:

Package of licorice: 230 calories; 0 milligrams calcium; 0 grams protein; 0 IU vitamin D

8-ounce (250 mL) fruit yogurt: 230 calories; 350 milligrams calcium; 8 grams protein; 1000 IU vitamin D

Opt for foods rich in nutrients.

Remember that serving sizes are approximations, so a guess is fine. If you have no idea what a serving looks like, you might want to measure it out once or twice for a future comparison. For example, measure a serving of cooked pasta ($^1/_2$ cup/125 mL) so that you are able to guesstimate that a restaurant entrée is probably about 4–5 servings.

Now that you have an idea of how many calories you should be taking in daily, look at the following chart to determine how many servings from each food group will be right for you. Keep in mind that these are only the servings for the four food groups, not the fats, oils, and sweets.

	1,600 calories	2,100 calories	2,700 calories
Grain food servings	6	9	12
Vegetable and fruit servings			
Vegetables	3	4	5
Fruit	3	3	4
Milk products servings	2–3*	2–3*	4
Meat and alternatives servings	2	2–3	3

*With recently increased calcium requirements, all people will benefit from 3 daily servings of low-fat dairy products.

Here are some handy sample menus for each caloric level.

	1,600 calories	2,100 calories	2,700 calories
Breakfast	1 bowl cereal with banana 1 cup (250 mL) low-fat milk 1 slice toast with jam 1 banana	3 pancakes 1 cup (250 mL) berries and some maple syrup 1 cup (250 mL) low-fat milk	Bowl of cereal with raisins and low-fat milk Large bagel with a smear of cream cheese Glass of orange juice
Lunch	Turkey breast (approx. 2–3 oz/60–90 g)	Turkey burger on a whole-grain kaiser roll	Large salad with 1 cup (250 mL) lentils, small amount of oil and vinegar

	1,600 calories	2,100 calories	2,700 calories
Lunch (cont'd)	2 slices low-fat Swiss cheese 2 slices whole-wheat bread Lettuce and tomato Carrot sticks	Green salad with vinaigrette	1 slice of broccoli and cheese pizza 1 apple
Snack	1 apple	3/4 cup (175 mL) low-fat fruit yogurt Banana	3 fig bars Strawberry yogurt smoothie
Dinner	Salad with vinaigrette Grilled salmon (approx. 3 oz/90 g) Rice (approx. 1 c/250 mL) Broccoli with Parmesan cheese	Sliced tomato and mozzarella (try low-fat) Linguini (approx. 2 c/ 500 mL) with shrimp (approx. 3 oz/90 g) and a lot of vegetables in tomato sauce Wedge of melon	1 dinner roll Lightly stir-fried chicken (approx. 5 oz/ 150 g) with a lot of vegetables (approx. 2 c/500mL) Brown rice (approx. 2 c/ 500 mL) 1 orange 3/4 cup (175 mL) carton low-fat yogurt

Adding more "other foods" (oil, margarine, dressings, and so on) will increase your daily calorie intake.

The Keys to Successful Eating: Variety, Moderation, and Balance

Now that we've covered the daily food requirements, let's find out what kind of eater you are. Are you one of those people who orders exactly the *same* thing, in the *same* restaurant, day after day? Have you packed the same lunch to bring to work for the last

15 years? Or do you skip eating lunch altogether? Do you define the four food groups as McDonald's, Pizza Hut, KFC, and Tim Horton's Donuts? If you answered "yes" to any of these questions, pay close attention to the next few paragraphs.

Eating a Variety of Healthy Foods

First, understand why variety is important. Varying your food provides a much greater range of nutrients. Eating the same foods day after day supplies your body with exactly the same vitamins and minerals over and over again. Although you might be consuming the recommended daily intake of many beneficial vitamins and minerals, *you miss out on many important nutrients and disease-fighting compounds that your body needs.*

Furthermore, variety can make your meals much more interesting! Forget about those humdrum standards; be adventurous!

> ➤ **Try new cookbooks.** Throw things together that you would never have dreamed of eating.

> ➤ **Give your palate a worldly kick.** Try a different ethnic restaurant or recipe each week.

> ➤ **Make a list...**of 20 different fruits, veggies, and grains, and try something new each day. Pick one day a week to create a meal that you've never had before. Your taste buds won't believe what they've been missing.

All Foods in Moderation

We need to place greater emphasis on healthy foods and downplay the not-so-healthy stuff. However, there is a place in *every* food plan for *all* kinds of foods (and let's face it—people cannot live on health food alone). Too many of us label high-fat, high-sugar foods as the enemy and, as a result, feel guilty when we allow ourselves to indulge. In fact, imposing limitations that are too strict may cause people to react by overindulging. Remember, Canada's Food Guide indicates that you should *limit* fat and sugar—not *avoid* it completely.

Take care of your mind, as well as your body: If you're absolutely crazy for chocolate cake, then you should have the pleasure of eating it once in a while. Obviously, you shouldn't eat high-fat foods all the time, but there is room for everything—*in moderation.* Even if you're trying to lose weight, you need to enjoy the occasional treat. I always tell my weight loss clients to include their favourite "splurge" food once a week. (People who have specific medical conditions such as heart disease, diabetes, food allergies, gastrointestinal ailments, and so on might have to avoid certain foods altogether. Check with your dietitian or doctor for more information.)

Eating in moderation also means controlling the *size* of your portions. Once you determine the number of servings that you should be eating from each food group, spread them throughout your daily meals. Proper planning will ensure that you are eating balanced meals in moderation and meeting your daily nutrient requirements.

Balancing Your Meals with Various Food Groups

Many people eat excessive amounts of food from one group and completely forget about other groups that offer important vitamins and nutrients. For instance, have you ever watched someone (not *you*, of course) reach for a couple of rolls from the breadbasket and then polish off a huge plate of pasta? The meal probably tasted delicious, but that's a lot of grain without much of anything else. What happened to the fruits, vegetables, and protein?

Once in a while a meal like that is fine, but, as a general rule, incorporate foods from different food groups into each meal. For example, choose a house salad, pasta with chicken and broccoli in tomato sauce, and a little Parmesan cheese. This balanced meal offers a significant amount of nutrition. All it takes is a little planning. To eat a balanced diet, aim to include foods from at least three food groups with each meal.

Food for Thought

Enjoy a variety of foods from and within each of the four main food groups.

Emphasize cereals, breads, other grain foods, vegetables, and fruit.

Choose lower fat dairy products, leaner meats, and foods prepared with little or no fat.

Achieve and maintain a healthy body weight by enjoying regular physical activity and healthy eating.

Limit salt, alcohol, and caffeine.

Developed by Health and Welfare Canada, 1990

Scheduling Time for Breakfast, Lunch, and Dinner

What kind of an eating schedule are you on? Do you make time in your day for breakfast, lunch, and dinner, or do you run on empty until dinner and then raid the cupboards in a nonstop frenzy as soon as you walk in the door? Everyone has his or her own eating regimen—some better than others. You should be fuelling your body *throughout* the day when you need the energy.

Breakfast with a Bang

You've heard it a million times: BREAKFAST IS IMPORTANT!

Think of your body as a car: It needs fuel to run properly. When you wake up from a good night's sleep, your body has been in a fasting state for about eight hours (if you're lucky enough to get that much sleep). "Break-fast" in the morning helps kick your system into gear by supplying food energy to your body. The process of digesting, absorbing, transporting, and storing nutrients from breakfast burns calories and revs your metabolism. Without food, you feel tired and sluggish.

Incidentally, breakfast also helps you control your weight: Eating a smart breakfast can help regulate your appetite throughout the day so you eat in moderation during lunch and dinner. Have you ever skipped breakfast to "save calories," only to find yourself so hungry by lunch that you overeat? So much for that diet. Start your day off smart: Schedule time for breakfast.

Fuelling Your Body All Day

Remember, breakfast alone won't give you enough fuel for the entire day. Your body needs to be constantly energized throughout the day to help keep you going. And you don't have to eat the standard three square meals to get proper energy. In fact, some people prefer six mini-meals (or grazing) each day. Do whatever works best for your schedule and eating style, but be sure that your daily food totals resemble the guidelines of Canada's Food Guide.

Food for Thought

Numerous studies have shown that children who eat breakfast perform better at school than children who miss the morning meal.

Source: Journal of the American Dietetic Association

The Least You Need to Know

➤ Make sure to eat a variety of foods from the four food groups.

➤ Don't get caught up with counting calories; it can drive you crazy! Simply focus on eating healthy foods in moderation.

➤ Get out of your food rut and be adventurous. Try new and exciting foods, recipes, and restaurants.

➤ Although Canada's Food Guide allows for "some" fat and sugar intake, don't overdo it.

➤ Schedule time to fuel your body throughout the day. Food can help keep you alert, energetic, and focused.

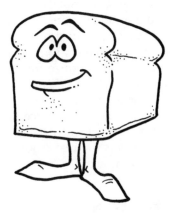

Chapter 2

A Close-Up on Carbohydrates

In This Chapter

➤ What's a carbohydrate?

➤ Simple carbs versus complex carbs

➤ How many carbohydrates should you eat?

➤ Do carbohydrates make you fat?

➤ To artificially sweeten or not

All the foods you eat are composed of three macronutrients known as carbohydrate, protein, and fat. Some foods consist primarily of only one macronutrient (in other words, bread is mainly carbohydrate, turkey is mainly protein, and butter is mainly fat), whereas other foods contain combinations of all three (for example, pizza, sandwiches, and stews).

Your body needs all three of these macronutrients to function properly, but not in equal amounts. Many leading health professionals recommend that we eat a daily diet made up of *approximately*

➤ 55 percent carbohydrate

➤ 15 percent protein

➤ No more than 30 percent total fat

By following the guidelines outlined in Canada's Food Guide, you'll automatically meet these proportions.

Nutri-Speak

Legumes belong to the bean and pea family and they are rich in complex carbohydrates, protein, and fibre. They supply iron, zinc, magnesium, phosphorous, potassium, and several B-vitamins, including folate. Because legumes provide both complex carbs and protein, they can fit into the meat and alternatives group *and* the grain foods group of Canada's Food Guide. Legumes include black beans, pinto beans, kidney beans, lima beans, navy beans, soybeans (tofu), black-eyed peas, chickpeas (garbanzos), split peas, lentils, and nuts and seeds, which are higher in fat.

Fifty-five percent of our recommended daily diet comes from carbohydrate; that's more than half your food coming from a single macronutrient. Thanks to growing consumer education about nutrition, many people now recognize the benefits of a carbohydrate-rich diet. Remember, carbohydrates provide us with important nutrients, and they are an excellent source of energy—specifically for those of us with active lifestyles. This chapter covers the real scoop on carbos, from simple to complex.

What Exactly Is a Carbohydrate?

Technically speaking, a carbohydrate is a compound made up of carbon, hydrogen, and oxygen. But chemistry aside, the most basic carbohydrates are called simple sugars and include honey, jams, jellies, syrup, table sugar, candies, soft drinks, fruits, and fruit juices. Glucose (also called dextrose) and fructose are two common simple sugars found in fruits, honey, and vegetables. Glucose is also the substance measured in blood. (In other words, blood sugar equals blood glucose.) As you can see from the figure, they are relatively small compounds. When several of these simple sugars are linked together, they form much more complicated molecules known as complex carbohydrates.

Complex carbohydrates that come from plants are called *starch* and are found in quality foods such as grains, vegetables, breads, seeds, and legumes (dried beans, peas, and lentils). Whether it's a handful of jellybeans or freshly sliced whole grain bread, it's all carbohydrate!

Simple sugar

Sweet Satisfaction: the Lowdown on Simple Sugars

Since your favourite sugary sweets are classified as carbohydrates—and you're supposed to eat a lot of carbohydrates—is it okay to load up on gummy bears and licorice?

Not a chance. Here's why: The *quality* of your carbohydrate matters tremendously. Simple sugars such as candy, pop, and sugary sweeteners found in cakes and cookies offer little in the form of nutrition except that they provide your body with energy and calories. These foods are literally "empty calories"—calories with no nutritional value. In moderation, simple sugars are perfectly fine (and, I admit, tasty), but people who consistently load up on the sweets often find themselves too full for, or uninterested in, the healthy foods their bodies require. The result is too much sugar and not enough nutrition.

Q & A

Does sugary candy promote dental cavities?

Actually, all foods that contain carbohydrates (rice, pasta, potato, cakes, cookies, and, yes, candy) can equally mix with the bacteria in plaque and increase your risk for tooth decay. But don't panic: By brushing a few times each day, flossing daily, and swishing water around in your mouth after eating, you can fight off your dentist's drill.

Where Do Fruits and Fruit Juices Fit In?

There are some exceptions to the "no sugar" rule. For example, fruits and fruit juices contain fructose (a natural simple sugar) and provide several vitamins and minerals. Eating a piece of fresh fruit or drinking unsweetened fruit juice is a far cry from snacking on jelly beans or drinking pop. When you can, choose whole fruit over fruit juice: You get the same nutrients, as well as more complex carbohydrates and dietary fibre. You'll read more about this in Chapter 6, "The Facts on Fibre."

As you can see in the following table, fruit juice and cola both contain simple sugars, but fruit juice provides a lot more nutrition.

8 ounces (250 mL) of unsweetened orange juice	8 ounces(250 mL) of cola
110 calories	100 calories
26 grams carbohydrate	26 grams carbohydrate
25 grams sugar	26 grams sugar
225% daily vitamin C	0% daily vitamin C
12% daily potassium	0% daily potassium
12% daily folic acid	0% daily folic acid

All About Complex Carbohydrates

Now that you know what you shouldn't load up on, let's take a look at the foods you should eat. By now, you should be clued in to which foods are rich in complex carbohydrates (pasta, rice, grains, breads, cereal, and legumes). Although they're actually made from hundreds—or even thousands—of simple sugars linked together, they react quite differently inside your body. After you ingest a complex carbohydrate (or starch), several enzymes break it down into its simplest form, called glucose. Glucose is the simple sugar that your body recognizes and absorbs. All carbohydrate (simple and complex) must be broken down and converted into glucose before your body can absorb and use it for energy.

If all carbs wind up as glucose, why can't we just eat simple sugars? I've already touched on the first reason: Many simple sugars lack vitamins, minerals, and fibre, whereas complex carbs are often a good source of these nutrients, depending on the food.

Check out this comparison: a small baked potato (complex carb) versus an 8-ounce (250 mL) glass of cola (simple carb). Although both provide about 100 calories, that's where the similarity ends. The potato supplies vitamin C, potassium, and fibre, along with several other vitamins and minerals. And the cola—you probably guessed—provides zilch. As you can see, eating complex carbs certainly does make a difference to your nutritional intake, even though the carbohydrate all ends up as glucose.

Another reason to choose complex carbohydrates is that the glucose created during digestion gets released into your blood more slowly. Simple carbohydrates are already broken down—they go straight into the blood, resulting in what is unofficially known as the "sugar rush"—whereas complex carbohydrates are larger molecules that must be broken down. As your body processes complex carbs, small glucose molecules are released into the blood over an extended period of time. This helps to regulate blood-sugar levels, especially in people who may have problems with their blood sugar (for example, people with hyperglycemia, hypoglycemia, or diabetes mellitus).

Carbohydrates and the Glycemic Index

Nutrition scientists are learning that not all complex carbohydrates are created equal. Some get converted to blood glucose as quickly (or more quickly) than simple sugars. For example, that bagel you ate for breakfast was absorbed into your bloodstream a little more quickly than the simple sugar in a can of pop! In fact, starchy foods vary widely in how quickly they're converted to blood glucose.

Nutri-Speak

Hyperglycemia is a condition resulting in an abnormally high blood-glucose (blood-sugar) concentration. *Hyper* means "too much," *glyce* means "glucose," and *emia* means "in the blood." **Hypoglycemia** is characterized by abnormally low blood sugar. Here, *hypo* means "too little." **Diabetes mellitus** is a disorder of blood-sugar regulation usually caused by the body's inability to either produce enough insulin or use it effectively.

Nutritionists now classify carbohydrate foods according to their "glycemic index" (GI), or their ability to cause a rise in blood sugar. Foods with a low GI raise your blood-sugar level more slowly than foods with a high GI. Foods with a low GI take longer to digest and lead to a gradual, slow rise in blood glucose. You don't get that sugar rush and the energy from food lasts longer. We are learning that eating a diet full of carbohydrates that are rapidly absorbed can increase feelings of hunger and cause you to overeat. And fast-acting carbohydrates may cause unstable blood-sugar levels in people with diabetes.

To keep your appetite satisfied and your energy levels up, use the list below to choose carbs with a low glycemic index.

Low Glycemic Index	High Glycemic Index
Pumpernickel bread (whole-grain)	Bagel
Rye bread (whole-grain)	White bread
Brown rice	Instant rice
Bulgur	
Barley	
Pasta	
Yams	Potato, mashed
	French fries
Oatmeal	Cream of Wheat
Red River Cereal	Corn Flakes
All-Bran	Rice Krispies

Low Glycemic Index	High Glycemic Index
Baked beans	
Chickpeas	
Lentils, green	
Kidney beans	
Soybeans	
Grapes	Watermelon
Oranges	Raisins
Apples	Fruit cocktail
Peaches	
Apricots, dried	
Plums	
Yogurt (with sugar added)	
Skim milk	
Yogurt (with sweetener)	

How Much Carbohydrate Should You Eat?

As mentioned earlier, Health Canada recommends that 55 percent of your total food calories for the day come from carbohydrates, specifically complex carbohydrates. In fact, 80 percent or more of your total carbohydrate intake should come from complex carbs and naturally occurring sugars in fruits and vegetables.

What exactly does this mean in terms of food? You'll need to fill more than half of your plate at each meal with carbohydrate-rich foods. Instead of bacon and eggs for breakfast, boost your carbohydrate intake with fresh fruit and whole-grain cereals or toast, whole-wheat waffles, pancakes, or hot oatmeal. For lunch, eat vegetable soups, salads with beans, whole-grain breads, and fresh fruit. With dinner, include a serving or two of rice, couscous, whole-wheat pasta, vegetables, legumes, or potatoes. The idea is to have *larger* amounts of carbohydrates and much *smaller* amounts of protein and fat.

Note: In extremely rare instances, due to medical conditions such as diabetes, some people cannot tolerate these recommended carbohydrate amounts and should be under a dietitian's supervision for dietary guidance.

Do you want to get more specific? Calculate the amount of carbohydrate you need:

1. Take your total calories for the day.

2. Multiply by .55 (or 55 percent).

3. Divide by 4 (which will convert your carbohydrate calories into grams because 1 gram carbohydrate = 4 carbohydrate calories).

Daily Calories	Cals from Carbs	Grams of Carbs
1,600 cals =	880	220
1,800 cals =	990	248
2,100 cals =	1,155	289
2,700 cals =	1,485	371

The amount of carbohydrate grams remains proportional to your caloric requirements. The more calories you require, the more carbohydrates you need to eat.

Do Pasta and Other Carbohydrates Make You Fat?

One day, you hear you should load up on carbs, and the next day, an article claims that pasta will make you fat. Ever feel like a nutrition yo-yo? What's the real story with carbs?

The story is that bread, pasta, and all other complex carbohydrates supply high-quality calories and should be included in every healthy food plan. Then why all the confusion? Well for starters, some people may confuse weight gain from fat with weight gain from carbohydrates. One gram of fat has more than double the number of calories of 1 gram of carbohydrate. What some people don't realize is that fat often accompanies the carbohydrates in a meal. For instance, people remember that they had pasta for dinner but forget that the pasta was swimming in oil, butter, cheese, or Alfredo sauce. Clearly, the culprit for weight gain was the fat (butter, oil, and so on), not the carbohydrate (pasta).

Another example has become our favourite staple—the bagel. Alone, a bagel is a wonderful complex carbohydrate. Add all that butter or cream cheese, and you'll wind up with a lot more calories and fat than you bargained for. The next time you question whether pasta or other carbos make you fat, reevaluate. It's more likely to be the fat that is making you fat.

But let's say you don't add much fat to your foods. You eat plain bagels, low-fat brownies, and pasta with tomato sauce, yet you still swear carbs are adding inches to your waistline. Well, there is some truth to the carbohydrate and weight story. Many people have gone overboard with the low-fat message, thinking that just because a bagel or pretzels are fat free they can eat as much as they want. Wrong! Too many calories from carbs add up, too! It doesn't matter if those extra calories come from carbohydrates, protein, or fat: Excess calories will be stored by your body as fat.

While it's true that carbohydrates supply only 4 calories per gram (less than half the amount in 1 gram of fat), just remember that a large bagel packs a lot of carbohydrate! And so do baked potato chips and fat-free muffins. What's more, studies suggest that too much high-GI carbohydrate can make you feel hungry and trigger overeating. The bottom line...you need to eat everything in moderation. Just because a food is fat free doesn't mean it's calorie free.

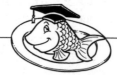

Food for Thought

Some excellent sources of carbohydrates include fruits, vegetables, legumes, pasta, rice, barley, couscous, oatmeal, pita bread, tortillas, unsweetened whole-grain cereal, potatoes, air-popped popcorn, fig bars, rice cakes, and low-fat, high-fibre muffins.

Adding Variety to Your Grain Foods

Expand your grain vocabulary:

➤ **Couscous**—A staple in Mediterranean countries, couscous is one of the easiest grains to cook and can be found in many grocery stores.

➤ **Quinoa** (pronounced "keen-wah")—Quinoa, a grain native to South America, is high in protein, calcium, and iron. It is good in puddings, soups, and stir-frys.

➤ **Barley**—Good in soups, stews, side dishes, puddings, and cereals, barley is found in grocery stores and is often called "pot" or "scotch barley."

➤ **Millet**—Millet is available in health food stores. It is good as a side dish or stuffing for poultry and is high in phosphorous and B-vitamins.

➤ **Wild rice**—This pseudo-grain is really a grass seed. It is high in protein and a good source of B-vitamins.

➤ **Amaranath**—High in protein, iron, and calcium, amaranath is native to South America and is available in health food stores and some upscale grocery stores. It serves as a good side dish or cereal.

➤ **Wheat berries**—Found in most grocery stores and health food stores, they make a good high-fibre cereal or substitute for rice.

To Artificially Sweeten or Not

Some people often have to use artificial sweeteners because of a medical condition. For example, sugar substitutes are often used by people with diabetes, who can't tolerate large amounts of *real* sugar because their bodies can't produce the hormone insulin. Insulin delivers the sugar (glucose) from our blood to our cells, where we use it as energy. When your body doesn't have enough insulin, or your cells are resistant to the action of insulin, sugar builds up in the blood and doesn't get into the cells. This condition is known as high blood sugar and can be extremely dangerous for people with diabetes.

Because sugar substitutes do not contain any glucose (and therefore do not require insulin), they can be effective sweeteners for people with diabetes.

A more popular reason for using artificial sweeteners is saving calories. However, this notion might not be as good as you think. Although it is true that diet soft drinks and other artificially sweetened foods can save you a lot of sugar calories, several studies have shown that people who "save calories" with these diet foods usually wind up eating those banked calories somewhere else. Other studies suggest that artificial sweeteners might, in fact, make you hungrier. Did you know that a packet of real sugar (that's 1 tsp/5 mL) has only 16 calories? You can easily burn that off walking an extra flight of stairs. It's certainly something to think about the next time you reach for the artificial sweetener. If you're watching your calorie intake, you're much better off to forgo the cream cheese on your bagel (which can run you 300 calories!) or limit your portion of salad dressing.

When it comes to your health, artificial sweeteners are the subject of much controversy. Before you tear open your next packet of a sugar substitute, read the following to become an informed consumer.

One of the first sugar substitutes to receive Health Canada's attention was *saccharin*, a sweetener derived from coal tar (mm, mm!). In 1977, the government released a study linking saccharin use to bladder cancer in rats. Since that time, manufacturers are not allowed to add saccharin to foods. But it is available in pharmacies and is sold over the counter as a tabletop sweetener. Although several studies have suggested that large quantities of saccharin can cause cancer in laboratory rats, no harmful effects have been shown in humans. For this reason, the artificial sweetener has not been banned in the United States.

Another controversial sweetener is *cyclamate*. Like saccharin, this compound is made from coal tar and its use has been associated with bladder cancer in animals. Although cyclamate is banned south of the border, it is available in Canada as a tabletop sweetener (Sucryl™, Sweet N' Low™, Sugar Twin™, and Weight Watchers™).

A very popular artificial sweetener is *aspartame*, better known as Nutrasweet™ or Equal™. Aspartame consists of two protein fragments (phenylalanine and aspartic acid) and has had Health Canada approval since 1981. It is currently found in more than 5,000 different products, and, despite the controversy, there is no scientific evidence to show it causes cancer. However, aspartame use has been reported to cause headaches and other reactions in sensitive people. And, because aspartame does contain phenylalanine, individuals with the metabolic disorder PKU (an inherited disease in which the body cannot dispose of excess phenylalanine) should consult their physicians before using this sweetener.

Sucralose, or Splenda™, is another artificial sweetener found in many diet foods and sold as a tabletop sweetener. This sweetener is made from sugar itself. Sucralose is relatively new to Canada, making its debut in 1991. So far, it has not been associated with cancer in laboratory studies.

23

The most recent artificial sweetener to come onto the market is called *acesulfame K*. This Health Canada–approved sweetener is sold under the brand name Sunett™, and it's found in drinks, fruit spreads, baked goods, candies, chewing gum, and tabletop sweeteners. Although our government has deemed it safe for human consumption, some experts argue that the data are inadequate to assess its cancer-causing potential.

The bottom line is that, while scientific studies have not proven a clear link between artificial sweeteners and human cancer, they don't rule it out either. Now, I don't want you to think that sipping the occasional diet pop will harm your health; it won't. But I do believe that you are entitled to know the facts before you make your decision to use these products. If you choose the artificial route to sweetness, don't overdo it. And remember the guidelines for healthy eating suggest eating real sugar *in moderation*, not avoiding it altogether.

The Least You Need to Know

➤ Approximately 55 percent of your total food for the day should come from carbohydrates (mostly complex carbohydrates). Carbohydrate-rich foods include fruit, legumes, bread, cereal, rice, pasta, and all other grain products.

➤ Limit your intake of candy, pop, and other sugary sweets. Although they are carbohydrates, simple sugars provide you with little more than "simply sugar."

➤ Fruit and unsweetened fruit juices are the exception to the "simple sugar" rule. Although considered simple carbohydrates, they provide a variety of important nutrients.

➤ Carbs aren't fattening; however, almost anything you consistently overeat will make you put on the pounds—including carbohydrates.

➤ In moderation, artificial sweeteners can be an effective sugar substitute for people with diabetes mellitus and for the general population. The choice between sugar and substitutes is yours.

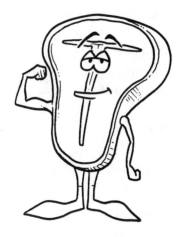

Chapter 3

The Profile on Protein

In This Chapter

➤ The importance of protein

➤ Amino acids—the building blocks

➤ Animal protein versus vegetable protein

➤ Combining incomplete proteins

➤ Your personal requirements

➤ The facts, the fallacies

It's time to learn the many powers of protein—one incredibly versatile molecule. Almost everyone seems to have a basic idea of which foods are rich in protein, but do you actually know your personal requirements or understand why protein is important and how it works? Stay tuned: This chapter presents the facts.

What's So Important About Protein?

First, protein is not just in food; it's also found *throughout* your body. Did you know that your bones, organs, tendons, ligaments, muscle, cartilage, hair, nails, teeth, and skin are all made up of protein? That's just the beginning. *Working proteins* are busy performing specific tasks in your body. These include the following:

➤ **Enzymes**—Proteins that facilitate and accelerate chemical reactions. They are also known as protein catalysts. Each enzyme has a specific function to perform in the body.

➤ **Antibodies**—Proteins that help fight illness and disease. They are made by special white blood cells.

➤ **Hemoglobin**—Proteins that transport oxygen all over the body.

➤ **Hormones (most)**—Proteins that regulate many body functions. Hormones signal enzymes to do their job, such as stabilizing blood-sugar levels, insulin levels, and growth.

➤ **Growth and maintenance proteins**—Proteins that serve as building materials for the growth and repair of body tissues.

The list is endless. But I promise not to take you back to high school biology.

Food for Thought

Protein got its name over 150 years ago from the Greek word *proteios*, meaning "of prime importance."

A Brief Return to Chemistry 101

Protein consists of carbon, hydrogen, oxygen, and nitrogen. The addition of nitrogen gives protein its unique distinction from carbohydrate and fat, along with establishing the signature name, amino acid. Much like simple sugars, which link together to form a *complex* carbohydrate (Chapter 2, "A Close-Up on Carbohydrates"), amino acids are the building blocks for the more complicated protein molecule.

Amino Acids: the Building Blocks of Protein

Nutri-Speak

Proteins are compounds composed of carbon, hydrogen, oxygen, and nitrogen arranged as strands of amino acids.

There are 20 different amino acids, and, depending upon the sequence in which they appear, they carry out a specific job or function in your body. Think of amino acids as similar to the alphabet—26 letters that can be arranged in a million different ways. These arranged letters create words, which then translate into an entire language. The arrangement of amino acids is your body's "protein language," which dictates the exact tasks that need to be carried out. Therefore, proteins that make up your enzymes will have one sequence, whereas those that form your muscles will have a completely different one.

Your Body: the Amino-Acid Recycling Bin

Your body continually gets the amino acids it needs from its own amino-acid pool and from a diet that meets your daily protein requirements. After you eat a food that contains protein, your body goes to work, breaking it down into various amino acids. (Different foods yield different amino acids.) When the protein is completely dissected, your body absorbs the amino acids (resulting from your digested food) and rebuilds them into the sequence that you need for a specific body task. In this way, your body is similar to a recycling bin.

Let's take this amino-acid talk a bit further. Out of 20 amino acids, 11 can actually be manufactured within your body. However, that means 9 cannot be manufactured. You cannot function without each and every amino acid. It is "essential" that you get these 9 from outside food sources. Therefore, they are appropriately called *essential amino acids*.

Essential Amino Acids	**Nonessential Amino Acids**
Histidine	Glycine
Isoleucine	Glutamic acid
Leucine	Arginine
Lysine	Aspartic acid
Methionine	Proline
Phenylalanine	Alanine
Threonine	Serine
Tryptophan	Tyrosine
Valine	Cysteine
	Asparagine
	Glutamine

Animal Protein Versus Vegetable Protein

In general, animal proteins (meat, fish, poultry, milk, cheese, and eggs) are considered good sources of *complete proteins*. Complete proteins contain ample amounts of all essential amino acids.

On the other hand, vegetable proteins (grains, legumes, nuts, seeds, and other vegetables) are *incomplete proteins* because

Nutri-Speak

Amino (a-MEEN-o) acids are the building blocks for protein that are necessary for every body function.

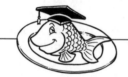

Food for Thought

Gelatin is the only animal protein that is not considered a complete protein.

they are missing, or do not have enough of, one or more of the essential amino acids. That's not such a big deal. You already know that grains and legumes are rich in complex carbohydrate and fibre. Now you learn that they can be a good source of protein as well; it just takes a little bit of work and know-how. By combining foods from two or more of the following columns—voilà—you create a self-made complete protein. You see, the foods in one column may be missing amino acids that are present in the foods listed in another column. When eaten in combination at the same meal (or separately throughout the day), your body receives all nine essential amino acids.

You can combine the following vegetable proteins to make complete proteins.

Sources of Complementary Proteins

Grains	Legumes	Nuts/Seeds
Barley	Beans	Sesame seeds
Bulgur	Lentils	Sunflower seeds
Cornmeal	Dried peas	Walnuts
Oats	Peanuts	Cashews
Buckwheat	Chickpeas	Pumpkin seeds
Rice	Soy products	Other nuts
Pasta		
Rye		
Wheat		

Combinations to Create Complete Proteins

Combine Grains and Legumes	Combine Grains and Nuts/Seeds	Combine Legumes and Nuts/Seeds
Peanut butter on whole-wheat bread	Whole-wheat bun with sesame seeds	Humus (chickpeas and sesame paste)
Rice and beans	Breadsticks rolled with sesame seeds	Trail mix (peanuts and sunflower seeds)
Bean soup and a roll	Rice cakes with peanut butter	

Combine Grains and Legumes	Combine Grains and Nuts/Seeds	Combine Legumes and Nuts/Seeds
Salad with chickpeas and cornbread		
Tofu-vegetable stir-fry over brown rice or pasta		
Vegetarian chili with bread		

Also, by adding small amounts of animal protein (meat, eggs, milk, or cheese) to any of the groups, you create a complete protein. Here are some examples:

➤ Oatmeal with milk

➤ Macaroni and cheese

➤ Casserole with a small amount of meat

➤ Salad with beans and a hard-cooked egg

➤ Yogurt with granola

➤ Bean and cheese burrito

Your Personal Protein Requirements

This chart presents the Recommended Nutrient Intakes (RNIs) of protein for a variety of age categories:

Infants	Up to 12 months	12 grams
Children	1 year	19 grams
	2–3 years	22 grams
	4–6 years	26 grams
	7–9 years	30 grams
Males	10–12 years	38 grams
	13–15 years	50 grams
	16–18 years	55 grams
	19–24 years	58 grams
	25–49 years	61 grams
	50–74 years	50 grams
	75+ years	57 grams

Nutri-Speak

Complementary proteins are two incomplete proteins in a food that compensate for one another's shortfalls when combined.

Food for Thought

Did you know that the mineral iron is best absorbed from the following animal proteins: liver, beef, pork, lamb, chicken, turkey, shellfish, and other fish?

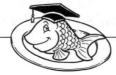

Food for Thought

Keep in mind that pregnant or lactating women have increased protein requirements. Pregnant women need an additional 5, 20, and 24 grams of protein a day during the first, second, and third trimesters respectively. Breast-feeding women need 20 extra grams a day.

Females	10–12 years	40 grams
	13–15 years	42 grams
	16–18 years	43 grams
	19–24 years	43 grams
	25–49 years	44 grams
	50–74 years	47 grams
	75+ years	47 grams
Pregnant	1st trimester	50 grams
	2nd trimester	65 grams
	3rd trimester	68 grams
Lactating		65 grams

Protein for the Day in a Blink of an Eye

The previous chart gave you a number; let's see how quickly 61 grams can translate into food. The following chart lists the protein content of commonly eaten foods.

Protein Content of Common Foods

Animal Proteins	Grams of Protein	Vegetable Proteins	Grams of Protein
Steak, sirloin	26	Peanuts (1 oz/30 g)	8
Ground meat	24	Walnut halves (1 oz/30 g)	4
Hamburger, 1 patty	21	Peanut butter (2 Tbs/25 mL)	8
Bologna, 3 slices (2 oz/60 g)	9	Sesame seeds (1 oz/30 g)	8
Hot dog, 1 small (1 oz/30 g)	4	Sunflower seeds (1 oz/30 g)	7
Bacon (1 slice)	2	Kidney beans ($^1/_2$ c/125 mL)	8
Ham	19	Lentils ($^1/_2$ c/125 mL)	8
Turkey breast	26	Chickpeas ($^1/_2$ c/125 mL)	8

Animal Proteins	Grams of Protein	Vegetable Proteins	Grams of Protein
Roast beef	28	Split peas (^{1}/2 c/125 mL)	8
Chicken, breast without skin	27	Tofu (3 oz/90 g)	7
Halibut	23	Oatmeal (1 c/250 mL)	6
Tuna, white, in water	30	Pasta (1 c/250 mL)	7
Salmon	25	Brown rice (1 c/250 mL)	5
Shrimp	22	White rice (1 c/250 mL)	3
Cottage cheese (^{1}/2 c/125 mL)	16	Whole-wheat bread (2 slices)	6
Cheddar cheese (1 oz/30 g)	7	Potato, baked (small)	5
Processed cheese (1 oz/30 g)	7	Broccoli (^{1}/2 c/125 mL)	2
Whole milk (1 c/250 mL)	8	Corn (^{1}/2 c/125 mL)	2
Skim milk (1 c/250 mL)	8	Spinach (^{1}/2 c/125 mL)	3
Low-fat plain yogurt (^{3}/4 c/175 mL)	10	Green peas (^{1}/2 c/125 mL)	4
Low-fat fruit yogurt (^{3}/4 c/175 mL)	8		
Egg (1)	7		

All are 3-ounce (90 g) servings (approximately the size of a deck of cards) unless otherwise indicated.
Source: 1987, Health Canada: Nutrient Value of Some Common Foods

You can imagine how quickly these numbers add up, especially because most people tend to eat much more than a 3-ounce (90 g) serving in one shot.

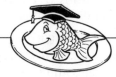

Food for Thought

The leanest protein sources include turkey breast, skinless chicken breast, egg whites, lean red meat, low-fat yogurt, skim or 1% milk, beans and lentils, all seafood and fish, split peas, chickpeas, and tofu.

Let's take a look at a typical day:

Breakfast:
2 scrambled eggs
3 strips of bacon
2 slices of toast with margarine
Glass of milk

Lunch:
A deli meat sandwich (4 oz/120 g)
2 slices of bread
Apple
Fruit-bottom yogurt

Snack:
Piece of cheese
Crackers

Dinner:
Steak or chicken breast (6 oz/180 g)
Some veggies and rice
Total protein = 137 grams (that's great if you're a male athlete!)

As mentioned earlier, people in industrialized countries don't have a problem meeting their protein requirements. In fact, as you can see, it's easy to *exceed* the amount you need because our society tends to focus on meat, fish, eggs, seafood, or dairy products with most every meal.

Should You Worry About Overeating Protein?

Well, maybe. The problem is that your body only uses what it needs. And the rest? Well, some protein from foods may be used for energy, but most is just extra calories, and usually not just protein calories. Many of these high-protein foods are also packaged with fat; therefore, excess calories, which can translate into weight gain, can be a major concern. Furthermore, filling up on large portions of animal protein might crowd out grains, fruits, and veggies. And that means you'll shortchange your body of many important nutrients, not to mention dietary fibre.

Go ahead and determine your personal protein needs—and then adjust your meals accordingly. You might want to prepare smaller pieces of animal protein (about 3 oz/ 90 g) and emphasize a variety of veggies and grains on your plate.

Also, watch out for "high-protein" diets, which promise quick weight loss by encouraging you to eat large amounts of protein while severely limiting carbohydrate intake (no bread, potatoes, rice, pasta, cereal, fruit, and so on). You might lose weight, but not from any magical combination of "high protein/low carbohydrates." One reason may be loss of water because the breakdown of excessive protein causes frequent urination. Another explanation may be that your total calorie intake usually decreases when you're limited to high-protein foods. How much plain protein can you really eat?

Furthermore, these high-protein/very low carb eating plans can be unhealthy (unless you are clinically diagnosed to be suffering from hyperinsulinemia by your physician). Your body cannot burn fat efficiently without adequate carbohydrates. As a result, you produce compounds called *ketones*, which can accumulate in the blood and leave you feeling dizzy, nauseated, fatigued, and headachy—and give you incredibly bad breath. High-protein diets usually mean people are eating a lot more fat, which can cause high blood cholesterol. Many people who try these diets complain of constipation from the missing fibre. What's more, excessive animal protein can also put an added strain on your kidneys. It's pretty ironic when the goal of losing weight should be to improve your health, not make it worse.

Does Excessive Protein Build Larger Muscles?

Okay, let's set the record straight. It's true that protein is needed for the development of muscle, but it's not true that "extra" protein will build bigger biceps. Body builders and other athletes do need more protein than the RNI; however, this increase is already accounted for in the typical North American diet. As mentioned earlier, we cannot store excess protein. Therefore, all those extra protein calories (and the fat that came along with them) will most likely wind up around your waist—not your quads!

In addition, anyone eating excessive protein will urinate more frequently because the breakdown of protein produces an increase in *urea*, a waste product in urine. You can imagine the inconvenience of running to the bathroom every 10 minutes, let alone your risk of becoming dehydrated. Furthermore, body builders who take tremendous amounts of protein tend to skimp on carbohydrates—the key energy-providing ingredient for an optimal workout.

The key to building muscle is the right combination of protein, carbohydrate, and, of course, weight training. You'll read more on this in Chapter 16, "Sports Nutrition."

The Scoop on Amino-Acid Supplements

Amino-acid supplements are unnecessary. Your body needs only a certain amount of each amino acid, and most of us receive far more than this amount from the food we eat (both animal and vegetable protein). Although the amount that you need is vital, there is nothing miraculous about megadosing. In fact, overkill can be expensive and inefficient. Think about it: For next to nothing, you can prepare a piece of grilled chicken with a meal instead of spending more than double the cost for one of those "amino-acid" shakes. If you do need to take a protein supplement to meet your protein requirements, pure amino acids are not the way to go. A protein powder made from whey (animal protein) or soy (vegetable protein) is less expensive and effective.

Should You Worry About Undereating Protein?

While most people don't have to fret over a lack of protein, getting enough of this powerful nutrient may be a challenge to some. If you're a strict vegetarian who doesn't eat beans or soy, or if you skimp on protein foods for fear of fat, you may be short-changing your body. Too little protein can zap your energy, weaken your immune system, and negatively affect your general health. If you suspect your diet is lacking, make a plan to eat a small portion of protein at each meal. Use Canada's Food Guide as your planning tool—meat and alternatives and milk products are the best food groups for protein.

The Least You Need to Know

➤ A total of 20 different amino acids act as building blocks for the more complicated protein molecules. Nine of these amino acids must be obtained from outside food sources and are called "essential amino acids."

➤ Animal proteins are considered to be "complete proteins" because they contain ample amounts of all nine essential amino acids. Vegetable proteins are "incomplete proteins" because they are missing one or more of the essential amino acids. By combining two or more incomplete vegetable proteins during the day, you can create a complete protein with all nine essential amino acids.

➤ Some people have a tendency to go *protein overboard*, which can also mean more fat and calories because foods high in protein may also be high in fat.

➤ Excessive protein and amino-acid supplements do not build larger muscles. In fact, these myths may lead to a host of problems, including dehydration, higher fat intake, and increased body fat.

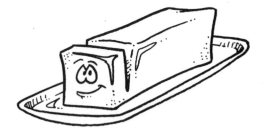

Chapter 4

Chewing the Fat

In This Chapter

➤ Various types of fat

➤ The heart disease connection

➤ Your cholesterol numbers and what they mean

➤ Gaining weight from excessive fat

➤ Living a low-fat lifestyle

Unless you've been living on another planet, you've heard that too much fat can create a lot of problems. Ironically, despite the "fat warnings" that bombard us every day, we remain an overweight society that eats too much. It's one thing to *know* what to eat (and I'm sure we would all do pretty well in the "Fat" category on *Jeopardy*), but it's a whole different ballgame to actually commit to eating healthy and follow through with it.

Let's not forget the flip side: Low fat does not mean no fat. Some people take this new "low-fat religion" to radical extremes. "I'll have a broiled fish, dry, no oil; salad with lemon juice on the side, no dressing; steamed veggies, nothing on them; and a baked potato, plain." You might as well remove your taste buds before digging into that meal! Food is supposed to be enjoyable, right?

This chapter shows that a high-fat diet can lead to a host of problems, including weight gain and disease. However, it will also emphasize to all the "fat-phobics" out there (some 20 percent of Canadians) that *some* fat is perfectly okay, in fact, necessary, and with some hard work and realistic planning, everyone can find his or her happy medium.

Why You Need a Little Fat...in Your Food and in Your Body

Before we talk about the downside of fat, let's look at all its positives. You heard right: There are actually good things about the three-letter macronutrient:

➤ Fat provides you with a ready source of energy.

➤ Children need fat to grow properly.

➤ Fat supports the cell walls within your body.

➤ Fat enables your body to circulate, store, and absorb the fat-soluble vitamins A, D, E, and K. Without any fat, you would become deficient.

➤ Fat supplies essential fatty acids that your body can't make and must therefore get from foods.

Nutri-Speak

Fat-soluble nutrients dissolve in fat. Some essential nutrients such as the vitamins A, D, E, and K require fat for circulation and absorption.

➤ Fat helps promote healthy skin and hair.

➤ Fat makes food taste better by adding flavour, texture, and aroma.

➤ Fat provides a layer of insulation just beneath the skin. People who are extremely thin are often cold because they lack this layer of subcutaneous fat. Overweight people tend to have too much of this insulation and become uncomfortably warm in hot weather.

➤ Fat surrounds your vital organs for protection and support.

Are All Fats Created Equal?

Dietary fat comes in a variety of forms; some are more harmful than others. In addition to watching your total fat intake, you must also pay attention to the *type* of fat you take in. Let's start from the beginning and figure out what's what in the world of fat.

First, here's the entire "fat vocabulary" you will need to speak like an expert (or a bore) at your next social function:

Nutri-Speak

If you don't like fish, **fish-oil supplements** may be a useful tool for helping to lower triglyceride levels and reducing the symptoms of rheumatoid arthritis. If you think you may benefit, ask your dietitian how to take these safely.

➤ **Triglyceride**—The general term used for the main form of fat found in food. The structure of a TG (that's the short form for triglyceride) is a *glycerol* (carbon atoms linked together) plus three fatty acids. There are several triglyceride categories, and, depending upon the fatty acid composition, a TG is classified as saturated, monounsaturated, or polyunsaturated.

You may also hear about your "triglyceride level" when the doctor takes your blood. That's because TGs, like cholesterol, are a storage form of fat in your body—circulating in the bloodstream and deposited in adipose tissue (better known as flab).

➤ **Monounsaturated fats**—As mentioned earlier, the molecular composition of a triglyceride can vary. When one double carbon bond is present in the fatty acid molecule (c=c) the fat is grouped as "monounsaturated" (one spot that is *not* saturated). Olive oils, peanut oils, sesame seed oils, canola oils, and avocados are high in monounsaturated fat. According to studies, these fats may help to lower blood cholesterol. But go easy with that olive oil if your weight is an issue. This "heart healthy" fat is still loaded with fat calories.

➤ **Polyunsaturated fats**—Another type of unsaturated fat is polyunsaturated. Where a "mono" has one double carbon bond, the "poly" fat has several (c=c=c, several spots that are *not* saturated). In corn oils, cottonseed oils, safflower oils, sunflower oils, soybean oils, and mayonnaise, polyunsaturated fat predominates. The fat in fish is also polyunsaturated (a type called omega-3 fatty acids). Didn't think fish had any fat? Well, it does (especially mackerel, salmon, albacore tuna, and sardines), but less than most meats. What's more, the poly-fats have also been shown to help reduce the risk of heart disease. So fish away—just don't fry it.

➤ **Saturated fats**—When triglyceride molecules contain only single carbon bonds (c-c-c, unlike the double bonds you saw in monosaturated and polyunsaturated fats), the fat is grouped as "saturated." Saturated fat can raise your blood cholesterol, which, in turn, can lead to heart disease. Hard to believe a simple molecular change can make such a difference, but it can, and eating too much of these fats can be destructive. Animal fats found in meat, poultry, and whole-milk dairy products are all high in saturated fats. Although most vegetable oils are unsaturated, some "saturated" exceptions include coconut, palm, and palm kernel oils (found in cookies, crackers, nondairy creamers, and other baked products). Do your body a favour: Make a concerted effort to cut back on these fats. You'll help protect yourself from heart disease, certain cancers, and other potential health problems.

Moo!

Overrated–Undercooked

All types of fat when eaten in excess can cause weight gain, but overloading on saturated fat, specifically, can also put you at risk for serious health problems, including heart disease.

➤ **Trans-fatty acids**—This type of fat is *not* naturally occurring but is created when innocent unsaturated fats undergo a manufacturing process called hydrogenation. Hydrogenation is the process of transforming a liquid or semisoft fat into a more solid state. Trans-fatty acids can be harmful because they act like saturated fats inside the body and raise blood cholesterol. What's more, these fats do not appear on a nutrition label since the government does not regulate them to date.

Why mess with a good thing and "hydrogenate?" The process can help preserve food or enable a food company to change the texture of a product. For example, margarine in the liquid form is unsaturated, but with some hydrogenation, it becomes semisoft (tub margarine). With further hydrogenation, it becomes hard (stick margarine). Unfortunately, most people prefer tub and stick over liquid margarines and end up paying the "trans-fatty" penalty. Other trans-fatty culprits include partially hydrogenated vegetable oils, commonly found in snack foods, french fries, cakes, crackers, cookies, and other baked goods. If you read the ingredients on food products, you'll see that trans-fats are everywhere.

What can you do? It would be almost impossible to avoid trans-fat completely. Reducing your total fat and limiting processed products that contain partially hydrogenated oils can significantly reduce your intake of trans-fatty acids.

Q & A

Is it better to use butter or margarine?

While butter is a concentrated source of saturated fat, many brands of margarine are packed with trans–fatty acids. Which one do you choose? Although both types of fat are bad for your arteries, studies suggest that trans-fat is worse. My advice—use a little butter, just go easy. If you're hooked on margarine, buy one that is "nonhydrogenated."

Most Fats Contain Combinations of All Three Types of Fat but Are Predominantly One Type

Saturated	Monounsaturated	Polyunsaturated
Beef fat	Canola oil	Corn oil
Butter	Olive oil	Cottonseed oil
Whole milk	Peanut oil	Safflower oil
Cheese	Sesame oil	Soybean oil

Saturated	Monounsaturated	Polyunsaturated
Coconut oil	Most nuts	Sunflower oil
Palm oil	Avocados	Margarine (soft)
Palm kernel oil		Mayonnaise
		Poultry fat
		Fish oils
		Sesame oil

The Cholesterol Connection and Heart Disease

If you have ever read a nutrition label, you know that dietary fat and cholesterol make up two very different categories. In fact, they are even measured in different units; fat is shown in grams, whereas cholesterol is shown in milligrams. We've already explored the facts on fat; now it's time to explore cholesterol.

Cholesterol is a waxy substance that contributes to the formation of many essential compounds, including vitamin D, bile acid, estrogen, and testosterone. At this point, you might be thinking, If cholesterol does so many great things, why can't I eat as much as I want? First of all, your liver makes all the cholesterol you'll ever need. And while experts agree that cholesterol in food has little effect on blood cholesterol, there are some people who are sensitive to a high-cholesterol diet. Excess cholesterol is transported in your blood and stored as plaque in your arteries. That's why our nutrition experts advise eating no more than 300 milligrams of cholesterol each day.

All animal-related foods and beverages contain cholesterol because all animals have livers. Eggs, meats, fish, cheese, milk, and poultry are all sources of cholesterol. Needless to say, a serving of liver is loaded with the stuff. What's more, plant foods do not contain cholesterol, simply because they never had a liver.

Q & A

How do you lower triglycerides?

Reduce your fat intake, specifically that of saturated fat; cut down on simple sugars such as candy, fruit juice, and so on; limit alcoholic beverages; and engage in regular aerobic exercise.

Don't Be Fooled by Misleading Labels

When a label reads "no cholesterol," the food in question is not necessarily low in calories and fat. Here is a perfect example. I walked into a famous cookie store and noticed these incredibly decadent peanut butter cookies. Next to them was a sign proclaiming "No-Cholesterol Cookies." Well, as far as I know, a peanut has never had a liver, and therefore, peanut butter doesn't have any cholesterol. But WOW, those cookies were packed with fat; the ingredients included peanut butter, margarine, and vegetable oil. Unfortunately, the majority of people mistook these cookies for low-calorie/low-fat cookies just because of the no-cholesterol label. The next time you grab something that reads "no cholesterol," check out the fat content; it might not be all it's cracked up to be.

How does saturated fat work its way into the cholesterol picture? This artery-clogging culprit can also raise blood-cholesterol levels. Eating large portions of high-fat animal foods such as marbled red meats, cheese, and whole-milk dairy products too often will send your blood cholesterol into an upward swing. Eating less saturated fat by choosing leaner meat, poultry breast, and low-fat dairy products is a key strategy to help lower high blood cholesterol.

Total Fat, Saturated Fat, and the Cholesterol Content of Common Foods

Food Name	Portion	Total Fat (g)	Saturated Fat (g)	Cholesterol (mg)
Beef, ground medium fat	3 oz (90 g)	13.3	5.7	79
Beef, ground lean	3 oz (90 g)	11.8	4.8	76
Beef, inside round steak	3 oz (90 g)	3.5	1.2	58.5
Wiener, beef and pork	1 (1$^{1}/_{3}$ oz/37 g)	11	4	19
Chicken breast, roasted no skin	3 oz (90 g)	3.0	trace	73
Turkey breast, no skin	3 oz (90 g)	3.0	trace	59
Liver, pan fried	3 oz (90 g)	7	2	415
Sole/flounder	3 oz (90 g)	1	trace	62
Swordfish	3 oz (90 g)	4.4	1.2	43
Salmon, Atlantic, farmed	3 oz (90 g)	10.5	2.1	54
Lobster	3 oz (90 g)	1	0	78
Shrimp	3 oz (90 g)	trace	trace	135
Whole egg	1	6	2	190
Egg yolk	1	6	2	190
Egg white	1	trace	0	0

Food Name	Portion	Total Fat (g)	Saturated Fat (g)	Cholesterol (mg)
Homogenized milk	1 cup (250 mL)	9	5	35
Skim milk	1 cup (250 mL)	trace	trace	5
Cheddar cheese	1 oz (30 g)	10	6.0	31
Processed cheese	1 oz (30 g)	9.3	6	28
Mozzarella, part skim	1 oz (30 g)	4.5	3.3	18
Peanuts	1/4 cup (50 mL)	38	5	0
Butter	1 Tbs (15 mL)	11	7	31
Margarine, tub	1 Tbs (15 mL)	11	2	0
Olive oil	1 Tbs (15 mL)	14	2	0

Sources: Health Canada: Nutrient Value of Some Common Foods, 1987; Food Values of Portions Commonly Used, Bowes & Church, 1998; The Beef Information Centre, 2000

Your Cholesterol Report Card

Yikes! The doctor just informed you that your blood cholesterol level is high. Are you now at risk for heart disease?

Although it's certainly not in your favour to have clogged arteries, that doesn't mean you'll wind up having a heart attack. In fact, most people have tremendous control over lowering their cholesterol value by limiting the fats and oils in their diet, increasing foods rich in soluble fibre and soy protein, losing weight if it's warranted, and becoming more physically active.

What do those numbers on the report card mean anyway?

➤ **Total blood cholesterol**—This number refers to the amount of cholesterol circulating in the bloodstream and provides a direct correlation to the amount of plaque deposited in your arteries. It is a combination of both types of cholesterol—HDL and LDL. Total cholesterol levels of less than 5.2 mmol/dL are considered desirable. To help remember which "DL" is which, just remember this: "L" in LDL stands for "lousy" and "H" in HDL stands for "helpful."

➤ **HDL**—The "good guys" actually help your body get rid of the cholesterol in your blood (sort of like garbage collectors taking

Food for Thought

Although shellfish contains a considerable amount of cholesterol, it has substantially less total fat and saturated fat than meat and is clearly a leaner choice.

Food for Thought

Some people are born with a genetic predisposition to high cholesterol and therefore might need the assistance of cholesterol-lowering medication.

away the garbage). Thus, the higher your HDL-cholesterol number, the better off you are. An HDL-cholesterol level of less than 0.9 mmol/dL is onsidered low and increases your risk for heart disease.

➤ **LDL**—This cholesterol tends to build up in the walls of your arteries. Thus, the higher your LDL-cholesterol number, the greater your risk for heart disease. A desirable LDL-cholesterol level is less than 3.4 mmol/dL.

Getting Fat from Eating Fat

The consequence of eating excessive fat is one that most of us know all too well: *weight gain*. Gram for gram, fat delivers more than twice as many calories as carbohydrate and protein. In other words, high-fat foods (such as french fries, donuts, cakes, and whole-milk dairy products) are more calorie dense than low-fat foods (grains, fruits, and veggies), and boy, those fat calories can add up quickly. A measly chocolate bar contains 240 calories; by contrast, so does an entire plateful of low-fat foods such as an apple, a banana, and a handful of pretzels. There is no comparison; you get a lot more quantity for the same number of calories when you go low-fat. Sure, the candy bar might sound more appealing, but consider the other fats you may have consumed that same day: salad dressings, fried foods, cheese, and fatty meats. That's a lot of fat, and those calories sure can accumulate!

Moo!

Overrated-Undercooked

Even though excess calories from carbohydrates and protein can put on pounds, it's a lot easier to get fat from eating a lot of fat. One gram of fat supplies more than twice the number of calories your body gets from carbohydrates and protein:

1 gram carbohydrate = 4 calories

1 gram protein = 4 calories

1 gram fat = 9 calories

Don't get me wrong: You shouldn't deprive yourself of the things you love; however, as with money, you must budget your fat so you don't go overboard by the end of the day. In this case, consistently going over budget won't leave you broke; it will leave you fat.

Filling up on fatty foods might also leave little room for the healthy foods that keep us fit. Great—chubby and malnourished! Believe me, I sympathize. It's tough limiting all those delicious donuts, cakes, and gooey, chocolate treats. I'm certainly not one of those "genetic lean machines" who can eat whatever she wants and not gain an ounce. (In my dreams.) For most people, maintaining an ideal weight means watching total fat intake.

How Much Fat and Cholesterol Should We Eat?

The Canadian Heart and Stroke Foundation recommends the following:

➤ Less than 30 percent of the day's total calories should come from fat.

➤ Less than 10 percent of the day's total calories should come from saturated fat.

➤ Less than 300 milligrams of dietary cholesterol is the total you should consume in a day.

A Guide to Recommended Daily Fat Intake

Daily Calories	Fat Calories	Total Fat Grams	Saturated Fat Grams
1,200	<360	<40	<13
1,500	<450	<50	<17
1,800	<540	<60	<20
2,000	<600	<67	<22
2,500	<750	<83	<28
2,800	<840	<93	<31
3,000	<900	<100	<33

Some Fats Are Easier to Spot Than Others

Although some fats and oils are rather obvious, others are hidden deep within our food. Take a look:

➤ **Visible fats**—butter*, cream cheese*, lard*, sour cream*, mayonnaise, oil-based salad dressings, cream-* or cheese-based salad dressings, animal shortenings*, guacamole, cooking oils, peanut butter, and margarine

➤ **Invisible fats**—whole-milk dairy products*, high-fat meats* (including bologna, pepperoni, sausage, bacon, pastrami, spareribs, and hot dogs), donuts*, cakes*, cookies*, nuts, candy bars*, chocolate chips*, avocado, ice cream*, fried foods, pizza*, cole slaw, pasta salad, and potato salad

Contains saturated fat

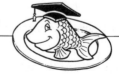

Food for Thought

Thirty to 40 percent of all cancers can be prevented by diet, physical activity, and maintaining a healthy weight. Evidence strongly suggests that people who eat low-fat diets have substantially less risk of certain types of cancer.

Slicing Off the Fat Without a Knife

These are tips to help you reduce the fat in your diet. Read through them and learn how to painlessly develop a low-fat lifestyle:

➤ Choose low-fat dairy products whenever possible: skim or 1% milk, low-fat cheese and yogurts, low-fat sour creams, and frozen yogurt.

➤ Prepare foods by roasting, baking, broiling, boiling, steaming, lightly stir-frying, or grilling.

➤ Use nonfat cooking sprays or nonstick pans when frying.

➤ Remove all skin from poultry and trim all visible fat from meats.

➤ Limit your portion of red meat to 3 ounces (90 g) and try to avoid completely the higher fat selections, including salami, bologna, sausage, pepperoni, bacon, and hot dogs.

➤ Use high-fat spreads like margarine, butter, mayonnaise, and cream cheese sparingly.

➤ Buy low-fat salad dressings, or make your own by mixing balsamic vinegar, Dijon mustard, spices, and a drop of olive oil.

➤ Instead of using butter and oily sauces, flavour your vegetables with herbs and seasonings. Also try lemon juice, spicy mustard, salsa, and flavoured vinegars.

➤ Watch out for pastas swimming in oil and cream sauce. Instead, substitute tomato-based sauces or broth.

➤ Opt for egg-white (or egg substitute) omelets rather than those made with whole eggs. If you can't live without eating whole eggs, limit yourself to five yolks per week.

➤ Pass on the ice cream, chips, and cookies. Instead, treat yourself to pretzels, fig bars, fresh fruit, low-fat yogurt, and fruit sorbets.

➤ Try extra-lean ground turkey breast instead of ground beef in your favorite recipes.

The "Fat-Phobic" Generation

Sure, a low-fat lifestyle is the way to go, but some people misinterpret this message and become utterly neurotic. Are you afraid to even touch anything that might have once possibly come in contact with fat? When ordering in a restaurant, do you create such chaos that your waiter is off and running out the back door?

It might sound funny, but it's no laughing matter to be completely preoccupied with fat. Certainly, a low-fat diet is an essential part of being healthy; however, taking this concept to the extreme can place major restraints on social eating and may set you up for a serious eating disorder. If your reason is weight control, think again. Some fat is fine, and I promise you can achieve and maintain your ideal body weight (within reason, of course) and still allow yourself to enjoy high-fat foods every once in a while.

In fact, joining a "fat-free cult" doesn't necessarily mean that you automatically lose weight. Quite frequently, I meet clients who cannot seem to drop an aggravating 5 or 10 pounds—even while following a strictly fat-free regimen. How can that be?

The answer is rather obvious: They simply overcompensate with fat-free products. For the most part, the explosion of lower fat foods on the market has been a wonderful tool, enabling people to lower their cholesterol and total fat intakes painlessly. Unfortunately for some people, the expression "low-fat" means carte blanche to eating huge amounts. Just because a product is fat free doesn't mean it's calorie free. As a matter of fact, many lower fat foods can pack in just as many calories as their original fat-containing counterparts.

Do you have a friend who will not go near a "real" chocolate-chip cookie but doesn't hesitate to inhale half a box of the fat-free version? Which is worse: the cookie with fat at 75 calories or 15 no-fat cookies at a whopping 750 calories? Remember, no matter where they come from, calories still count in the battle of the bulge.

The Least You Need to Know

➤ Fats perform vital roles in the body, including providing stored energy, storing and circulating fat-soluble vitamins, and providing a layer of insulation underneath the skin.

➤ All types of fat, when eaten in excess, can cause a variety of health problems, including weight gain.

➤ Saturated fat can increase blood cholesterol and therefore promote heart disease.

➤ Live a "low-fat lifestyle" by limiting your intake of higher fat red meats, whole-milk dairy products, fried foods, high-fat spreads, oily sauces, and high-fat snack foods. Switch to low-fat milk, yogurts, and cheese while jazzing up foods with herbs, spices, lemon juice, and Dijon mustard. Munch on popcorn, pretzels, and baked tortilla chips, and when you do, remember that fat-free foods can still pack on the calories.

➤ Although low-fat and fat-free foods are great for your diet, every diet must have some sort of fat in it. A totally "fat-free diet" is dangerous because fat is responsible for vital body functions.

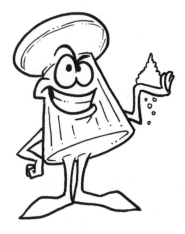

Chapter 5

Don't As-*salt*
Your Body

In This Chapter

➤ All about salt

➤ Sodium and water retention

➤ The high blood pressure connection

➤ How much is recommended

➤ Decreasing your intake

True story: I had a friend in university who would buy a large bucket of salted popcorn at the movie theatre. Once in her seat, she'd whip out a salt shaker hidden in her jacket and heavily salt each handful before popping it into her mouth. The sign of a true salt addict!

Much of your salt habit has to do with the way you grew up and your cultural background. (Some cuisines are loaded with salty condiments and seasonings.) Were your parents into the salt shaker? Were the first three ingredients in Grandma's secret recipes salt, salt, and salt? If so, you were clearly "salt corrupted" as a kid. What about our convenience-food generation? Nowadays, people are so happy to buy prepared, prepackaged, frozen, micro-wavable, and take-out meals, they don't realize the colossal amounts of salt they're putting into their bodies.

So what's the problem? Well, using excessive amounts of salt might lead to uncomfortable water retention and the more serious problem of high blood pressure. Although it has been proven that *not* everyone is "salt sensitive," there is no way to tell who is—and it is certainly better to be safe than sorry when your health is at stake. Read on and learn how to give up the shaker without giving up taste.

All About Salt

Salt is composed of 40 percent sodium and 60 percent chloride. When most people speak of the problems associated with salt, they are usually referring to the part of salt called sodium. What exactly is sodium and what does it do?

Sodium is a mineral that is essential for many important functions, such as

➤ Controlling the fluid balance within your body

➤ Transmitting electrical nerve impulses

➤ Contracting muscles (including your heart)

➤ Absorbing nutrients across cell membranes

➤ Maintaining your body's acid/base balance

Nutri-Speak

Hyponatremia is the excessive loss of sodium and water due to persistent vomiting, diarrhea, or profuse sweating. In this case, both water and salt must be replenished to maintain the correct balance for your body.

With such a wonderful résumé for sodium, why worry about your sodium intake? Here's the reason: Although sodium is essential for good health, it only takes about 115 mg (or $1/20$ of a teaspoon) of salt to cover the needs of sedentary people living in temperate climates. The average Canadian consumes about $1^3/4$ teaspoons of salt each day, almost 40 times more than we need! This is one salty society we live in. In fact, most people could stand to cut back substantially on their salt intake.

Feeling a Bit Waterlogged?

Have your fingers ever been so swollen that it's literally impossible to get your rings on or off? Oh, the uncomfortable effects of excess salt.

Food for Thought

Although your salt intake might vary from day to day, the amount of sodium in your body doesn't generally vary by more than 2 percent. Your body is efficient at conserving sodium if you need it and at excreting it if you have a surplus.

It's common to experience a temporary bloating or swelling after eating highly salted foods. You see, your body requires a certain balance of sodium and water at all times. Extra salt requires extra water, resulting in water retention. Where does this extra water or fluid come from? Usually your glass. Salt triggers your thirst response to balance out the sodium-water concentration. Ever wonder why you're so thirsty after munching on salty pretzels or nuts? It's no coincidence that the snacks offered in drinking establishments are covered with salt. What a strategy: The more you eat, the more you drink!

Try performing this test: Record your weight one morning. Then, before going to bed that night, eat a large serving of heavily salted popcorn or other food (drink a lot of water). Weigh yourself again the next morning. It is amazing how much water that salt can retain. All you dieters out there, remember that this is water weight—not fat weight. Don't panic; it will be gone by the end of the day.

Note: Do not, under any circumstances, try the preceding test if you have any medical condition.

Can't Take the Pressure!

For reasons that are not completely understood, salt can play an active role in raising the blood pressure in people who are salt sensitive.

What Exactly Is High Blood Pressure?

When your heart beats, it pumps blood into your arteries and creates a pressure within them. High blood pressure (also known as hypertension) occurs when too much pressure is placed on the walls of the arteries. This can occur if there is an increase in blood volume or the blood vessels themselves constrict or narrow.

People who are genetically sensitive to salt can't efficiently get rid of extra sodium through their urine. Therefore, that extra sodium hangs around, drawing in extra water, which means an increase in blood volume. This increased blood volume can then stimulate the vessels to constrict, creating increased pressure.

Imagine a garden hose with a normal flow of water running through it. No problem. Now, think about the increased pressure on the hose when you drastically increase the amount of water rushing out. What if you were to pinch off spots of this hose, like a constricted blood vessel? A garden hose might endure the wear and tear, but your arteries can become extremely damaged by such constant pressure—so damaged that the result might include a heart attack, stroke (a brain attack), or kidney disease.

Nutri-Speak

Hypertension is the medical term for sustained high blood pressure. It has nothing to do with being tense, nervous, or hyperactive.

Food for Thought

A person whose high blood pressure is not successfully treated faces up to a 40 percent risk of stroke within 10 years.

After the age of 55, the risk of stroke doubles every 10 years.

Stroke is the fourth leading cause of death in Canada.

Source: Canadian Heart and Stroke Foundation

What Causes High Blood Pressure?

According to recent statistics, one out of every five Canadian adults—nearly 5 million people—has high blood pressure. In a small percentage of people, this increased pressure is from an underlying problem such as kidney disease or a tumour of the adrenal gland. However, in 90 to 95 percent of all cases, the cause is unclear. That's why it is known as the *silent killer*; it just creeps up without any warning. Whereas some of the contributing factors are *not* controllable, others can be quite controllable.

Risk factors that cannot be controlled are

> ➤ **Age**—The older you get, the more likely you are to develop high blood pressure.

> ➤ **Race**—African-Americans tend to have high blood pressure more often than white people. They also tend to develop it earlier and more severely.

> ➤ **Heredity**—High blood pressure can run in families. If you have a family history of high blood pressure, you're twice as likely to develop it than people who do not have such a history.

Risk factors that can be controlled are

> ➤ **Obesity**—Being extremely overweight is clearly related to high blood pressure. In fact, nearly 60 percent of all high blood pressure cases concern overweight patients. By losing weight—even a small amount—obese individuals can significantly reduce their blood pressure.

> ➤ **Sodium consumption**—Reducing the intake of salt can lower blood pressure in people who are salt sensitive.

> ➤ **Alcohol consumption**—Regular use of alcohol can dramatically increase blood pressure in some people. Fortunately, alcohol's effect on blood pressure is completely reversible. Limit yourself to a maximum of two drinks a day.

> ➤ **Smoking**—Although the long-term effect of smoking on blood pressure is still unclear, the short-term effect is that it can raise blood pressure briefly. However, given that both smoking and high blood pressure have been linked to heart disease, smoking compounds the risk.

> ➤ **Oral contraceptives**—Women who take birth control pills may develop high blood pressure.

> ➤ **Physical inactivity**—Lack of exercise can contribute to high blood pressure. By becoming more active with moderate exercise, an inactive person can get into better shape, feel terrific, and help keep his or her blood pressure in check.

Investigating Your Blood Pressure Numbers

Your doctor measures two numbers when checking your blood pressure, systolic and diastolic. *Systolic pressure* is the top, larger number. This represents the amount of

Q & A

What's a normal blood pressure reading?

Normal blood pressure readings fall within a range. It is not one set of numbers; however, it should be less than 140/90 if you are an adult.

How do you know if you have high blood pressure?

You don't! High blood pressure is known as the "silent killer" because it has no symptoms. In fact, many people can have hypertension for years without knowing it; by that time, their body organs may have already been damaged. Stay on top of your health and have your blood pressure checked regularly by a qualified health professional.

pressure that is in your arteries while your heart contracts (or beats). During this contraction, blood is ejected from the heart and into the blood vessels that travel throughout your body.

Diastolic pressure is the bottom, smaller number. This represents the pressure in your arteries while your heart is relaxing between beats. During this relaxation period, your heart is filling up with blood for the next squeeze. Although both numbers are critically important, your doctor might be more concerned with an elevated diastolic number because this indicates that there is increased pressure on the artery walls even when your heart is resting.

How to Lower High Blood Pressure

If your blood pressure is high, don't panic. Most people can significantly lower their numbers with know-how and determination. A diagnosis of high blood pressure often requires reducing salt intake, losing excess weight, increasing exercise, and in some instances, taking medication:

➤ **Diet**—Lose weight if you are overweight by cutting back on calories and fat. Reduce your consumption of sodium by avoiding salty foods, and limit the amount of alcohol you drink. Better yet, avoid alcohol completely.

➤ **Exercise**—Become physically active and get some type of exercise at least four times a week. Check with your doctor before beginning any diet or exercise program.

➤ **Medication**—For some people, diet and exercise are just not enough. In this case, your doctor might give you medication to help lower your blood pressure.

➤ **If you smoke—QUIT!**

How Much Sodium Is Recommended?

Food for Thought

Studies suggest that calcium, potassium, and magnesium may also play a beneficial role in the regulation of blood pressure. Consult with your dietitian for further information on how to boost your intake of these minerals.

Many question the "one size fits all" recommendation because not everyone is salt sensitive. However, there is no test for salt sensitivity; therefore, it makes sense for *everyone* to play it safe and follow a prudent approach. Most health professionals recommend limiting your intake of sodium to no more than 2,400 milligrams per day. This includes both the salt you add and the sodium that is already present in foods you eat. You might want to know that 75 percent of the salt we eat comes from processed foods, not the salt shaker. Become familiar with the following list of high-sodium foods, and learn to balance your diet so you don't go sodium overboard. Note, if you have high blood pressure, your doctor might prescribe a more severe sodium restriction.

Common Foods That Are High in Sodium

Seasonings and Cooking Aids	Portion Size	Sodium (mg)
Baking powder	1 tsp (5 mL)	426
Baking soda	1 tsp (5 mL)	1,259
Table salt	1 tsp (5 mL)	2,300
Garlic salt	1 tsp (5 mL)	2,050
Bouillon cube, chicken	1 item	1,152
Bouillon cube, beef	1 item	864
Monosodium glutamate (MSG)	1 Tbs (15 mL)	1,914
Salad dressing, Italian	1 Tbs (15 mL)	116
Soy sauce	1 Tbs (15 mL)	1,029
Low-sodium soy sauce	1 Tbs (15 mL)	660
Canned Food Items	**Portion Size**	**Sodium (mg)**
Tuna, canned	3 oz (90 g)	303
Sardines, canned	3 oz (90 g)	261
Caviar, black and red	1 Tbs (15 mL)	240
Chicken noodle soup	1 cup (250 mL)	1,106
Vegetable soup	1 cup (250 mL)	795
Veg. beef soup (low-sodium)	1 cup (250 mL)	57
Corn, canned	1/2 cup (125 mL)	266
Asparagus, canned	1/2 cup (125 mL)	472
Sauerkraut, canned	1/2 cup (125 mL)	780

Processed/Cured and Smoked Meats	Portion Size	Sodium (mg)
Bologna	3 oz (90 g)	832
Salami	3 oz (90 g)	1,922
Hot dog	1 item	639
Smoked turkey	3 oz (90 g)	916
Smoked fish	3 oz (90 g)	619
Smoked sausage	3 oz (90 g)	853

Snack Foods	Portion Size	Sodium (mg)
Salted nuts	1 oz (30 g)	230
Pretzels	1 oz (30 g)	476
Corn chips	1 oz (30 g)	164
Potato chips	1 oz (30 g)	133
Popcorn	1 oz (30 g)	179
Saltines	5 crackers	180
Peanut butter	1 Tbs (15 mL)	76

Dairy Products	Portion Size	Sodium (mg)
Processed cheese	1 oz (30 g)	336
Cheddar cheese	1 oz (30 g)	176
Parmesan cheese	1 oz (30 g)	527
Cottage cheese	1/2 cup (125 mL)	459
Butter	1 Tbs (15 mL)	116
Margarine	1 Tbs (15 mL)	132

Common Breakfast Cereals	Portions Size	Sodium (mg)
Rice Krispies	1 oz (30 g)	294
Corn Flakes	1 oz (30 g)	351
All-Bran	1 oz (30 g)	320
Cheerios	1 oz (30 g)	307
Special K	1 oz (30 g)	306
Raisin Bran	1 oz (30 g)	155

Source: First Databank, 1996 and Bowes & Church's Food Values of Portions Commonly Used, 15th ed., 1989

Salt-Less Solutions

Giving up salt doesn't mean giving up the pleasure of eating. However, you'll need to be a bit more selective with certain food products and much more creative in the seasoning department. The following guidelines can show you how to drastically cut the amount of salt in your food and body:

Overrated-Undercooked

Be aware that some over-the-counter medicines contain a lot of sodium. For example, two tablets of dissolvable Alka-Seltzer (plop plop fizz fizz) have a whopping 1,134 milligrams of sodium. (Each single tablet provides 567 milligrams.) Instead, opt for the caplets that you swallow; they contain *only* 1.8 milligrams. Quite a difference.

➤ Enhance the flavour of your foods with spices and herbs. Try allspice, basil, bay leaves, chives, cinnamon, curry powder, dill, garlic (not garlic salt), onion (not onion salt), rosemary, nutmeg, thyme, sage, turmeric, mace, and salt substitutes.

➤ Avoid putting a salt shaker on your table.

➤ Choose fresh and frozen vegetables when possible. (The canned versions generally contain a lot of salt.) When canned is the only option, reduce the salt by draining the liquid and rinsing the vegetables in water before eating.

➤ Here I go with another plug for fresh fruit: It's naturally low in sodium.

➤ Go easy on condiments that contain considerable amounts of salt, including ketchup, mustard, monosodium glutamate (MSG), salad dressings, sauces, bouillon cubes, olives, sauerkraut, and pickles. Stock your kitchen with low-sodium versions of soy sauce, teriyaki sauce, steak sauce, and anything else you might find in your travels.

➤ Select unsalted (or reduced salt) nuts, seeds, crackers, popcorn, and pretzels.

➤ Take it easy with processed cheese slices and cheese spreads. Unfortunately, they have not only a lot of fat, but also a lot of sodium.

➤ Read labels carefully and choose foods lower in sodium, especially when choosing frozen dinners, canned soups, packaged mixes, and combination dishes.

➤ Beware of processed luncheon cold cuts, as well as cured and smoked meats, because they are saturated with sodium. This includes bacon, bologna, salami, sausages, hot dogs, smoked turkey, fish, and beef. Also be aware that most varieties of canned fish (tuna, salmon, and sardines) are extremely high in sodium. Whenever you can, choose low-sodium varieties.

➤ When dining in Asian restaurants, ask for meals without MSG or added salt. Nowadays, you can also request low-sodium soy sauce for your table. If they don't have any, dilute the regular by adding a tablespoon of water.

The Least You Need to Know

➤ Salt consists of 40 percent sodium and 60 percent chloride. The mineral sodium is essential for many important functions. It maintains body fluids and the contraction of muscles and transmits nerve impulses.

➤ Eating a high-sodium diet can increase blood pressure in people who are "salt sensitive."

➤ People diagnosed with high blood pressure often need to reduce their salt intake, lose excess weight, increase exercise, and in some instances, take blood pressure–lowering medication.

➤ Because salt sensitivity is *not* something we are tested for, everyone should limit his or her sodium intake to less than 2,400 milligrams per day.

➤ Reduce your sodium intake by using herbs, spices, and other seasonings instead of salt. Limit canned food items, salty snack foods, luncheon cold cuts, and meats that have been smoked or cured. Go easy on high-sodium condiments such as soy sauce, teriyaki sauce, mustard, ketchup, olives, pickles, and sauerkraut. Also read labels carefully and opt for the lower sodium foods.

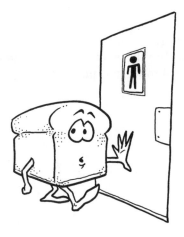

Chapter 6

The Facts on Fibre

In This Chapter

➤ What is fibre?

➤ The different kinds of fibre

➤ Benefits of a fibre-rich diet

➤ How much fibre do you need?

➤ Increasing your daily fibre intake

Say you're a little constipated? Have high cholesterol? Want to reduce your risk of colon cancer? Have I got a food for you! What is this magical food? Where can you get some? Well, the nice part is that you don't have to buy any special potions or formulas or seek the advice of your local medicine man or woman. This incredible healer is conveniently found in some of your favourite carbohydrate-rich foods.

Fibre Facts: What Is Fibre Anyway?

Fibre is a mix of many different substances found in plant cell walls and is not digestible by the human body. *In it comes and out it goes*. How can a substance we cannot even digest (and which, by the way, has no nutritional value) be so beneficial? Might sound crazy, but once inside your body, fibre does some pretty amazing things. The term *dietary fibre*, when listed on a nutrition label, simply refers to the amount of these indigestible substances in a specific food product. By reading nutrition labels, you can identify a food rich in fibre.

Fibre fits in one of two categories, insoluble and soluble, depending upon its ability to dissolve (or not dissolve) in water. Some foods contain *both* soluble and insoluble fibre, whereas in others, only one predominates. The key is to eat a variety of fibre-rich foods each day and receive the beneficial effects from both types.

Soluble Fibre

Water-soluble fibre readily dissolves in water. Technically speaking, soluble fibres include pectins, gums, and mucilages. It's obvious, however, that these terms won't be of any help to you in your grocery store. Translated into "real-food" terminology, you'll find soluble fibre in the following:

- ➤ Oats
- ➤ Brown rice
- ➤ Barley
- ➤ Oat bran
- ➤ Psyllium
- ➤ Dried beans and peas
- ➤ Rye
- ➤ Seeds
- ➤ Vegetables (especially carrots, corn, cauliflower, green peas, and sweet potatoes)
- ➤ Fruits (especially apples, strawberries, oranges, cantaloupe, nectarines, and pears)

Why all the hoopla? Well for starters, foods rich in soluble fibre have been shown to help decrease blood cholesterol, therefore reducing the risk of heart disease. Another benefit of fibre comes from its ability to slow the absorption of glucose (sugar in the blood), which might in turn help control blood sugar levels in people with diabetes.

Insoluble Fibre

The type of fibre that does not readily dissolve in water is called *water-insoluble* fibre. Insoluble fibre includes lignin, cellulose, and hemicellulose. Once again, converted into understandable food terms, we are talking about the following:

- ➤ Wheat bran
- ➤ Corn bran
- ➤ Whole-wheat breads and cereals
- ➤ Fruits
- ➤ Vegetables (especially potatoes with skin, parsnips, green beans, and broccoli)

As you can see, some foods are mentioned on both lists, indicating that they provide both soluble *and* insoluble fibre.

Insoluble fibre is primarily responsible for accelerating intestinal transit time, along with increasing and softening stools. In other words, insoluble fibre is responsible for "moving things along," if you know what I mean. In addition to promoting regularity, insoluble fibre has been shown to decrease your risk for colon cancer and diverticulosis.

Reducing Your Risk of Colon Cancer

Can a diet rich in fibre actually lower your chance of developing colon cancer? Several studies say yes, and it makes perfect sense. Think about it. *Insoluble fibre* helps move waste material through your intestines more quickly. Therefore, there is less time for suspicious substances to lurk around and possibly damage your colon and rectal area. In addition, fibre may bind with possibly harmful bacteria, transporting it through the intestines and out of your body. While we're down there, it's a perfect time to point out that softer, more regular bowel movements can also prevent constipation and reduce your chance of getting hemorrhoids.

Lowering Your Cholesterol Level

If your cholesterol tends to be a bit high, or you'd just like to maintain an already low number, you might want to increase your *soluble fibre*. Soluble fibres have been shown to bind with cholesterol and pull it out of the body. Fruits, vegetables, legumes, oats, oat bran, and cereals enriched with psyllium can therefore reduce your risk for heart and artery disease by lowering blood cholesterol. Another thought is that high-fibre foods can displace some of the high-fat, artery-clogging foods in your diet— a double impact!

Feeling Fuller with Less Food

Did you ever feel as though a plate of vegetables expanded in your stomach after you ate it? Well, it did! Eating fibre-rich foods can make you feel full because they absorb water and swell inside you. You might also feel full longer if you choose a meal with some soluble fibre. Unlike insoluble fibre, which quickly moves food through your body, soluble fibre tends to stick around a while, keeping you full and satisfied.

Does this mean you'll lose weight from eating a lot of fibre? It does if you eat these foods *instead* of the high-fat, high-calorie stuff. If you eat them in addition to all the junky food, your chance of becoming slim is slim.

Nutri-Speak

Diverticulosis is an illness or condition where tiny pouches (called diverticula) form in the wall of the colon. The condition is often without symptoms, but when the pouches become infected or inflamed, it can be painful. When this happens, the condition is known as diverticulitis, which can cause fever, abdominal pain, and diarrhea.

Overrated-Undercooked

Just because a food sounds healthy doesn't necessarily mean that it is. Some commercial bran muffins are loaded with fat and sugar—certainly not worth the small amount of fibre they provide.

How Much Fibre Do You Need?

Although there's no Recommended Nutrient Intake (RNI) for fibre, most health experts agree that we should aim for 25–35 grams of dietary fibre each day (a mix of both soluble and insoluble). On the following page are a few ideas to help you raise your intake of fibre.

> **Ready-Made Menu**
> This sample day provides about 35 grams of fibre:
>
> Breakfast   Bowl of **bran cereal** with milk
> **Banana**
> Glass of unsweetened fruit juice
>
> Lunch   Roast beef sandwich on **100% whole-wheat bread**
> Cup of **vegetable barley soup**
> **Apple with skin**
> A lot of water
>
> Snack   **Chewy fruit bar**
> Low-fat yogurt
>
> Dinner   **Mixed green salad**
> Grilled fish with **sautéed carrots**
> **Baked sweet potato**
> **Fresh strawberries**
> Club soda with lemon

Tips to Increase the Fibre in Your Diet

As you read the following tips, keep these points in mind. It's important to increase your fibre *gradually* (sometimes over several weeks) because your body needs time to adjust. For example, if you are a newcomer to the world of fibre, start with 20 grams each day for the first week. Increase to 25 grams per day the second week, and—if your stomach can handle it—graduate to 30+ grams per day by week three. Also, drink plenty of fluids. Fibre acts as a bulking agent by absorbing some of the fluid in your body. Extra fluids will prevent you from becoming dehydrated, and most importantly, help that bulk to move merrily on its way.

➤ Read nutrition labels. Generally, a high source of fibre should have at least 4 grams per serving. A very high source of fibre has at least 6 grams.

➤ Start your day with a high-fibre breakfast cereal. Supermarkets are flooded with them. Read the nutrition label and select a cereal that offers at least 4 grams per serving.

➤ Add a few tablespoons of wheat bran to your hot cereal, cottage cheese, yogurt, and salads.

➤ Include plenty of fresh or frozen vegetables in your day. Add them to soups, pizza, sandwiches, stir-frys, pastas, omelets, rice, and anything else you can think of.

➤ Eat breads and pasta made from whole-wheat, rye, and oat products, along with brown rice, barley, and bulgur.

➤ Add fruit to your cereal (hot or cold), top off your pancakes and waffles with fruits, mix fruits into yogurts and salads, or simply enjoy them plain. Remember, whole fruit, with seeds and peel intact, provides more fibre than most fruit juice.

➤ Cook with beans and lentils. They are loaded with fibre. Enjoy them in soups, pastas, stews, salads, burritos, and a million other creative entrees.

➤ Get your fibre from food sources, not supplements. Food is a natural provider not only of fibre, but of other essential nutrients as well.

Q & A

How much fibre do kids need?

Just tack on an extra 5 grams to their age; this works for healthy kids from age 3 to 18. Your child's age plus five equals the grams of dietary fibre he or she requires each day.

The following table lists foods rich in fibre:

Foods Rich in Fibre

Fruits	Grams of Fibre
Raspberries (1 c/250 mL)	5.50
Pear (1)	4.65
Blueberries (1 c/250 mL)	4.00
Prunes (5)	3.00
Apple (1)	3.00
Orange (1)	3.00
Strawberries (1 c/250 mL)	2.70
Grapes (1^1/2 cups/375 mL)	2.30
Banana (1)	2.00
Peach (1)	2.00
Grapefruit (^{1}/2)	1.70
Nectarine (1)	1.60

Vegetables (All Servings ¹/₂ Cup/125 mL Cooked)	Grams of Fibre
Green Peas	4.00
Broccoli	3.60
Brussels sprouts	3.00
Sweet potato (small)	3.00
Baked potato with skin (small)	2.50
Carrots	2.50
Spinach	2.20
Corn	1.70

Breads and Grains	Grams of Fibre
Barley (1 c/250 mL cooked)	8.80
Whole wheat bread (2 slices)	3.20
Brown rice (³/₄ c/175 mL cooked)	2.50
Bran muffin (1)	2.50

Cereals (Measured by Weight; Serving Sizes Will Vary)	Grams of Fibre
Fibre One (¹/₂ c/125 mL)	12.90
100% Bran (¹/₂ c/125 mL)	9.75
All-Bran (¹/₃ c/75 mL)	8.40
Bran Buds (¹/₃ c/75 mL)	7.70
Bran Flakes (³/₄ c/175 mL)	5.00
Raisin Bran (³/₄ c/175 mL)	4.50
Shredded Wheat (³/₄ c/175 mL)	4.00
Oatmeal (¹/₂ c/125 mL cooked)	2.20
Wheat bran (4 Tbs/50 mL)	2.00
Wheat germ (2 Tbs/25 mL)	1.50

Beans (All Servings Equal; ¹/₂ Cup/125 mL Cooked)	Grams of Fibre
Pinto	6.40
Navy	4.70
White	4.40
Kidney	4.30
Black	3.60

Sources: First Databank, 1996 and Bowes & Church's Food Values of Portions Commonly Used, 15th Ed., 1989

Don't Overdo It!

Can you ever eat too much fibre? You sure can, especially if your body is not used to it. I remember a friend who ate a large bowl of All-Bran cereal the night before his first 10-kilometre race, and spent the entire run looking for a gas station. Overloading on fibre can cause severe bloating, cramping, gas, diarrhea, and other abdominal discomforts. Furthermore, excessive amounts of fibre (generally 50 grams or more per day) can decrease the absorption of important vitamins and minerals—specifically calcium, zinc, magnesium, and iron. With all this in mind, once again, be sure to increase your fibre gradually, over a period of several weeks, and drink plenty of extra fluids to help the fibre pass through your system. The key is to pay attention to your body's response so you can figure out the amount you can handle at one time.

Food for Thought

Watch how the amount of fibre can decrease as food changes form:

Apple with peel = 3.0 grams

Apple without peel = 2.4 grams

$1/2$ cup/125 mL apple juice = 0 grams

The Least You Need to Know

➤ Fibre is the indigestible substance found in plants and is classified in two categories: water soluble and water insoluble.

➤ Most foods contain combinations of both fibres. Foods particularly rich in soluble fibre include oats, oat bran, psyllium-enriched breakfast cereals, legumes, rye, fruits, and vegetables. Foods rich in insoluble fibre include wheat bran, whole-wheat breads and cereals, fruits, and vegetables.

➤ Studies show that soluble fibre can help lower blood cholesterol and improve the control of blood sugar in people with diabetes. Insoluble fibre has been reported to decrease the risk for colon cancer and diverticulosis, and to prevent hemorrhoids and constipation.

➤ The recommended fibre intake is 25–35 grams a day and is an important part of every well-balanced food plan for the average adult.

➤ Increase your fibre gradually to give your body time to adjust. Also, be sure to drink plenty of extra fluids.

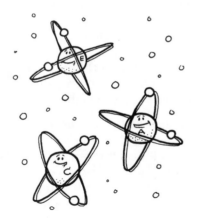

Chapter 7

Vitamins and Minerals: the Micronutrients

In This Chapter

➤ All about vitamins and minerals

➤ Recommended nutrient intakes (RNIs) and dietary reference intakes (DRIs)

➤ Choosing foods that supply what you need

➤ How antioxidants improve your health

A woman walked into my office for an initial consultation. After introducing herself, she pulled open a large duffel bag filled to the rim with vitamin and mineral bottles. "I take one of each, every day," she claimed. "Why?" I asked. "Well, a neighbour told me about extra Bs, and my hairdresser recommended extra iron, and the others I can't seem to remember."

Unfortunately, this story is not uncommon. Popping pills has certainly become a popular morning ritual throughout Canada and the United States. And why not? We've all heard the dramatic tales of vitamins and minerals. Everywhere from health food stores to infomercials, the buzz seems to be about megadosing on one thing or another. Needless to say, the vitamin industry is big business, with annual sales reaching the *multibillion dollar* level.

Do you really need all of the pills? Chances are you don't. With so much misinformation floating around, it's no wonder some people swallow exorbitant amounts of supplements they don't need. By the way, some of those extra supplements are literally money down the toilet because your body usually filters out the extra stuff. What's worse, some vitamins do not get flushed out and can potentially become toxic.

Don't get me wrong, vitamins and minerals are essential for normal functioning, and without them, you could not survive. However, your body requires only minute amounts of these micronutrients, and most nutrition experts agree that the best way to get the vitamins and minerals you need is to eat a varied diet. Whole foods contain not only vitamins and minerals, but also natural chemicals that fight disease. A supplement pill can't give you this entire package of protective ingredients.

Some groups of people *can* benefit from supplements, though. I admit that it's not easy to eat a balanced diet brimming with healthy foods every single day. Surveys show that many Canadians fall short on important nutrients such as calcium, iron, and zinc. If you're on the go, under stress, or a haphazard eater, chances are you don't always eat right. In this case, a multiple vitamin and mineral is a wise idea. I think of multivitamins as a form of nutritional insurance. In Chapter 8, "Mighty Minerals: Calcium and Iron," I help you determine if you need to take a supplement.

Even if you are getting the recommended nutrient intake (RNI), there are certain vitamins you probably should get more of. Vitamins such as C, E, and folate may reduce your risk for cancer, heart disease, and other age-related illness if taken in amounts greater than the official RNIs. It may be a challenge, or in some cases impossible, to get these amounts from your diet. Vitamin E is a good example. The RNI is a mere 13 international units (IU), yet studies have found that much more may prevent a heart attack. Before you rush off to your local health food store, it's important to check with a competent health professional about supplementing your diet safely.

But first, let's boost your diet with micronutrients! This chapter will help clear up the facts on vitamins and minerals and help you find out whether you are getting what your body needs.

What Are Vitamins and Minerals?

In previous chapters, you became familiar with the *macronutrients* carbohydrate, protein, and fat. Now it's time to understand the *micronutrients* (in other words, vitamins and minerals), which exist within the macronutrients. Although the macronutrients receive top billing, micronutrients are equally important in our diets because they perform specific jobs that enable your body to operate efficiently.

Think about carbohydrate, protein, and fat as the rock stars on stage. Now, imagine the vitamins and minerals as the backup singers, the band, and all the people who help produce the concert. Everyone works together to get the job done, and the result is one amazing show.

That's how your body works. You eat the carbohydrate, protein, and fat, which in turn supply your body with the 13 vitamins and at least 22 minerals you need. Although tiny in size and quantity, these nutrients accomplish the mighty tasks that keep your body going. Furthermore, a lack of any one will cause a unique deficiency that can be corrected only by supplying that particular nutrient.

The RNIs: Recommended Nutrient Intakes

The recommended nutrient intakes (RNIs) are standards set by an expert committee known as the Scientific Review Committee of Health and Welfare Canada. These recommendations list the average daily requirements for a variety of nutrients (in other words, vitamins and minerals) and are intended for healthy people. The RNIs represent the amount of a nutrient that's needed to prevent your body becoming deficient.

Note: People with certain illnesses might require more or less of specific nutrients. The RNI guidelines are set slightly higher than the level your body actually needs, building in a precautionary safety net.

The DRIs: Dietary Reference Intakes

Because scientific knowledge regarding diet and health has increased, a panel of Canadian and American experts (called the Food and Nutrition Board of the National Academy of Sciences) has recently expanded its framework and developed the dietary reference intakes (DRIs) for several vital nutrients. It is forecasted that over the next three to four years, additional groups of nutrients, including antioxidants, phytoestrogens, and phytochemicals, will also be slated for review aimed at developing DRIs. These new DRI standards include the recommended dietary allowances (RDAs) (this term will replace recommended nutrient intakes) as goals for intakes, plus three new reference values; the estimated average requirement (EAR), the tolerable upper limit (UL), and the adequate intake (AI). On the two reference charts provided here, you'll notice that some nutrients are listed as DRIs, some as RDAs, and some as AIs—a bit confusing—but all you'll need to understand is the actual recommended amount.

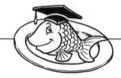

Food for Thought

For your personal nutrition profile, visit my Web site at www.lesliebeck.com. Simply fill out your food for a typical day (and list your height, weight, and age), and I'll show you how you measure up to your daily requirements for vitamins, minerals, calories, carbohydrate, protein, fat, sugar, fibre, and much more.

Fat-Soluble Vitamins

Vitamins are organic compounds (compounds that contain carbon), and of the 13 that your body needs, 4 are called fat soluble (A, D, E, and K). Fat-soluble vitamins do not dissolve in water and are stored in your body's fat and liver. As a result, these vitamins can build up in the tissues and become toxic (specifically vitamins A and D).

FOOD AND NUTRITION BOARD, NATIONAL ACADEMY OF SCIENCES–NATIONAL RESEARCH COUNCIL
RECOMMENDED DIETARY ALLOWANCES,[a] Revised 1989 (Abridged)
Designed for the maintenance of good nutrition of practically all healthy people in the United States

Category	Age (years) or Condition	Weight[b] (kg)	Weight[b] (lb)	Height[b] (cm)	Height[b] (in)	Protein (g)	Vitamin A (µg RE)[c]	Vitamin E (mg α-TE)[d]	Vitamin K (µg)	Vitamin C (mg)	Iron (mg)	Zinc (mg)	Iodine (µg)	Selenium (µg)
Infants	0.0–0.5	6	13	60	24	13	375	3	5	30	6	5	40	10
	0.5–1.0	9	20	71	28	14	375	4	10	35	10	5	50	15
Children	1–3	13	29	90	35	16	400	6	15	40	10	10	70	20
	4–6	20	44	112	44	24	500	7	20	45	10	10	90	20
	7–10	28	62	132	52	28	700	7	30	45	10	10	120	30
Males	11–14	45	99	157	62	45	1,000	10	45	50	12	15	150	40
	15–18	66	145	176	69	59	1,000	10	65	60	12	15	150	50
	19–24	72	160	177	70	58	1,000	10	70	60	10	15	150	70
	25–50	79	174	176	70	63	1,000	10	80	60	10	15	150	70
	51+	77	170	173	68	63	1,000	10	80	60	10	15	150	70
Females	11–14	46	101	157	62	46	800	8	45	50	15	12	150	45
	15–18	55	120	163	64	44	800	8	55	60	15	12	150	50
	19–24	58	128	164	65	46	800	8	60	60	15	12	150	55
	25–50	63	138	163	64	50	800	8	65	60	15	12	150	55
	51+	65	143	160	63	50	800	8	65	60	10	12	150	55
Pregnant						60	800	10	65	70	30	15	175	65
Lactating	1st 6 months					65	1,300	12	65	95	15	19	200	75
	2nd 6 months					62	1,200	11	65	90	15	16	200	75

NOTE: This table does not include nutrients for which Dietary Reference Intakes have recently been established (see *Dietary Reference Intakes for Calcium, Phosphorus, Magnesium, Vitamin D, and Fluoride* [1997] and *Dietary Reference Intakes for Thiamin, Riboflavin, Niacin, Vitamin B₆, Folate, Vitamin B₁₂, Pantothenic Acid, Biotin, and Choline* [1998]).

[a] The allowances, expressed as average daily intakes over time, are intended to provide for individual variations among most normal persons as they live in the United States under usual environmental stresses. Diets should be based on a variety of common foods in order to provide other nutrients for which human requirements have been less well defined.

[b] Weights and heights of Reference Adults are actual medians for the U.S. population of the designated age, as reported by NHANES II. The median weights and heights of those under 19 years of age were taken from Hamill et al. (1979). The use of these figures does not imply that the height-to-weight ratios are ideal.

[c] Retinol equivalents. 1 retinol equivalent = 1 µg retinol or 6 µg β-carotene.

[d] α-Tocopherol equivalents. 1 mg d-α tocopherol = 1 α-TE.

FOOD AND NUTRITION BOARD, INSTITUTE OF MEDICINE-NATIONAL ACADEMY OF SCIENCES
DIETARY REFERENCE INTAKES: RECOMMENDED INTAKES FOR INDIVIDUALS

Life-Stage Group	Calcium (mg/d)	Phosphorus (mg/d)	Magnesium (mg/d)	Vitamin D (µg/d)[a,b]	Fluoride (mg/d)	Thiamin (mg/d)	Riboflavin (mg/d)	Niacin (mg/d)[c]	Vitamin B_6 (mg/d)	Folate (µg/d)[d]	Vitamin B_{12} (µg/d)	Pantothenic Acid (mg/d)	Biotin (µg/d)	Choline[e] (mg/d)
Infants														
0–6 mo	210*	100*	30*	5*	0.01*	0.2*	0.3*	2*	0.1*	65*	0.4*	1.7*	5*	125*
7–12 mo	270*	275*	75*	5*	0.5*	0.3*	0.4*	4*	0.3*	80*	0.5*	1.8*	6*	150*
Children														
1–3 yr	500*	460	80	5*	0.7*	0.5	0.5	6	0.5	150	0.9	2*	8*	200*
4–8 yr	800*	500	130	5*	1*	0.6	0.6	8	0.6	200	1.2	3*	12*	250*
Males														
9–13 yr	1,300*	1,250	240	5*	2*	0.9	0.9	12	1.0	300	1.8	4*	20*	375*
14–18 yr	1,300*	1,250	410	5*	3*	1.2	1.3	16	1.3	400	2.4	5*	25*	550*
19–30 yr	1,000*	700	400	5*	4*	1.2	1.3	16	1.3	400	2.4	5*	30*	550*
31–50 yr	1,000*	700	420	5*	4*	1.2	1.3	16	1.3	400	2.4	5*	30*	550*
51–70 yr	1,200*	700	420	10*	4*	1.2	1.3	16	1.7	400	2.4[f]	5*	30*	550*
>70 yr	1,200*	700	420	15*	4*	1.2	1.3	16	1.7	400	2.4[f]	5*	30*	550*
Females														
9–13 yr	1,300*	1,250	240	5*	2*	0.9	0.9	12	1.0	300	1.8	4*	20*	375*
14–18 yr	1,300*	1,250	360	5*	3*	1.0	1.0	14	1.2	400[g]	2.4	5*	25*	400*
19–30 yr	1,000*	700	310	5*	3*	1.1	1.1	14	1.3	400[g]	2.4	5*	30*	425*
31–50 yr	1,000*	700	320	5*	3*	1.1	1.1	14	1.3	400[g]	2.4	5*	30*	425*
51–70 yr	1,200*	700	320	10*	3*	1.1	1.1	14	1.5	400	2.4[f]	5*	30*	425*
>70 yr	1,200*	700	320	15*	3*	1.1	1.1	14	1.5	400	2.4[f]	5*	30*	425*
Pregnancy														
≤18 yr	1,300*	1,250	400	5*	3*	1.4	1.4	18	1.9	600[h]	2.6	6*	30*	450*
19–30 yr	1,000*	700	350	5*	3*	1.4	1.4	18	1.9	600[h]	2.6	6*	30*	450*
31–50 yr	1,000*	700	360	5*	3*	1.4	1.4	18	1.9	600[h]	2.6	6*	30*	450*
Lactation														
≤18 yr	1,300*	1,250	360	5*	3*	1.5	1.6	17	2.0	500	2.8	7*	35*	550*
19–30 yr	1,000*	700	310	5*	3*	1.5	1.6	17	2.0	500	2.8	7*	35*	550*
31–50 yr	1,000*	700	320	5*	3*	1.5	1.6	17	2.0	500	2.8	7*	35*	550*

NOTE: This table presents Recommended Dietary Allowances (RDAs) in bold type and Adequate Intakes (AIs) in ordinary type followed by an asterisk (*). RDAs and AIs may both be used as goals for individual intake. RDAs are set to meet the needs of almost all (97 to 98 percent) individuals in a group. For healthy breastfed infants, the AI is the mean intake. The AI for other life-stage and gender groups is believed to cover needs of all individuals in the group, but lack of data or uncertainty in the data prevent being able to specify with confidence the percentage of individuals covered by this intake.

a As cholecalciferol. 1 µg cholecalciferol = 40 IU vitamin D.
b In the absence of adequate exposure to sunlight.
c As niacin equivalents (NE). 1 mg of niacin = 60 mg of tryptophan; 0–6 months = preformed niacin (not NE).
d As dietary folate equivalents (DFE). 1 DFE = 1 µg food folate = 0.6 µg of folic acid (from fortified food or supplement) consumed with food = 0.5 µg of synthetic (supplemental) folic acid taken on an empty stomach.
e Although AIs have been set for choline, there are few data to assess whether a dietary supply of choline is needed at all stages of the life cycle, and it may be that the choline requirement can be met by endogenous synthesis at some of these stages.
f Because 10 to 30 percent of older people may malabsorb food-bound B_{12}, it is advisable for those older than 50 years to meet their RDA mainly by consuming foods fortified with B_{12} or a supplement containing B_{12}.
g In view of evidence linking folate intake with neural tube defects in the fetus, it is recommended that all women capable of becoming pregnant consume 400 µg of synthetic folic acid from fortified foods and/or supplements in addition to intake of food folate from a varied diet.
h It is assumed that women will continue consuming 400 µg of folic acid until their pregnancy is confirmed and they enter prenatal care, which ordinarily occurs after the end of the periconceptional period—the critical time for formation of the neural tube.

Vitamins fall into two classes: fat soluble and water soluble.

Fat-Soluble Vitamins	Water-Soluble Vitamins
Vitamin A	B-vitamins:
Vitamin D	Thiamin
Vitamin E	Riboflavin
Vitamin K	Niacin
	Vitamin B-6
	Folate
	Vitamin B-12
	Pantothenic acid
	Biotin
	Vitamin C

Vitamin A (Retinol)

Like your parents always said, eat plenty of carrots and you'll see in the dark. That's because carrots contain beta-carotene, a substance that is converted into vitamin A by your body. Vitamin A promotes good vision, as well as healthy skin and the normal growth and maintenance of your bones, teeth, and mucous membranes. What they didn't tell you was that beta-carotene is also found in most orange-yellow fruits and vegetables, and in dark green vegetables.

Your body converts beta-carotene into vitamin A only when you need it, so eating foods rich in beta-carotene cannot cause vitamin A toxicity. However, eating huge amounts might turn your skin slightly orange. Not to worry, this condition isn't serious. Simply lay off the orange veggies for a few days and the colour will disappear.

Although your body controls the creation of vitamin A from beta-carotene, it has no control when you ingest straight vitamin A, which can be found in vitamin tablets. Oversupplementation can be extremely toxic, resulting in general fatigue and weakness, severe headaches, blurred vision, insomnia, hair loss, menstrual irregularities, skin rashes, and joint pain. In extreme cases, liver and brain damage may result. Huge doses taken in the prenatal period can cause birth defects.

What happens if you don't get enough? Vitamin A deficiency can cause night blindness, total blindness, and lowered resistance to infection because vitamin A plays a key role in the structural integrity of your cells. Here come the germs!

These foods are rich in vitamin A:

Liver	Butter
Eggs	Margarine
Milk	Cheese

These foods are rich in beta-carotene:

Cantaloupe	Winter squash
Carrots	Spinach
Sweet potato	Broccoli

Vitamin D: the Sunshine Vitamin

Vitamin D plays an indispensable role in building and maintaining strong bones and teeth. In fact, vitamin D is responsible for the body's absorption and use of the mineral calcium. Insufficient amounts of this key vitamin can lead to serious bone abnormalities, including rickets (bones that are soft and malformed) in children and osteoporosis or osteomalacia (softening of the bone) in adults.

On the other hand, vitamin D is fat soluble, so taking large supplemental doses can be dangerous. Some of the toxic effects are drowsiness, diarrhea, loss of appetite, headaches, high blood pressure, high cholesterol, fragile bones, and calcium deposits throughout your body (including your heart, kidneys, and blood vessels). If you are taking supplements, make sure you're not getting much more than the recommended amount for your age category; you'll notice that adults over 50 need more. The adequate intake (AI) for vitamin D is given in international units (IU).

These foods are rich in vitamin D:

Fortified milk	Margarine
Fortified soy and rice beverage	Egg yolk
Tuna	Salmon
Canned sardines	Cod-liver oil
Shrimp	Mackerel

Your body can also synthesize its own vitamin D when your skin is exposed to sunlight for 10 to 20 minutes. In fact, three sunny days per week can provide you with all the vitamin D you need. During the long, dark winter months, however, be sure to include vitamin-D–rich foods in your daily diet.

Vitamin E (Tocopherols)

Talk about a hot nutrient! Later, I explain vitamin E's tremendous role as an antioxidant, but for now, let's investigate its traditional side.

Vitamin E aids the formation and functioning of your red blood cells, muscle, and other tissues and protects essential fatty acids (special fats that are needed by your body). Because vitamin E is found in a variety of foods, vitamin E deficiency is rare. However, an extreme case of vitamin E deficiency involves wasting of the muscles and neurological disorders. To date, no shown toxic effects from taking doses well over the RNI have been shown.

These foods are rich in vitamin E:

Vegetable oils	Margarine
Salad dressings	Whole-grain cereals
Green leafy vegetables (kale!)	Nuts and seeds
Peanut butter	Wheat germ

Vitamin K

Thanks to vitamin K, you won't bleed to death after an injury. That's because vitamin K is essential for normal blood clotting. Current research also suggests that this vitamin might play a role in maintaining strong bones in adults. Where do you get this vitamin? Interestingly enough, bacteria that live in your intestines help to make 80 percent of the vitamin K that you need, and the rest can be found in a variety of foods listed here.

A vitamin K deficiency can cause hemorrhaging (uncontrollable bleeding), mainly in newborn infants because their immature intestinal tracts might not have enough bacteria to make this vitamin. In addition, people taking antibiotics might temporarily lose the ability to make vitamin K because the medication destroys all bacteria, good and bad.

These foods are rich in vitamin K:

Turnip greens	Cauliflower
Spinach	Beef liver
Broccoli	Kale
Cabbage	Lettuce

Water-Soluble Vitamins

Unlike fat-soluble vitamins, water-soluble vitamins can easily dissolve in the watery fluids of your body. Because excessive amounts are generally excreted in the urine, there is less chance for toxic side effects but more chance for deficiencies. Therefore, it is important to regularly replenish these vitamins by eating healthy foods that supply ample amounts. Be extra careful when preparing food. Because some of these vitamins are easily washed away or destroyed by light, air, and heat, use small amounts of water, avoid overcooking, and cut your fruits and vegetables right before you eat them. The following sections provide a quick rundown on each of the nine water-soluble vitamins—eight B vitamins and vitamin C.

Thiamin (B-1)

Thiamin is needed for the conversion of carbohydrate-rich foods into energy. B-1 also plays a role in keeping your brain, nerve, and heart cells healthy. A deficiency will lead to loss of energy, nausea, depression, muscle cramps, nerve damage, and muscular weakness. Although rare in Canada, a severe depletion of thiamin can result in the disease beriberi, causing potential muscle wasting and paralysis.

These foods are rich in thiamin (B-1):

Pork	Beef
Liver	Peas
Seeds	Legumes
Whole-grain products	Oatmeal
Lamb	

Riboflavin (B-2)

Like its buddy thiamin, riboflavin plays a key role in the metabolism of energy. Furthermore, this vitamin is involved in the formation of red blood cells and is necessary for healthy skin and normal vision.

A riboflavin deficiency will cause dry, scaly skin, accompanied by cracks on your lips and in the corners of your mouth. If that's not enough, getting insufficient amounts can also make your eyes extremely sensitive to light.

These foods are rich in riboflavin (B-2):

Milk	Yogurt
Cheese	Whole-grain breads and cereals
Green leafy vegetables	Meat
Eggs	Beef liver

Note: This vitamin is easily destroyed with exposure to sunlight; therefore, store these foods in the fridge, a cabinet, or the pantry.

Niacin (B-3)

This B-vitamin is also involved in energy-producing reactions in the cells that convert food to energy. In addition, niacin helps maintain healthy skin and nerves, and your digestive system. In some instances, you can use large doses of niacin as a cholesterol-lowering medication. However, you should only do this under the supervision of your doctor. Megadoses can cause hot flashes, itching, ulcers, high blood sugar, and liver damage.

In the rare case of a niacin deficiency, symptoms include diarrhea, mouth sores, changes in the skin, nervous disorders, and pellagra disease known to cause the "four Ds": diarrhea, dermatitis, dementia (mental confusion), and death.

These foods are rich in niacin (B-3):

Meat	Poultry
Liver	Eggs
Nuts	Enriched breads and cereals
Brown rice	Baked potato
Fish	Peanut butter
Milk	Whole grains

Pyridoxine (B-6)

Vitamin B-6 is a vital component for chemical reactions involving proteins and amino acids. (Remember those protein building blocks?) It also participates in the formation of red blood cells, antibodies, and insulin, in addition to maintaining normal brain function. Deficiency causes skin changes, convulsions in infants, dementia, nervous disorders, and anemia.

These foods are rich in pyridoxine (B-6):

Lean meats	Fish
Legumes	Green leafy vegetables
Raisins	Corn
Whole-grain cereals	Pork
Bananas	Lentils
Mango	Poultry

Cobalamin (B-12)

Vitamin B-12 assists in the formation of red blood cells and the normal functioning of your nervous system and is required for the synthesis of DNA (your genetic résumé). Because B-12 is found only in foods of animal origin, strict vegetarians might need to take a supplement or eat fortified foods to avoid a deficiency. Furthermore, this unique vitamin needs the help of another substance called *intrinsic factor* to be absorbed. Because intrinsic factor is made by the lining of the stomach, people with gastrointestinal disorders (especially the elderly) might need to get B-12 shots directly into the blood-stream. Symptoms of B-12 deficiency include nervous disorders and pernicious anemia.

Because a good amount of vitamin B-12 can be stored in the liver, it might take years for a deficiency to be recognized. As a result, people should have their B-12 levels checked starting at age 60 and every decade thereafter.

These foods are rich in cobalamin (B-12):

Meat	Fish
Poultry	Eggs
Milk products	Clams
Fortified soy and rice beverages	

Folate (Folacin, Folic Acid)

Folate appropriately gets its name from the word *foliage* because it's primarily found in leafy, dark green vegetables. In addition to playing a vital role in cell division and red blood cell formation, this vitamin is needed to make the genetic material DNA.

In recent years, folate has gained a lot of attention for its ability to reduce neural-tube birth defects in newborn babies. Needless to say, getting appropriate amounts of folate from both food and supplementation is imperative for pregnant women and women of childbearing age (because some women may not know they are pregnant). For this reason, folate is a key ingredient in most prenatal vitamins (folate is called folic acid when it's in a supplement). Because this nutrient is involved in cell division, a deficiency will leave you vulnerable to anemia and an abnormal digestive function because your blood cells and cells of the intestinal tract divide most rapidly.

These foods are rich in folate:

Spinach	Liver
Beans (all types)	Peas
Asparagus	Lentils
Oranges and orange juice	Brussels sprouts
Collard greens	Avocado

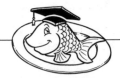

Food for Thought

Folate has recently been shown to decrease your risk of colon cancer. If you have ulcerative colitis or feel that you are at high risk for colon cancer, speak to your dietitian about supplementation.

Folate may also reduce the risk of heart disease by lowering the levels of a harmful substance called homocysteine in the blood.

Pantothenic Acid and Biotin

Pantothenic acid and biotin are both part of the B vitamin group that participates in the metabolism of energy. Pantothenic acid also plays a role in the formation of certain hormones and brain chemicals called neurotransmitters. Although both of these vitamins are vital for normal functioning, as of today there isn't a set RNI for either one. This is because deficiencies are so rare, and both pantothenic acid and biotin are found in a wide variety of plant and animal foods.

Vitamin C (Ascorbic Acid)

Now for the million dollar question: Can vitamin C ward off the common cold? The scientists say no. To date, there is no documented evidence supporting this notion. However, this vitamin can lessen the severity and duration of those lousy symptoms experienced *during* a cold. That's because vitamin C has a mild antihistaminic effect and it increases the body's production of *interferon*, a natural virus fighter.

What else can vitamin C do? Let's just say that if all the vitamins and minerals were on a pay scale according to the jobs they perform, vitamin C would be rolling. Vitamin C wears many hats, from helping to keep your bones, teeth, and blood vessels healthy to healing wounds,

Nutri-Speak

Scurvy is a disease resulting from a deficiency of vitamin C and is characterized by bleeding and swollen gums, joint pain, muscle wasting, and bruises. Scurvy is now very rare, except among people with alcoholism, and can be cured by as little as 5–7 milligrams of vitamin C.

boosting your resistance to infection, and participating in the formation of collagen (a protein that helps support body structures). Another benefit from eating vitamin C–rich foods is that you increase the absorption of the mineral iron—good news for people with deficiencies or greater iron requirements.

Although vitamin C deficiency is uncommon, it can cause a lowered resistance to infection, sore gums, hemorrhages, and in severe cases, the disease scurvy.

On the flip side, some studies have shown that megadosing on vitamin C might help reduce the risk of certain diseases. (This is further discussed in the section on antioxidants.) However, large doses might also lead to uncomfortable side effects, including diarrhea and nausea.

These foods are rich in vitamin C:

Melon	Strawberries
Tomatoes and tomato juice	Potatoes
Broccoli	Fortified juices
Guava	Kiwi
Mango	Papaya
Citrus fruits (oranges, grapefruits, etc.)	Red pepper
Brussels sprouts	Green pepper

A Day in the Life of an Antioxidant

We've all heard the news: Antioxidants help reduce your risk of heart disease and certain cancers and boost your immune system. So what exactly are antioxidants and how do they work?

As you know, every cell in your body needs oxygen to function normally. Unfortunately, the use of this oxygen produces harmful by-products called *free radicals*. Free radicals are also created from environmental pollution, certain industrial chemicals, and smoking.

Outside the body, the process of oxidation is responsible for the browning of a sliced apple and the rusting of metal. Inside the body, oxidation contributes to heart disease, cancer, cataracts, aging, and a host of other degenerative diseases. In other words, free radicals are bad news.

So why isn't everyone falling apart? Your cells have their own special defence technique to fight off these harmful free radicals. What's more, scientists have found compelling evidence suggesting that certain vitamins (specifically C, E, and beta-carotene) can actually enhance your body's ability to ward off these free radicals and therefore prevent oxidation. Appropriately, we call these vitamins antioxidants.

What Can Antioxidants Do?

To date, numerous studies have shown that antioxidants may protect against the following:

➤ **Cardiovascular disease**—Findings from studies suggest that vitamins C and E might play a role in preventing heart disease by reducing the amount of LDL-cholesterol lodged in the arteries and protecting LDL-cholesterol from free-radical damage. When LDLs become oxidized, they stick more readily to your artery walls. (Remember LDLs from Chapter 4, "Chewing the Fat"?)

➤ **Cancer**—Studies suggest that vitamins E and C and beta-carotene might have a protective effect against several types of cancers. Keep in mind that certain factors appear to influence the development of cancer, including heredity, smoking, nutritional excesses and deficiencies, and the environment.

➤ **Cataracts**—Scientists suspect that cataracts develop from the oxidation of the proteins in the lens of the eye. Antioxidants, particularly vitamin C, might help to reduce the risk of developing this disease.

➤ **Immunity**—Researchers theorize that antioxidants might help to strengthen the immune system by preventing the action of free radicals.

Nutri-Speak

Free radicals can be described as unstable, hyperactive atoms that circulate in your body and damage healthy cells and tissue.

Overrated-Undercooked

Although beta-carotene is still considered a powerful antioxidant, it is no longer recommended in supplemental form. Several years ago, a study found that male smokers who took beta-carotene supplements showed an increased risk of lung cancer. However, these findings certainly do not mean that beta-carotene has lost any importance among the antioxidant world. It does mean that until we have further information, people (especially smokers) should solely focus on getting beta-carotene from food sources rather than supplemental megadoses.

➤ **Exercise-induced free-radical damage**—Recent studies have shown increased free-radical activity following strenuous exercise. Therefore, vitamin E might play a role in reducing muscle inflammation and soreness after bouts of vigorous exercise.

How Much Should You Take?

Your primary focus should be on eating *foods* rich in antioxidant vitamins. Contrary to what people might think, there are no magic bullets (or pills) to good health. Another plug for food is that scientists are constantly discovering new food substances that might help with the quest for well-being. Furthermore, scientists believe that it's not just one isolated vitamin but interactions between several food ingredients that enhance disease prevention.

To date, no harmful side effects have been reported from supplemental doses well above the RNI for vitamins E and C. However, the science of nutrition is constantly being challenged with new discoveries —something to think about before popping the next pill. We know that getting your nutrients from food sources is safe and effective, but we don't know everything about supplemental megadosing.

The bottom line: If you decide to take antioxidant supplements, stay on top of the current research and speak with a competent health professional.

Food for Thought

Popeye was sure on to something. With just one can of spinach (2 c/500mL), he swallowed about 29,000 IU of beta-carotene, 50 milligrams of vitamin C, and 12 milligrams of vitamin E. That's one heck of a healthy sailor!

The Scoop on Minerals

Together with vitamins, at least 22 minerals are needed by your body to make things happen. Major minerals such as calcium and potassium are needed in large amounts, whereas trace minerals such as iron and zinc are required in only minute amounts. Just because a mineral is classified as a trace mineral doesn't mean it is any less important. The small RNI for iron is just as important to your body as the large RNI for calcium. It's sort of like bread—a lot of flour with a drop of yeast...both are equally important for that perfect baked loaf.

Food for Thought

What most people *do* know is that in large quantities, arsenic becomes a lethal poison. What most people *don't* know is that in very small amounts, arsenic is an essential mineral that your body needs to function properly.

Here's the master list of minerals. The following chapter focuses on two powerhouse players: calcium and iron.

Major Minerals	Trace Minerals
Calcium	Iron
Chloride	Zinc
Magnesium	Iodine
Phosphorous	Selenium
Potassium	Copper
Sodium	Manganese
Sulphur	Fluoride
	Chromium
	Molybdenum
	Arsenic
	Nickel
	Silicon
	Boron
	Cobalt

The Least You Need to Know

➤ More than 13 vitamins and 22 minerals are essential for normal body function. Eating a well-balanced, varied diet will supply your body with all the right ingredients.

➤ Water-soluble vitamins (eight B-complex vitamins and vitamin C) can easily dissolve in the watery body fluids, and excessive amounts are generally excreted through the urine.

➤ Fat-soluble vitamins (A, D, E, and K) do not dissolve in water and are stored in the body's fat. As a result, these vitamins (specifically A and D) have the potential to build up in tissues and become toxic when large supplemental doses are taken for a period of time.

➤ Antioxidants can help to prevent certain cancers, heart disease, cataracts, exercise-induced soreness, and other degenerative diseases by protecting against free-radical damage. Eat plenty of foods rich in vitamins C and E and beta-carotene to reap the benefits.

➤ Some people may benefit from taking supplements. To learn how to get more vitamins and minerals from food and supplements, visit the Dietitians of Canada Web site (www.dietitians.ca) to find a dietitian in your community.

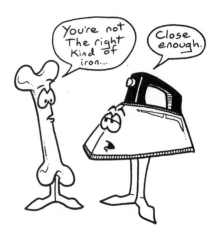

Chapter 8

Mighty Minerals: Calcium and Iron

In This Chapter

➤ All about calcium and iron

➤ How much you need

➤ Where to find the best food sources

➤ Are you a candidate for a vitamin or mineral supplement?

As you've learned from the preceding chapter, at least 22 minerals are essential for a number of vital functions and body processes. Because not a day goes by without a client or friend asking for some sort of information regarding calcium or iron, I've dedicated this entire chapter to these powerhouse minerals.

Calcium and Healthy Bones

Calcium is by far the most abundant mineral in your body, with about 99 percent of the stuff stored in your bones. The other 1 percent is located in your body fluids, where it helps to regulate functions such as blood pressure, nerve transmission, muscle contraction (including the heart beat), the clotting of blood, and the secretion of hormones and digestive enzymes. Make no bones about it: Calcium, along with vitamin D, fluoride, and phosphorous, is best known for its ability to promote strong, healthy bones. Calcium serves a vital role in bone structure, providing integrity and density to your skeleton. In turn, your bones act as a "calcium bank," releasing calcium into your blood when your diet might be deficient (which we hope is not too often).

Many people think that once you're past a certain age, you don't have to worry about getting enough calcium. Wrong! Adequate calcium is important *throughout* your life, first and foremost for optimal bone building, and later on for bone maintenance. Generally, the first 24 years are important because your body is laying down the foundation for strong bones and teeth. In the first three decades of life, your bones reach their *peak adult bone mass*. (At this time bones are done growing in size and density.) Children who drink plenty of milk and eat other dairy products will enter adulthood with stronger bones than those who skimp on calcium-rich foods.

Calcium intake in the later years is equally important for maintaining healthy bones. (I hope you already did all the right things in your first 30 years.) With age, your bones gradually lose their density (that is, calcium), which is especially true in menopausal women. People who take in adequate amounts of calcium can help slow down this process and defy those brittle bones of old age.

Q & A

Why bother with calcium?

Imagine your bones as your calcium bank. Over the years, you can develop quite an extensive savings account by taking in plenty of calcium-rich foods and supplementing your diet with calcium pills. Keep up the good work as an adult and your bones stay calcium-rich!

On the other hand, regularly skimp on this mineral, and you'll wind up calcium broke! Your body fluids still need calcium to regulate normal body functions. What these fluids don't get from food must be borrowed from the calcium bone bank. Borrowing day after day, year after year, will deplete the savings account and leave you at risk for osteoporosis (brittle bones that break easily).

How Much Calcium Is Recommended?

The Dietary Reference Intakes for calcium were revised in 1997. The updated DRIs for various age categories are shown below.

Group	DRI (mg/d)
Infants	
Birth–6 months	210
6 months–1 year	270
Children	
1–3 years	500
4–8 years	800

Males

9–13 years	1,300
14–18 years	1,300
19–30 years	1,000
31–50 years	1,000
51–70 years	1,200
>70 years	1,200

Females

9–13 years	1,300
14–18 years	1,300
19–30 years	1,000
31–50 years	1,000
51–70 years	1,200
>70 years	1,200

Pregnancy/Lactation

18 years or less	1,300
19–30 years	1,000
31–50 years	1,000

Are You Getting Enough Calcium? The Foods to Choose

Browse through the following chart and notice that dairy foods, along with fortified juice and sardines, provide the most calcium hands down. One more thing: Don't be put off by the high amounts of fat in cheese. Simply shop for the low-fat brands in your local store. They have less fat but still retain ample amounts of calcium.

The Best Sources of Calcium in Various Foods

Milk Group	Amount	Calcium in mg
Yogurt, plain (low-fat)	³/₄ cup (175 mL)	311
Yogurt, fruit-flavoured (low-fat)	³/₄ cup (175 mL)	259
Milk, nonfat (dry)	¹/₄ cup (50 mL)	377
Milk, skim	1 cup (250 mL)	302
Milk, 1%–2%	1 cup (250 mL)	300
Milk, whole*	1 cup (250 mL)	291
Buttermilk	1 cup (250 mL)	285
Milk, chocolate (low-fat)	1 cup (250 mL)	284
Cheese, Parmesan (grated)	¹/₄ cup (50 mL)	338
Cheese, Swiss*	1 oz (30 g)	272
Cheese, Monterey Jack*	1 oz (30 g)	212

83

Milk Group	Amount	Calcium in mg
Cheese, mozzarella, part skim	1 oz (30 g)	207
Cheese, cheddar*	1 oz (30 g)	204
Cheese, colby*	1 oz (30 g)	194
Cheese, processed slices*	1 oz (30 g)	174
Ice cream*	1/2 cup (125 mL)	88
Cottage cheese, creamed 1%	1/2 cup (125 mL)	63

Fruit and Vegetable Group	Amount	Calcium in mg
Collards, cooked	1/2 cup (125 mL)	168
Turnip greens, cooked	1/2 cup (125 mL)	134
Kale, cooked	1/2 cup (125 mL)	103
Spinach, cooked	1/2 cup (125 mL)	84
Broccoli, cooked	1/2 cup (125 mL)	68
Chard, cooked	1/2 cup (125 mL)	64
Carrot, raw	1 medium	27
Orange	1 medium	60
Dates, chopped	1/4 cup (50 mL)	26
Raisins	1/4 cup (50 mL)	22

Protein Group (Meat, Beans, Eggs)	Amount	Calcium in mg
Sardines (canned, w/bones)	3 oz (90 g)	372
Salmon, pink (canned, w/bones)	3 oz (90 g)	165
Tofu (processed, w/calcium)	4 oz (120 g)	145
Almonds, shelled*	1 oz (30 g)	66
Soybeans, cooked	1/2 cup (125 mL)	66
Soy beverage, fortified	1 cup (250 mL)	3–330
Dried beans, cooked (lima, navy, kidney)	1/2 cup (125 mL)	35–60
Egg	1 large	27
Peanut butter*	2 Tbs (25 mL)	18
Beef patty, cooked*	3 oz (90 g)	9

Grain Group	Amount	Calcium in mg
Farina, enriched (instant, cooked)	1 cup (250 mL)	189
Tortilla, corn	1 medium	60
Bread, whole-wheat	1 slice	25

Calcium-Fortified Foods	Amount	Calcium in mg
Orange juice and grapefruit juice (Tropicana, Minute Maid, Oasis)	1 cup (250 mL)	300
Soy beverage, fortified	1 cup (250 mL)	3–330

*Denotes foods that are also high in fat

Source: Calcium Information Center, USA

Q & A

Should I take calcium supplements?

If you are having a problem consistently getting enough calcium from food sources, you might want to speak with your dietitian or doctor about supplementation. Stick with a calcium supplement in the form of calcium carbonate or calcium citrate, and do not take more than 500–600 milligrams in one dose. Also be aware that some calcium carbonate supplements need to be taken with food or juice for proper absorption. That's because this form of calcium needs plenty of stomach acid to make it ready for absorption.

If you're over 50, choose a calcium citrate supplement. They're better absorbed than pills made from calcium carbonate. Many older adults produce less stomach acid and will do better with a more absorbable form of calcium.

Be sure to choose a supplement with added vitamin D. Just remember that your daily totals of vitamin D (from your multivitamin/mineral and calcium supps and food) should not exceed 2000 IU. This is the upper limit for vitamin D.

Iron Out Your Body

Iron deficiency is the most widespread type of vitamin or mineral deficiency in the world. Do you constantly experience sluggishness, irritability, and headaches? Perhaps you suffer from this condition. Let's take a closer look and find out.

About 70 percent of the iron in your body is located in a portion of your red blood cells known as *hemoglobin*. Hemoglobin is your oxygen delivery service, supplying every cell with the oxygen it needs to perform essential metabolic functions. Iron is also a component of *myoglobin*. Like the hemoglobin in red blood cells, myoglobin ensures adequate oxygen delivery to all your muscles. At this point, you're probably starting to

85

understand the importance of iron in this equation: too little iron, too little oxygen. The result is fatigue, irritability, weakness, headaches, a tendency to feel cold, and, in the case of severe depletion, iron-deficiency anemia.

Fortunately, iron is found in a variety of animal and plant foods, making it easy to get your daily requirement. *Heme* iron, the type found in animal products (red meats, liver, poultry, and eggs), is more readily absorbed than *nonheme* iron, which can be found in vegetables and other plant foods (beans, nuts, seeds, dried fruits, and fortified breads and cereals). Interestingly enough, the body adjusts the amount it absorbs according to the body's need. In other words, a person with iron-deficient anemia will absorb about two to three times more iron after eating exactly the same meal than a person with normal iron status.

Certain groups of people are at increased risk for developing an iron deficiency. If you think you might fall into one of the following categories, ask your doctor to check your iron status before you self-prescribe supplementation. (A simple blood test can tell if you are deficient.)

Groups at risk for iron deficiency include

➤ Infants and children: Their rapid growth and finicky eating habits demand that they get iron in a variety of ways.

➤ Women who bleed heavily during menstruation: They lose iron-rich blood each month.

➤ Pregnant women with increased blood volume: They are supporting their growing babies' needs as well as their own.

➤ Strict vegetarians who take in only nonheme sources of iron: Remember, nonheme plant foods are *much* less absorbent than iron-rich animal foods.

➤ People who lose a lot of blood during surgery or other bleeding injuries.

➤ "Chronic dieters" who bounce from one crash diet to another: People suffering from eating disorders might not eat enough iron-rich foods to meet their requirements.

Tips to Boost Your Dietary Iron Intake

Here's information that will help you increase your iron intake and its absorption within your body.

➤ Make a point of eating iron-rich foods, both animal (heme) and non-animal (nonheme) sources each day.

➤ When eating nonheme foods, couple them with some vitamin C. (See the list of vitamin-C–containing foods.) Vitamin C can increase the absorption of iron.

➤ Avoid drinking coffee or tea with an iron-rich meal; they inhibit the absorption of iron.

➤ Calcium interferes with the absorption of iron, so if you take calcium supplements do not take them with an iron-rich meal. Try them with a snack or some juice because you usually do need some food with your calcium pills.

➤ Cook casseroles, stews, and sauces in cast iron cookware. Believe it or not, some of the iron will seep into the food.

➤ The presence of heme iron (even very small amounts) at a meal with nonheme iron will enhance the absorption of the nonheme iron.

The best sources of iron (heme) are

Lean red meats
Turkey
Chicken
Pork
Lamb
Veal
Egg yolk
Liver

Good sources of iron (nonheme) are

Beans
Lentils
Whole grains
Dried fruit
Broccoli
Spinach
Collard greens
Nuts and seeds
Chickpeas
Fortified cereals
Blackstrap molasses
Barley
Wheat germ

Nutri-Speak

Although not very common, **iron toxicity** is a serious problem that occurs from either a genetic abnormality causing the body to store excessive amounts or the unnecessary oversupplementation of iron. The result can be liver and other organ damage.

Are You a Candidate for a Vitamin or Mineral Supplement?

Ideally, you should be getting your daily supply of vitamins and minerals from your diet, not from pill popping. There are exceptions to this rule, but don't abandon good eating habits for a little brown bottle; it just doesn't work that way. Generally speaking, nutrients from food are absorbed more readily by your body, the way nature intended. And food provides you with energy in the form of calories—something you don't get from pills.

As I mentioned earlier, some people do need assistance to obtain the required daily intakes for vitamins and minerals. Check out the following list to see if you fall into one of the categories that require a little help. If you do, speak with a registered dietitian (a registered dietitian, or RD, is a board-certified nutritionist with the proper education and credentials) or your doctor about appropriate supplementation.

Groups at nutritional risk include people with these qualities:

➤ Do you constantly skip meals, grabbing only snack foods throughout the day? Do you eat fewer than five fruits and vegetables each day? You might benefit from a multivitamin/mineral supplement (supplying 100–300 percent of the RNIs) to fill in the nutrition gaps.

➤ Are you a vegan, a strict vegetarian who consumes absolutely no meat, dairy, or other animal products? You might benefit from a supplement that supplies the RNI for vitamins D and B-12 and the mineral calcium.

➤ Are you over 50 years old? People in this category might have a decline in the absorption of the following vitamins: B-6, B-12, C, D, E, folic acid, and the mineral calcium. A one-a-day multivitamin/mineral might provide some extra backup. Also, think about some extra calcium if you are not eating enough calcium-rich food.

➤ Do you regularly drink alcohol or smoke? Excessive amounts of alcohol and smoking interfere with the body's ability to absorb and use certain vitamins and minerals. In this case, a supplement recommendation is not the advice. You get the picture!

➤ Are you a professional dieter—on and off of every wacky fad diet out there? Chances are you're cheating your body of important nutrients and would probably benefit from the support of a one-a-day multivitamin/mineral supplement.

➤ Do you completely avoid specific types of foods? Some people stay away from certain foods for reasons such as food allergies, intolerances, or just plain dislikes. In these cases, supplements of specific nutrients might be needed.

For women only, ask yourself these questions:

➤ Do you experience heavy bleeding during menstruation? If so, you might lose iron-rich blood. Check with your doctor about whether you will benefit from taking a supplement with iron. Note: Iron supplements tend to cause constipation.

➤ Are you currently pregnant or breast-feeding? Women in this category have greater needs for the vitamins A, C, B-1, B-6, B-12, and folic acid, as well as the minerals iron and calcium. These extra amounts are usually included in prenatal vitamins—although, you might need more calcium than the prenatal supps supply, so speak with your dietitian if you aren't eating enough calcium-rich food.

Are Your Vitamin and Mineral Supplements Absorbable?

Most people automatically assume that their supplements will be absorbed completely after they swallow them. It's a fair assumption. Unfortunately, it doesn't always work that way. Here are a two ways to help you assess whether your vitamin and mineral supplements stand a good chance of being absorbed and used by your body.

Home Testing

You can always test your own supplements at home by immersing the individual pill or capsule in about $1/4$ cup (50 mL) of household vinegar and letting it stand for one to two hours. (You should stir it a bit.) During this time, the vinegar should cloud up and the pill or capsule should disintegrate (fall into pieces). If it remains intact, there's a chance that it won't disintegrate in your stomach but will pass right through you undigested.

This type of home testing is only a rough approximation of what happens in the stomach, but it will give you a good sense of whether a product will be available in your intestine for absorption. No guarantee.

Look for "GMP" on the Label

This notation on a product label stands for "good manufacturing practices" and means that the company manufacturers vitamin supplements using methods acceptable to Health Canada. These high-standard practices ensure that the manufacturing plant is clean, the raw ingredients are pure, and the product is stable and works! In a nutshell, GMP on a product label means that the company makes high-quality, safe supplements that do their job in the body. If your supplement label doesn't have a statement regarding the use of GMP, call the company and ask. You may also find this information on product pamphlets or by visiting the company Web site.

Unfortunately, at this time vitamins and minerals do not have to conform to GMP standards to be sold in this country. Many brand-name vitamins are not labeled GMP because the manufacturer either doesn't want to spend the money to perform the tests or prefers to guarantee the vitamin through the brand name. However, it's expected that over the next few years Health Canada will demand that all supplement companies follow GMP. In the meantime, my recommendation is to buy products made by companies that enforce these higher standards.

The Least You Need to Know

➤ Adequate calcium intake is required throughout the life cycle: the early years for bone building and the later years for bone maintenance. Make it a habit to load up on low-fat dairy products and other calcium-rich foods.

➤ The mineral iron is responsible for delivering oxygen to every cell in your body and is found in a variety of foods.

➤ *Heme* iron, the most absorbable type, is found in animal products such as meat, liver, and poultry. *Nonheme* iron, found in plants, is less absorbable and is found in dried fruits, nuts, beans, seeds, and fortified grains.

➤ Boost the absorption rate of nonheme iron by combining foods high in vitamin C with an iron-rich meal (such as iron-fortified cereal with a glass of orange juice).

➤ Although certain groups of people can benefit from vitamin and mineral supplementation, a well-balanced diet should be your primary focus for optimal nutrition. If used, vitamin pills should *supplement* a healthy diet.

➤ If you think you might be a candidate for supplementation, speak with a registered dietitian (a nutritionist with the proper education) or family doctor. Visit www.dietitians.ca, the Web site of Dietitians of Canada, to find a registered dietitian in your area.

Part 2
Making Savvy Food Choices

Decisions, decisions! With the hundreds and hundreds of foods offered in grocery stores, restaurants, delis, and even your own kitchen, it's can be a real challenge trying to decide what to eat, let alone choose something nutritious to eat. But it shouldn't be that way. In fact, thanks to the growing number of health-conscious consumers, most grocery stores and restaurants are now well equipped to cater to your special food concerns. You simply need to know what to look for.

Part 2 of this book covers every angle. You'll learn how to decode the information on nutrition labels so you can make informed food choices in your local grocery store. Then, we'll put your know-how into action by scouting out the supermarket, aisle by aisle, introducing you to the smart food items to load into your shopping cart. You'll also master low-fat cooking techniques so you're ready to wow your friends, family, and taste buds with some knockout meals at home. You certainly won't need to give up dining out. This section fills you in on the best bets for most all ethnic cuisine. Bon appétit!

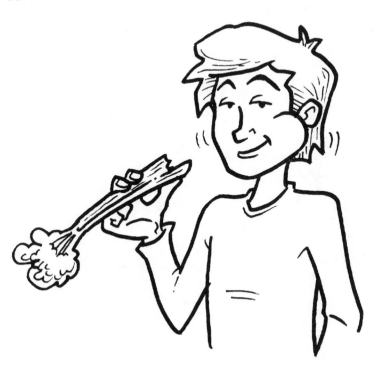

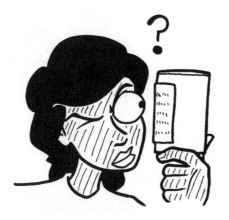

Chapter 9

Decoding a Nutrition Label

In This Chapter

➤ How to read a nutrition label

➤ Understanding the percentage of recommended daily intake

➤ Testing your label savvy

➤ Using the ingredient list

Now that you have some solid nutrition know-how, let's put this knowledge to work and decode all that mumbo-jumbo written on packaged food products. Once you can interpret the information on nutrition labels, you'll become quite a detective in your local grocery store, which will further enhance your skills as a healthy eater. You'll be able to make more informed food choices, as well as compare similar food products to see which brand is nutritionally superior.

At this time, nutrition labelling isn't mandatory in Canada so you won't find nutrition facts on every food package. But if you're like most Canadians (a whopping 93 percent!) who want to see nutrition information on *all or most* food products, you'll be pleased to hear that our labelling laws are under review. It's anticipated that sometime over the next few years new regulations will be gradually phased in and you'll start to see revamped, user-friendly nutrition labels on most food packages. Until that happens, this section will give you a crash course on how to read and use our current nutrition labels.

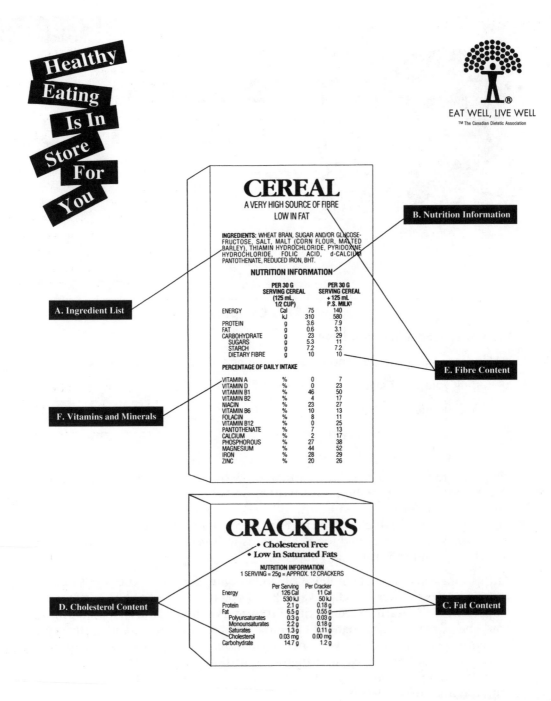

Healthy Eating Is In Store For You

EAT WELL, LIVE WELL
™ The Canadian Dietetic Association

CEREAL
A VERY HIGH SOURCE OF FIBRE
LOW IN FAT

INGREDIENTS: WHEAT BRAN, SUGAR AND/OR GLUCOSE-FRUCTOSE, SALT, MALT (CORN FLOUR, MALTED BARLEY), THIAMIN HYDROCHLORIDE, PYRIDOXINE HYDROCHLORIDE, FOLIC ACID, d-CALCIUM PANTOTHENATE, REDUCED IRON, BHT.

A. Ingredient List

B. Nutrition Information

E. Fibre Content

F. Vitamins and Minerals

NUTRITION INFORMATION

		PER 30 G SERVING CEREAL (125 mL, 1/2 CUP)	PER 30 G SERVING CEREAL + 125 mL P.S. MILK†
ENERGY	Cal	75	140
	kJ	310	580
PROTEIN	g	3.6	7.9
FAT	g	0.6	3.1
CARBOHYDRATE	g	23	29
SUGARS	g	5.3	11
STARCH	g	7.2	7.2
DIETARY FIBRE	g	10	10

PERCENTAGE OF DAILY INTAKE

VITAMIN A	%	0	7
VITAMIN D	%	0	23
VITAMIN B1	%	46	50
VITAMIN B2	%	4	17
NIACIN	%	23	27
VITAMIN B6	%	10	13
FOLACIN	%	8	11
VITAMIN B12	%	0	25
PANTOTHENATE	%	7	13
CALCIUM	%	2	17
PHOSPHOROUS	%	27	38
MAGNESIUM	%	44	52
IRON	%	28	29
ZINC	%	20	26

CRACKERS
- **Cholesterol Free**
- **Low in Saturated Fats**

NUTRITION INFORMATION
1 SERVING = 25g = APPROX. 12 CRACKERS

	Per Serving	Per Cracker
Energy	126 Cal	11 Cal
	530 kJ	50 kJ
Protein	2.1 g	0.18 g
Fat	6.5 g	0.55 g
Polyunsaturates	0.3 g	0.03 g
Monounsaturates	2.2 g	0.18 g
Saturates	1.3 g	0.11 g
Cholesterol	0.03 mg	0.00 mg
Carbohydrate	14.7 g	1.2 g

D. Cholesterol Content

C. Fat Content

94

Serving Size

First, figure out how much food was analyzed by the company that prepared the nutrition label, such as the one shown here. "Serving" clearly describes the set amount of food for which the nutrition information is given. For example, the cereal label shown here reports that a serving is 30 grams or $1/2$ cup (125 mL). The nutrition information for cereal is always based on a 30-gram serving. Since 30 grams of a dense cereal may be a much smaller portion than 30 grams of a lighter, flake-type cereal, it's important always to look at the household measure.

Do you eat the amount of food defined as one serving? Remember, if your portion size is more than this amount, you're getting more calories, fat, and other nutrients. And for some foods, it's certainly easy to eat more than one measly serving. Here's a perfect example of the difference between serving size and the actual servings eaten: 1 serving of ice cream ($1/2$ cup/125 mL) has approximately 12 grams of fat. Most of the people I know can easily eat 1 cup (250 mL) in a sitting—and you know what that means. When you double the serving size, you double everything: the calories, protein grams, carbohydrate grams, and, of course, the fat grams. Pay close attention to the amount per serving. If you go over (or under) on servings, keep that in mind when reading the remaining information on the nutrition label.

Energy

"Energy" tells you how many calories a single serving contains (one calorie equals roughly 4.2 kilojoules). The sample cereal label shows 75 calories (310 kJ) per serving. What about those "low-cal" claims frequently displayed on the packaging? Luckily, the following key words are defined by the government and must mean what they say:

> ➤ **Calorie-free**—less than 1 calorie per 100-gram serving
> ➤ **Low-calorie**—15 calories or fewer per serving
> ➤ **Calorie-reduced**—contains 50 percent fewer calories than the regular (not calorie-reduced) version of that food item

Protein

As you know from Chapter 3, "The Profile on Protein," most Canadians eat more protein than they actually need (0.8 grams per kilogram of body weight). Some of the best protein sources (such as beef, poultry, eggs, and fish), unfortunately, do not carry a nutrition label. On the other hand, most dairy products and some prepackaged food items do list the grams of protein in a single serving. It's interesting to see that there are even small amounts of protein in foods you might not expect.

Carbohydrate

In Chapter 2, "A Close-Up on Carbohydrates," you became well versed in the various types of carbohydrates. Now you can use the label information to identify whether a food contains a lot of simple sugar or complex carbohydrate (starch).

Look for the "Carbohydrate" listing. This will reveal the amount of *all types* of carbs (simple, complex, and fibre) in a single serving of a food. Sometimes this is all the information you'll get. For other foods, such as breakfast cereal, you get a complete breakdown of carbs. Look for the smaller listings located under "Carbohydrate"— "Sugars", "Starch," and "Dietary Fibre."

Let's look at the cereal label for an example:

Carbohydrate	23 g
Sugars	5.3 g
Starch	7.2 g
Dietary Fibre	10 g

These numbers indicate that the majority of carbohydrates are coming from starch and dietary fibre, not simple sugars.

Dietary fibre is predominantly found in carbohydrate-rich foods and includes both soluble and insoluble fibre sources. Because fibre promotes regularity, and reduces the risk of heart disease and certain cancers, choose cereals with at least 4 grams of dietary fibre per serving, and aim for a total intake of 25–35 grams each day.

Here's what claims about dietary fibre mean:

➤ **Source of dietary fibre**—at least 2 grams of dietary fibre per serving

➤ **High source of dietary fibre**—at least 4 grams of fibre per serving

➤ **Very high source of dietary fibre**—at least 6 grams of fibre per serving

Fat

This section of the label titled "Fat" lists the total number of fat grams from all types of fat—saturated, monounsaturated, and polyunsaturated. As you can see, the cereal label reveals that there are 0.6 grams of fat per serving. If you look at the nutrition label for the crackers, you'll find 6.5 total fat grams per serving (12 crackers).

Use the fat gram information to compare similar products. You might pull another box of crackers off the grocery store shelf and find 12 grams of fat per serving. If the serving sizes are similar for the two brands of crackers your choice is clear! If you have read chapter 4, "Chewing the Fat," I'm sure you'll opt for the lower fat cracker. Right?

Here are some of the common "fat" phrases that appear on packaged food products and how they are defined by the government:

> ➤ **Fat-free**—no more than 0.1 grams of fat per 100-gram serving
> ➤ **Low in fat**—3 grams of fat (or less) per serving

Saturated Fat

When a manufacturer makes a claim about fat or cholesterol on the label (like the cracker company), the amounts of all types of fat must be presented on the label. The saturated-fat number reveals the amount of artery-clogging fat in a food product. As you can see, the sample label shows 1.3 grams of saturated fat—that's low! In general, avoid foods that are high in saturated fat. This type of fat is responsible for increasing your risk of heart disease and other illnesses.

Here's how the government defines a claim about saturated fat:

> ➤ **Low in saturated fat**—no more than 2 grams in a serving size and no more than 15 percent of calories coming from saturated fat

Cholesterol

Remember this waxy substance? I told you earlier that dietary cholesterol can raise blood cholesterol in some people who are sensitive and can therefore increase their risk for heart disease. You'll notice that the cholesterol content of a food product is measured in milligrams. Budget your daily foods and eat less than 300 milligrams of dietary cholesterol per day.

Understand the following claims when they appear on food labels:

> ➤ **Cholesterol-free**—no more than 3 milligrams of cholesterol and 2 grams of saturated fat (or less) per 100-gram serving
> ➤ **Low in cholesterol**—no more than 20 milligrams of cholesterol and 2 grams of saturated fat (or less) per serving

These cholesterol claims are allowed only when a food product contains 2 grams (or less) of saturated fat as well.

Sodium

You won't always find the sodium content on a nutrition label. That's because companies don't have to disclose the salt content unless they claim their product is a sodium-reduced product. Let's hope that will change when the new labelling laws are established. Sodium is responsible for water retention and high blood pressure in salt-sensitive people. Limit the amount of high-sodium foods in your diet, and aim for a daily intake of 2,400 milligrams or less.

Here's some sodium lingo and what it means:

➤ **Sodium-free/Salt-free**—no more than 5 milligrams of sodium per 100-gram serving

➤ **Low sodium**—50% less sodium than the regular product and no more than 40 milligrams of sodium per 100-gram serving; no salt added

➤ **No added salt/unsalted**—no salt added; none of the ingredients contain a large quantity of salt

Percentage of Recommended Daily Intake

Now for the confusing part: What are those "%" signs at the bottom of the cereal label? Vitamins and minerals are listed as percentages. If you are interested in one nutrient, such as calcium, then this information might be useful to you. The percentages are based on a 2,000-calorie reference diet. In other words, these percentages indicate how much of the RNI for each nutrient is present in a single serving. Of course, your job is ultimately to eat a variety of foods that supply 100 percent of all nutrients needed. For example, one serving of the sample breakfast cereal provides 46 percent of your daily vitamin B-1 (thiamin) and 0 percent of your daily vitamin B-12. Adding milk boosts the vitamin B-12 to 25 percent of the recommended daily intake.

What happens if you eat more or less than 2,000 calories? You can adjust the percentages up or down slightly if you're good with numbers (and extremely motivated). In general, the 2,000-calorie reference diet provides appropriate guidelines for almost everyone (adults and children over 4) to follow.

The following are the set recommended daily intakes for vitamins and minerals used on food labels. At this time, many Canadian manufacturers use American values, since many foods are packaged in the United States. For the most part, though, our recommendations are quite similar. These numbers are used specifically for food labels and are based on a 2,000-calorie reference diet.

Recommended Daily Intakes for Vitamins and Minerals

Food Component	Daily Intake
Sodium	2,400 mg
Potassium	3,500 mg
Vitamin A	5,000 IU
Vitamin C	60 mg
Calcium	1,000 mg
Iron	18 mg
Vitamin D	400 IU
Vitamin E	30 IU

Food Component	Daily Intake
Vitamin K	80 mcg
Thiamin	1.5 mg
Riboflavin	1.7 mg
Niacin	20 mg
Vitamin B-6	2.0 mg
Folate	400 mcg
Vitamin B-12	6.0 mcg
Biotin	0.3 mg
Pantothenic acid	10 mg
Phosphorous	1,000 mg
Iodine	150 mcg
Magnesium	400 mg
Zinc	15 mg
Copper	2.0 mg
Selenium	70 mcg
Manganese	2.0 mg
Chromium	120 mcg
Molybdenum	75 mcg
Chloride	3,400 mg

mg = milligrams; mcg = micrograms; IU = international units
Source: Title 21 "Code of Federal Regulations" Parts 100–169, April 1, 1995, Section 101.9

Take the Nutrition Label Challenge

Put your know-how to the test and answer the following questions according to the nutrition label shown on the next page:

1. For what serving size is the nutrition information presented?

2. How many calories are there in two servings of this food product?

3. How much of your daily recommended intake of iron does one serving of this food provide?

4. Knowing the daily percentage of iron in one serving, calculate the amount of iron in milligrams that this product supplies.

5. How many grams of unsaturated fat are in one serving of this product?

6. Would you consider this food a good source of calcium?

7. Do you think that eating a lot of this food has artery-clogging potential?

8. How many grams of protein are there in one serving?

9. Any idea what this food may be?

Answers to Quiz:

1. Nutrient content is for 2 tablespoons (25 mL).

2. Two servings contain 190 × 2 = 380 calories.

3. One serving provides 4% of the daily recommended iron.

4. This product supplies 4% of 18 milligrams = 0.72 milligrams.

5. Add the polyunsaturated fat grams (4 g) and monounsaturated fat grams (10 g) to get a total of 14 grams of unsaturated fat.

6. This product is not a good source of the mineral calcium. At the bottom of the label, notice "Calcium 0%." To be considered a good source of a nutrient, a food must provide at least 25 percent of the daily recommended intake for that nutrient.

Nutrition Information	
Information nutritionnelle	
Per 32 g serving (2 Tbs/25 mL)	
Energy	190 Calories
	792 kJ
Protein	10 g
Fat	16 g
Saturates	2 g
Polyunsaturates	4 g
Monounsaturates	10 g
Carbohydrate	6 g
Dietary Fibre	2 g
% of Recommended Daily Intake	
% de l'apport quotidien recommandé	
Vitamin A	0%
Vitamin C	0%
Calcium	0%
Iron	4%

7. This food is *not* an artery-clogging one because the majority of the fat it contains is unsaturated.

8. One serving contains 10 grams of protein.

9. Did you guess peanut butter?

Ingredient Lists

What happens if your favourite food products don't have nutrition information labels? Well, if you want to get a feel for the fat, sugar, or sodium content, you can always use the ingredient list. By law, all packaged foods in Canada must list the ingredients in descending order according to their weight. This means that the ingredients closest to the end of the list are present in the smallest amounts. In the cereal example, wheat bran is the first ingredient listed and therefore is present in the largest amount. If your favourite brand of cookies lists vegetable shortening near the top, you might want to shop for a lower fat treat!

Now that you're a true nutrition detective, here are some key words to be on the lookout for:

➤ **Fat**—butter, lard, vegetable oil, vegetable shortening, hydrogenated vegetable oil, partially hydrogenated vegetable oil

➤ **Sugar**—sucrose, glucose, dextrose, fructose, maltose, lactose, sorbitol, mannitol, honey, corn syrup, corn syrup solids, molasses, maple syrup

➤ **Sodium**—salt, onion salt, celery salt, garlic salt, seasoned salt, monosodium glutamate, baking powder, baking soda, meat tenderizer, bouillon, sodium benzoate, sodium caseinate, sodium citrate, sodium phosphate, sodium propionate

Buyer Beware!

Nutrition labels and ingredient listings are great tools to help you shop for healthy foods, but there are a few things you need to watch out for. For starters, remember that nutrition information is based on the food *as sold*. What you do when you get the product home can change the nutritional content. Putting three heaping spoonfuls of sugar on your breakfast cereal will send the carbohydrate numbers out of whack.

I already told you to pay attention to the serving size stated on the label. Is it realistic? Or do you usually down twice as much and get double the calories and nutrients?

Finally, heads up when you see the claim "light" or "lite" on a food package. These words can be used to describe a number of properties of the food. The food might be light in colour, light tasting, light in sodium, or light in fat when compared to the regular product.

So there you have it, Sherlock. Consider yourself ready to tackle the supermarket!

The Least You Need to Know

➤ The nutrition information provided on prepackaged food labels can help you make more informed food choices and compare similar food items, and by doing so make healthier buying choices.

➤ All the nutrition information provided is based on one serving size. Check to see how much of a particular food is considered one serving, and if you eat more or less, adjust the nutrition information accordingly.

➤ Choose foods for which there is a big difference between the number of total calories and the number of fat calories. This indicates that a food is not primarily made of fat.

➤ Percentage of recommended daily intake refers to how much of a day's recommended amount for vitamins and minerals is supplied in one serving of a food product.

➤ When a food product doesn't have a nutrition label, use the ingredient list to get a sense of the fat, sugar, or salt content. Ingredients are listed in descending order, according to their weight.

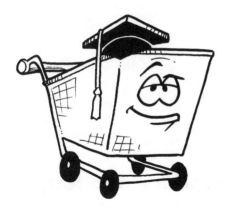

Chapter 10

Shopping Smart

In This Chapter

➤ Scouting the supermarket aisle by aisle

➤ Selecting fresh fruits and vegetables

➤ Best bets for dairy products, grains, and protein

➤ Shopping for fats, spreads, and condiments

➤ Filling your cupboards with healthy snacks

How many times have you eaten unhealthy food just because you didn't have any nutritious food in the house? Are cookies, cakes, and chips constantly on display on your shelves, or do you fill your pantry with fresh fruit and whole grains? Let's face it: When you get those midday munchies, the last thing you want to do is drive to a supermarket to buy an apple. You're going to grab whatever's closest to the couch—and who knows what that might be.

Half the battle of healthy eating is having a variety of nutritious foods on hand so that when the "food mood" strikes, you've got the supplies to satisfy that growling stomach with some savvy food choices. Grab a cart and read on; you're about to go grocery shopping.

The Shopping List

The nice part about food shopping today is that supermarkets are responding to nutrition-conscious consumers and shelving more and more healthy foods. Start by getting organized—set up a shopping list by different food categories:

➤ Vegetables

➤ Fruits

➤ Dairy products

➤ Grains (bread, cereal, pasta, and others)

➤ Protein foods (meats, poultry, fish, eggs, and legumes)

➤ Frozen meals and canned items

➤ Snack foods

➤ Condiments

➤ Fats, oils, dressings, and other spreads

Aisle One: Starting with the Produce Section

The produce aisle will provide you with a lot of nutritional bang for your buck. Spend a lot of time walking through, and load up your cart.

Voluptuous Veggies

Vegetables are naturally low in calories and fat and provide an array of vitamins, minerals, and fibre. Bundles of fresh produce don't carry nutrition labels, but you might see posters in the produce area revealing the benefits of specific items. Rest assured: Label or no label, you can never eat too many vegetables!

Most fresh veggies can be judged for freshness and quality by their appearance; closely examine your produce and avoid any that show decay or bruising. Buy only what you need for the next few days. Fresh veggies will go bad if they sit around for a long time. If you don't shop often, or you don't have the time to wash and chop your vegetables, your best bet is to fill your freezer. Frozen vegetables come in a variety of combinations (cut, whole, chopped, and puréed, along with medleys of premixed veggie concoctions), and all you have to do is pop them in a pot or wok to cook. Even lazy people have no excuse. What's more, the freezer keeps the nutrients locked in, so there's no rush to eat them before they go bad.

Here are some general shopping tips for buying produce:

➤ Buy fresh fruits and vegetables that are in season so prices are reasonable.

➤ Examine your fruits and vegetables for freshness; avoid those with bruises and other deformities.

➤ Because fresh produce is perishable, buy only what you need. If you're buying groceries for an extended period of time, load up on the frozen varieties.

➤ Read the labels on frozen and canned vegetables to make sure they don't contain a lot of added fat or salt. Read labels on frozen and canned fruits to make sure there isn't a lot of added sugar or heavy syrup.

➤ If you're into "super convenience," buy bags of prewashed, precut salad, carrots, celery, broccoli, and other produce offered at your supermarket. Look for premade fruit salads in either the fresh or frozen sections of your grocery store.

➤ Check out the salad bar in your grocery store. You can get the exact amount of anything you need, and it's already precut and prewashed for you.

➤ Speak with the person in charge of produce at your local supermarket; ask about unfamiliar fruits and vegetables, and then try something new!

Getting to Know Vegetables

Here is a quick rundown on some common vegetables and what to look for when buying fresh selections:

➤ **Artichokes** provide potassium and folate. Look for artichokes that are plump and heavy in relation to size. The many leaf-like parts are called "scales" and should be thick, green, and fresh looking. Avoid artichokes with any brownish discoloration or mouldy growth on the scales.

➤ **Asparagus** provides vitamins A and C, niacin, folate, potassium, and iron. Look for closed, dense tips with smooth, deep green spears. Avoid tips that are spread open or have any mould or decay.

➤ **Broccoli** provides calcium, potassium, iron, fibre, vitamins A and C, folate, and niacin. Look for stalks that have compact, firm, bud clusters and are dark green or sage green in colour. Avoid broccoli with a wilted appearance, yellowish-green discoloration, or bud clusters that are spread open. These are all signs of overripeness.

➤ **Brussels sprouts** provide vitamins A and C, folate, potassium, iron, and fibre. Look for Brussels sprouts with a bright green colour and tight-fitting outer leaves. Avoid Brussels sprouts that appear wilted or blemished.

➤ **Cabbage** provides vitamin C, potassium, folate, and fibre. Whether it's green or red, cabbage can be used in coleslaw, salads, and a variety of cooked dishes. Look for a dense head of cabbage that is heavy relative to its size, with outer leaves that display a green or red colour (depending on the type). Avoid cabbages with wilted or blemished outer leaves.

➤ **Carrots** provide vitamin A, potassium, and fibre. Look for smooth, firm, well-formed carrots that have a rich orange colour. Avoid roots that are discoloured, soft, or flabby.

➤ **Cauliflower** provides vitamin C, folate, potassium, and fibre. Look for compact, firm curds (the edible creamy-white portion), and don't worry about green leaflets that may be scattered throughout a bunch. Although most grocers sell cauliflower without the outside jacket leaves; in the rare instance that they are left on, a nice green colour reveals freshness. Avoid cauliflower that shows severe discoloration, blemishes, or spreading of the white curd.

➤ **Corn** provides vitamin A, potassium, and fibre. Although yellow-kernel corn is the most popular, there are varieties of white-kernel and mixed-kernel (peaches-and-cream) corn as well. Look for fresh green husks (the outer covering) and make sure that the silk ends are free of decay or injury by worms. If the corn has already been husked (had the outside covering removed), choose ears of corn that are heavily covered with bright yellow, plump kernels. Avoid kernels that appear dried or lacking in colour.

➤ **Eggplant** provides potassium. Look for firm, heavy, dark purple eggplants (although there are other coloured varieties). Avoid any that are shrivelled, soft, or lacking in colour or that reveal decay in the form of brownish spots.

➤ **Lettuce** comes in several varieties: Among them are iceberg, butter, romaine, and leaf lettuce. Lettuce provides vitamin C and folate. Look for bright colour and crisp leaf texture when buying romaine. For other leafy varieties, select those with succulent, tender leaves and avoid any that are seriously discoloured or wilted. Remember, the greener the lettuce, the more nutrients it contains.

➤ **Mushrooms** provide potassium, niacin, and riboflavin. Look for mushrooms on which the cap is closed around the stem and the gills (the rows of paper-thin tissue located underneath the caps) are pink or light tan in colour. Avoid mushrooms with wide-open caps and dark, discoloured gills.

➤ **Okra** provides vitamin A, potassium, and calcium. Look for bright green, tender pods that are under $4^1/2$ inches long. Avoid pods that have stiff tips (those that resist bending) or are a lifeless, pale green colour.

➤ **Onions** are not a significant source of nutrition, but they can certainly enhance the flavour of the foods you eat. They also provide natural sulphur compounds, which may give some protection from certain types of cancer. With all types (red, white, and yellow), look for hard, dry onions that are free of blemishes. Avoid onions that are wet or mushy.

➤ **Peas** (green) provide vitamin A, folate, potassium, protein, and fibre. Look for firm, fresh, bright green pods. Avoid flabby, wilted pods and any sign of decay.

➤ **Peppers** (sweet) provide vitamins A and C, potassium, and fibre. Although green peppers are the most common, other delicious varieties are yellow, orange, red, purple, and white. Look for firm peppers with deep characteristic colour. Avoid very lightweight, flimsy peppers that have punctures or signs of decay on the outside.

➤ **Potatoes** provide potassium, most B-vitamins, vitamin C, protein, and fibre. Look for reasonably smooth, firm, blemish-free potatoes. Avoid potatoes with large bruises or soft spots and those that have sprouted or are shrivelled.

➤ **Rhubarb** provides vitamin A, calcium, and potassium. Look for firm but tender stems with a decent amount of pink/red colour. Avoid rhubarb that appears wilted or flabby.

➤ **Spinach** provides vitamin A, calcium, folate, potassium, and fibre. Look for healthy, fresh leaves that have a dark green colour. Avoid spinach leaves that appear wilted or show significant discoloration.

➤ **Squash** (summer) provides vitamins A and C, potassium, and fibre and includes several varieties such as the yellow crookneck, large straightneck, greenish-white pattypan, and slender green zucchini. Look for firm, well-developed, tender squash. Check for a glossy (not dull) skin, which indicates that the squash is tender. Avoid dull, tough, or discoloured squash.

➤ **Squash** (winter) includes acorn, butternut, buttercup, green and blue hubbard, delicious, and banana, which all provide vitamins A and C, potassium, and fibre. Look for squash that is heavy for its size and has a tough, hard rind. Avoid squash with any signs of decay, including sunken spots, bruising, or mould.

Overrated–Undercooked

Generally, canned vegetables tend to be loaded with salt. If you do buy cans occasionally, be on the lookout for labels that read "low-sodium" or "no added salt."

➤ **Sweet potatoes** provide vitamins A and C, folate, potassium, and fibre. Look for firm, smooth sweet potatoes with uniformly coloured skins. The moist type known as yams should have orange flesh, whereas dry sweet potatoes have a more pale appearance. Avoid discoloration, worm holes, and any other indication of decay.

➤ **Tomatoes** provide vitamins A and C and potassium. Look for well-ripened, smooth tomatoes with a rich red colour. If you're not planning to eat them within the next few days, choose slightly less ripe, firm tomatoes with a pink or light red colour. Refrigerate only fully ripe tomatoes because the cold temperature might prevent immature tomatoes from ripening. Avoid tomatoes that are overripe and mushy or show any signs of decay.

Fabulous Fruits

For a quick nutritious snack, a deliciously healthy dessert, or even part of a creative meal, reach for fruit. Just like its vegetable neighbours in the produce section, fruit is naturally low in calories and fat (except for avocado and coconut), and is chock-full of nutrients and fibre. Get in the habit of keeping a bowl of fresh fruit on your table. Although dried fruit is another tasty option, keep in mind that it is more concentrated in calories because it has less water than its fresh counterparts. Also, beware of canned (and sometimes frozen) fruit with "heavy syrup added"; these products are packed with calories and sugar. When buying canned or frozen fruit, read labels and look for key phrases such as "no added sugar," "packed in its own juice," "packed in 100% fruit juice," or "unsweetened."

What about fruit juice? It's certainly not a substitute for whole fruit (in fact, even the brands with pulp added will be lacking in dietary fibre), but unsweetened fruit juice does provide nutrients and is clearly better than colas, sweetened iced-teas, or fruit punch. Put a couple of containers of juice in your shopping cart; when available, opt for the brands with added vitamin C or the calcium-fortified varieties.

Here are some helpful hints for shopping for fresh fruits:

➤ **Apples** provide potassium and fibre and are available in many varieties, including Red Delicious, McIntosh, Granny Smith, Empire, Spy, and Golden Delicious. Although each kind differs in seasonal availability, taste, and appearance, some general shopping savvy is to look for crisp, firm apples with a rich colour (depending upon the type). Avoid apples with bruising, soft spots, or mealy flesh.

➤ **Apricots** provide a lot of vitamin A, iron, and some potassium and fibre. Look for apricots that have a golden-orange colour and appear to be plump and juicy. Avoid apricots that are dull looking, mushy, or overly firm or that have a yellowish-green colour.

➤ **Avocados** provide vitamin A, potassium, folate, and fibre. Look for avocados that are slightly tender to the touch if you plan to eat them immediately. Otherwise, buy firm avocados and let them ripen at room temperature for a few days. Avoid any with broken surfaces or prominent dark spots.

➤ **Bananas** provide a lot of potassium and some vitamin A and fibre. Look for firm bananas that are either yellow green (and will ripen in a few days) or fully yellow and ready to eat. In general, bananas have their best flavour when the solid yellow colour is speckled with some brown. Avoid bananas that are bruised or have a grey appearance.

➤ **Blueberries** provide vitamin C, potassium, and fibre. Look for plump, firm blueberries that are dark blue in colour. Avoid berries that are mushy, mouldy, or releasing their liquid.

➤ **Cantaloupes** provide vitamins A and C and potassium. Look for cantaloupes with rough skin that are slightly soft and flexible when you press on the top or bottom and that have a sweet, fresh odour. Avoid extremely hard cantaloupes (unless you want to wait for them to ripen) and any with mouldy spots.

➤ **Cherries** provide vitamin A and potassium. Look for cherries that are dark red and plump and have fresh stems. Avoid cherries that appear dull, shrivelled, or dried.

➤ **Grapefruits** provide vitamins A and C and potassium. Look for firm, compact grapefruits that are heavy for their size. Don't worry about slight discoloration or scars on the skin; usually such blemishes do not interfere with the quality of the taste. Avoid grapefruits that look extremely dull and lack colour.

➤ **Grapes** provide some fibre and come in several colour varieties. Look for richly coloured, plump grapes that are tightly attached to the stem. Avoid grapes that are shrivelled and soft or that have brown, brittle stems.

➤ **Kiwi fruit** provides a lot of vitamin C and potassium. Look for plump kiwi fruit that yields slightly to the touch; this means it's ripe. You can ripen firm kiwi fruit at

108

home by leaving it at room temperature for a few days. Avoid kiwi fruits that are very soft or shrivelled.

➤ **Lemons** provide vitamin C. Look for firm lemons with a rich, glossy yellow colour. Avoid lemons with mould, punctures, or a dull, dark yellow colour.

➤ **Mangos** provide vitamins A and C, potassium, and fibre. Look for orange-yellow to red mangos that are well developed and barely soft to the touch. Avoid mangos that are rock hard or overripe and mushy.

➤ **Nectarines** provide vitamin A and potassium. Look for brightly coloured, plump nectarines with orange, yellow, and red colour combinations. Nectarines that are hard will ripen in a few days at room temperature. Avoid nectarines that are overly soft, lack colour, or show signs of decay.

➤ **Oranges** provide a lot of vitamin C, potassium, and folate. Look for firm, heavy oranges (because these characteristics indicate juiciness) with relatively smooth, bright-looking skin. Avoid oranges that are very light in weight (they contain little juice) or that have thick, coarse, or spongy skins.

➤ **Peaches** provide vitamin A and potassium. Look for peaches that are firm but slightly soft to the touch. Avoid greenish, hard peaches that are underripe and mushy peaches that are overripe.

➤ **Pears** provide potassium and fibre. Look for pears that are firm but not too hard. The colour depends on the variety. Bartletts are pale yellow to rich yellow, Anjou or Comice pears are light green to yellowish-green, Bosc are greenish-yellow to brownish-yellow, and Winter Nellis are medium to light green. Avoid wilted or wrinkled pears with any distinct spots.

➤ **Pineapples** provide vitamin C and fibre. Look for pineapples that are fragrant, plump, firm, and heavy for their size. Avoid pineapples that appear dull, bruised, or dried or those that have an unpleasant smell.

➤ **Raspberries** provide vitamin C, potassium, and fibre. Look for plump, tender berries with a rich, uniform scarlet colour. Avoid berries that are mushy or mouldy.

➤ **Strawberries** provide a lot of vitamin C, along with potassium, folate, and fibre. Look for firm, red berries that still have the cap attached. Avoid berries that have large uncoloured or excessively seedy areas. Also avoid strawberries that are shrunken or mouldy.

➤ **Tangerines** provide vitamins A and C. Look for deep yellow or orange tangerines with a bright lustre (which indicates freshness and maturity). Avoid tangerines that have a pale yellow or greenish colour or punctures in the skin.

➤ **Watermelon** provides vitamin A and some vitamin C. For uncut watermelons, look for a smooth surface, well-rounded ends, and a pale green colour. For cut watermelons, look for juicy flesh with a rich, red colour that is free from white streaks. Avoid melons with a lot of white streaks running through pale flesh and those with light-coloured seeds.

Aisle Two: Down Dairy Lane

Milk products supply you with calcium (responsible for healthy bones) and provide protein, several B-vitamins, and vitamins D and A. The problem is that whole milk also contains a lot of saturated fat, which can increase your risk of heart disease, weight gain, and other serious illnesses. What can you do? Simple: When you're at home and have control over the type of dairy products that go on your cereal and into recipes and sandwiches, use the lower fat versions that are available in all supermarkets today.

Don't throw in the towel if you don't like some of the reduced-fat items; different brands taste different. Just try another brand or version the next time you shop. Another thing to keep in mind is that some fat-free dairy products are literally "taste free." (Some brands even resemble plastic.) You don't have to use fat-free products if you can't stand the taste; low-fat products are fine, and have a mere 3–5 extra grams of fat per serving.

Here's your lower fat dairy shopping list. Browse through the section and pick out the items that sound appealing:

1% milk

Yogurts with 1% milkfat or less (plain and flavoured)

Skim milk (no fat)

Buttermilk

Nonfat varieties of processed cheese

Skim milk powder

Part-skim varieties of all cheese (15–19% milkfat)

Evaporated skim milk

Reduced-fat cream cheese

Dry-curd cottage cheese

Reduced-fat sour cream (5–7% milkfat)

1% cottage cheese

Low-fat/no-fat ice creams

Low-fat/no-fat frozen yogurts

Food for Thought

Contrary to its name, buttermilk is actually a low-fat dairy product. In fact, buttermilk is simply skim or low-fat pasteurized milk with some added lactic acid. The consistency is thicker than that of regular milk and the sodium is also higher at 257 milligrams per cup (250 mL) (about double the amount of regular low-fat milk).

Nutri-Speak

Pasteurized milk is briefly heated to kill harmful bacteria and then is rapidly chilled.

Homogenized milk has been processed to reduce the size of the milkfat globules so that the cream does not separate and the milk stays consistently smooth and uniform. Its milkfat content is 3.3 percent.

Aisle Three: Shopping for the Whole Grains

Here are some shopping tips for buying breads and cereals:

➤ Stick with whole grain products, including those containing whole wheat, multi-grain, rye, millet, oat bran, oat, and cracked wheat. (This goes for all types of bread: sliced bread, pita, bagels, English muffins, crackers, and so on.)

➤ Although "wheat" bread might sound just as healthy as "whole-wheat" bread, don't be fooled; wheat bread merely contains a blend of white and whole-wheat flour. A product labeled "whole-wheat" must be made from 100 percent whole-wheat flour.

➤ Check the label and choose breads with at least 2 grams of fibre per slice.

➤ If you're looking to save calories, try the whole-wheat, reduced-calorie bread (approximately 40 calories per slice with 2 grams of fibre), although I personally think there are more important places to cut calories.

➤ Don't forget to check the expiration date on the label.

➤ Take advantage of the fibre that some cereals pack in, and choose varieties that have at least 4 grams of fibre per serving. You can usually (not always) get a sense of whether a cereal has fibre from the name on the box (Bran Flakes, All-Bran, 100% Bran, Raisin Bran, Fibre-One, Shredded Wheat, and Corn Bran).

➤ Some cereals pack in more sugar and salt than most people realize. Check "Sugars" (on the nutrition label) to make sure sugar is not a main component of the total carbohydrates. In fact, opt for the brands that report 6 grams of sugar or less per serving. If your kids (or spouse) insist on the sugary brands, mix them with half a bowl of a healthier look-alike (for instance, try half Frosted Flakes and half Bran Flakes).

➤ Check the serving size. Some of the denser, heavier cereals allot only a minuscule amount for one serving. Take this into consideration if you plan to eat a normal-size bowl (and you're watching your weight). Remember, double the serving size means double the calories.

➤ Don't forget to throw some hot cereal into your cart. Whether you opt for the instant variety or the kind that requires cooking, stick with unsweetened varieties of oatmeal, cream of rice, oat bran, and cream of wheat. You can sweeten them with some of the fresh fruit you bought in the produce section.

➤ Most cereals are low in fat, with the exception of granola and other cereals that contain nuts, seeds, coconut, and oils. Read the label and choose cereals with no more than 2 grams of fat per serving.

➤ Read the list of ingredients on your cereal box and make sure that wheat, rye, corn, or oats are listed first. Items are listed in the order in which they are highest by weight.

Pasta, Rice, and More

Pasta is one of those Canadian staple foods that everyone seems to enjoy. What's more, pasta is high in complex carbohydrates, easy to make, and inexpensive. Don't stop at a box of spaghetti; try elbow macaroni, ziti, rigatoni, penne, fusilli, orzo, shells, bow ties, and lasagna noodles. If your supermarket has any whole-grain varieties, throw them in your basket; they're a great source of fibre.

Rice is another excellent source of complex carbohydrates and tends to be a popular standard in many homes. The most nutritious is brown rice, with a bit more fibre than the white varieties. Next in the nutrition lineup is polished white rice, and last is instant white rice, with the fewest nutrients of all.

Try some of the not-so-common grains. Pile your cart with couscous, barley, buckwheat, bulgur, kasha, millet, polenta, wheat berries, and cracked wheat. They are all brimming with complex carbohydrates—so jazz up your dinners and impress your family!

Aisle Four: Best Bets for Protein

Meat

When buying beef, pork, lamb, and veal, look for lean, well-trimmed cuts. Agriculture Canada grades meats according to their fat content and texture. In other words, grading refers to eating quality. Each type of meat has its own unique set of criteria for grading. Chances are, you're most familiar with the grading symbols for beef. Canada's top grades of beef are AAA, AA, and A. Look for these grades at the meat counter; they're your assurance that you are buying the best.

The difference between the three "A" grades relates to the amount of marbling, or fine white streaks of fat running throughout the lean meat. AAA is the most marbled and has the best overall eating quality. Marbling contributes to tenderness, taste, and juiciness, therefore resulting in a more consistent product. There's no need to fret over the extra fat in the AAA grade. In fact, the average fat content of about 3 ounces (90 g) of cooked, trimmed beef is 8.2 grams. A cooked, trimmed 3-ounce (90 g) portion of AAA grade beef contains 8.6 grams of fat, a difference of only 0.4 grams or 4 calories.

In order for any cut of meat to be classified as "lean" it must contain no more than 10 percent fat when it's raw. With the exception of short ribs, all cuts of beef are considered lean.

Your leanest beef choices are

Inside round steak	Sirloin steak
Rump roast	Eye of round roast
Outside round steak/roast	Sirloin tip/inside round roast
Eye of round teak	Strip loin steak

Blade roast

Cross rib/rib eye

Blade Steak

Flank

Ground beef, extra lean

Tenderloin

T-bone/porterhouse

Brisket

Rib roast

Your leanest lamb and veal choices are

Leg of lamb

Foreshank

Lean loin chop

Veal loin chop

Lamb roast

Arm chop

Veal roast

Veal cutlet

Your leanest pork choices are

Tenderloin

Centre loin chops

Centre loin roast

Lean ham

Loin, rib end roast

Top loin roast

Peameal bacon

Leg, inside round

Shoulder blade steak

Poultry

Let's not forget about poultry. Poultry can be one of your leanest animal protein sources, but lose the skin if you want to save fat! You can buy poultry with the skin if it's more reasonably priced. You can even cook poultry with the skin for some added moistness; just be sure to remove the skin before eating.

Your leanest poultry choices are

Skinless chicken breast

Turkey breast (white meat, no skin)

Cornish game hen (no skin)

Ground chicken or turkey breast (look for white meat only/no skin added)

Duck and pheasant (no skin)

Fish and Seafood

When choosing seafood and fish, scout the aisle and pick up anything that looks fresh and appealing. Fresh fish should have bright skin and bulging eyes (for whole fish), and both fish and seafood should have firm flesh and no fishy smell. You might have heard that some fish are fattier than others. It's true, but the amount of fat is so small that all fish and seafood remain great choices nutritionally. In addition, the type of fat found in fish is polyunsaturated (more specifically, omega-3 fatty acid), which has been shown to do positive things in the fight against heart disease and cancer. What's more, all types of fish supply excellent, high-quality protein, along with other vitamins and minerals.

Your leanest fish choices are

Cod	Haddock
Flounder	Monkfish
Sea bass	Perch
Whiting	Tuna
Halibut	Mullet
Red snapper	Swordfish
Sole	Shark
Mollusks (abalone, clams, mussels, oysters, scallops, and squid)	Shellfish (crab, lobster, and shrimp)

Fish higher in Omega-3 fats include

Salmon	Albacore tuna
Mackerel	Bluefish
Herring	Shad
Eel	Catfish
Pompano	Trout

Eggs

Eggs are a good source of high-quality protein, iron, and vitamin A—but they also provide a lot of cholesterol, about 190 milligrams, to get technical. There are approximately 5 grams of fat in just one egg yolk. If you eat eggs everyday, you might think about using only the whites, or grab a carton of egg substitute (which has no cholesterol and is low in fat), available in the frozen foods section. Also, many grocery stores carry preseparated egg whites in refrigerated cartons right next to the whole eggs.

Legumes (Dried Beans, Peas, and Lentils)

Definitely add some legumes to your shopping list. Legumes supply protein, calcium, iron, zinc, magnesium, and B-vitamins. Most impressive is that dried beans, peas, and lentils are the only high-protein foods that provide ample amounts of fibre. Get creative and make a meatless meal a couple of times each week.

Look for these beans:

Baked beans	Great northern beans
Pinto beans	Black beans
Kidney beans	Split peas
Black-eyed peas	Lentils
Tofu	Cannelloni beans
Lima beans	Vegetarian chilis
Navy beans	White beans
Garbanzo beans (chickpeas)	

Aisle Five: Frozen Meals, Canned Soups, and Sauces

As mentioned earlier, frozen and canned items can be convenient and tasty. Just remember to read the labels carefully and keep the following tips in mind:

➤ For full frozen meals, always read the label and look for those that contain less than 400 calories, 15 grams of fat, and 800 milligrams of sodium.

➤ When choosing soups, avoid the creamy varieties unless you have the option of mixing in your own low-fat milk. When you can, buy soups that say "reduced-sodium," "low-sodium," or "no added salt." Some nutritious selections include minestrone, garden vegetable, chicken noodle, split pea, tomato rice, Manhattan clam chowder, and the lentil-bean combinations.

➤ To cut fat, buy sauces that are tomato or vegetable based.

Aisle Six: Savvy Snacks

Most of us love to nibble between meals. If you plan to stock up your kitchen, do so with these low-fat items:

Plain popcorn kernels for air poppers
Fruit and fig bars
"Lite" or "reduced-fat" microwave popcorn
Low-fat granola bars and chewy cereal bars
Pretzels and baked chips
Lower fat whole-grain crackers
Animal crackers, ginger snaps, and graham crackers
Raisins and other dried fruit
Frozen fruit pops and sorbet
Flavoured rice cakes

Aisle Seven: Condiments for the Health Conscious

The following low-fat condiments can help add pizzazz to your meals. But keep in mind that many of these flavour enhancers are also high in sodium. Salt-sensitive people need to pay close attention to the salt contents listed on the package:

Ketchup	Cider vinegar
Mustard	Lemon juice
Jams	Fruit preserves
Low-sugar spreads	Worcestershire sauce
Soy sauce (low sodium)	Cocktail sauce
Teriyaki sauce(low sodium)	Chutney
Balsamic vinegar	Salsa

Aisle Eight: Heart-Smart Fats, Spreads, and Dressings

When purchasing fats, remember to stick with those that are predominantly unsaturated. If you like to add a lot of these products to your food, opt for the reduced-fat or fat-free versions of the original dressings and spreads. You'll cut down substantially on your fat intake.

Here's a master list to select from:

Monounsaturated

Olive oil   Canola oil

Peanut oil

Polyunsaturated

Safflower oil   Sunflower oil

Corn oil   Soybean oil

Others That May Come in Handy...

Nonstick cooking sprays

Fat-free and low-fat salad dressings

Low-fat dips, soft-tub margarines (nonhydrogenated)

Butter substitutes (sprays or granules)

Low-fat mayonnaise

Peanut butter (it may be high in fat, but it also provides a lot of protein)

The Least You Need to Know

➤ The first step to a well-stocked kitchen begins with a comprehensive, healthy shopping list. Organize your list according to the food categories discussed.

➤ Load up your cart with fresh vegetables and fruit, but buy only what you need because fresh produce is perishable. Frozen and canned fruits and vegetables are good options for people who do not shop frequently; just check to make sure there is not a lot of added fat, sugar, and salt.

➤ Buy lower fat dairy products and lean cuts of meat, poultry, and fish, and don't forget about legumes for those meatless meals. Also, look in the freezer section of your market for egg substitutes; if you eat eggs regularly, you'll save some fat and plenty of cholesterol by using such products.

➤ Scout out the grain products made with whole-grain flour. When choosing cereals, read the labels and select brands that are low in sugar and provide at least 4 grams of fibre per serving.

➤ Read labels on salad dressings, fats, and other spreads. Opt for products that are made with monounsaturated or polyunsaturated oils. Try reduced-fat, low-fat, or fat-free dressings and spreads.

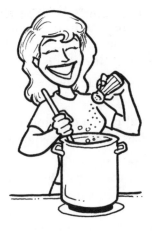

Chapter 11

Now You're Cooking

In This Chapter

➤ Simple cooking modifications

➤ Great recipes for breakfast, lunch, and dinner

➤ Finding a good cookbook

Mealtime is the perfect opportunity to bond with your family, converse with friends, relax in private, or impress your date with a fabulous dish. The hardest part is already done: You've stocked your kitchen with the right ingredients. So grab some pots and pans and turn on some inspiring music; this chapter offers helpful hints for recipe remodelling, and it provides you with recipes for easy-to-make, tasty breakfasts, lunches, dinners, and desserts.

The Recipe Makeover: Remodelling Family Favourites

Skimming the fat in your recipe means more than just using leaner ingredients. It also means using healthful cooking techniques and tools. Here are some quick tips and tricks of the trade:

1. Use low-fat and no-fat cooking methods, such as steaming, poaching, stir-frying, broiling, grilling, microwaving, baking, and roasting as alternatives to frying.

2. Get a good-quality set of nonstick saucepans, skillets, and baking pans so you can sauté and bake without adding fat.

3. Use nonstick vegetable sprays or 1–2 tablespoons of defatted broth, water, juice, or wine to replace cooking oil.

4. Be aware that low-fat cheeses have slightly different cooking characteristics than their fattier counterparts. For the most part, low-fat cheeses don't melt as smoothly. To overcome this, shred these cheeses very finely. When making sauces and soups, toss the cheese with a small amount of flour, cornstarch, or arrowroot.

5. Trim all visible fat from steaks, chops, roasts, and other meat cuts before preparing them.

6. Replace one-quarter to one-half the ground meat or poultry in a casserole or meat sauce with cooked brown rice, bulgar, couscous, or cooked and chopped dried beans to skim the fat and add fibre.

7. Deciding to remove the skin from poultry before or after cooking depends upon your cooking method. Skin helps prevent roasted or baked cuts from drying out, and studies have shown that the fat from the skin doesn't penetrate the meat during cooking. However, if you do leave the skin on, make sure any seasonings you've applied go under the skin or you'll lose the flavour when the skin is removed.

8. Skim and discard the fat from hot soups and stews, or chill the soup or stew and skim off the solid fat that forms on top.

9. Use puréed cooked vegetables, such as carrots, potatoes, and cauliflower, to thicken soups and sauces instead of cream, egg yolks, or a butter and flour roux. Also, use soft tofu to thicken sauces.

10. Select "healthier" fats when you need to add fat to a recipe. That means replacing butter, lard, or other highly saturated fats with oils such as canola, olive, safflower, sunflower, corn, and others that are low in saturated fats. Remember, it takes just a few drops of a very flavourful oil, such as extra-virgin olive oil or dark sesame, walnut, or garlic oil, to really perk up a dish, so go easy.

11. Skim the fat where you won't miss it, but keep the characteristic flavour of fatty ingredients such as nuts, coconut, chocolate chips, and bacon by reducing the quantity you use by 50 percent. For example, if a recipe calls for 1 cup (250 mL) of walnuts, use $^{1}/_{2}$ cup (125 mL) instead.

12. Toast nuts and spices to enhance their flavour and then chop them finely so they can be distributed more fully throughout the food.

13. If sugar is the primary sweetener in a fruit sauce, beverage, or other dish that is not baked, scale the amount down by 25 percent. Instead of 1 cup (250 mL) of sugar, use $^{3}/_{4}$ cup (175 mL). If you add a pinch of cinnamon, nutmeg, or allspice, you'll increase the perception of sweetness without adding calories.

14. In baked goods, add puréed fruit instead of fat. One of the reasons fat is included in baked products is to make them moist. The high concentration of natural sweetness in puréed fruit will actually help hold on to the moisture during the baking process.

Fat has flavour, but so does fruit. Fat adds liquid volume and moisture to bread or cake batter, but so does fruit. When substituting fruit for fat, if the recipe calls for $^1/_2$ cup (125 mL) of fat, simply add $^1/_2$ cup (125 mL) of puréed fruit. Use applesauce in apple bran muffins or cakes. Puréed, crushed pineapple works well in pineapple upside down cake. Here are some other tips:

➤ Dark-coloured fruits, such as blueberries and prunes, are best used in dark coloured batters. You can add lighter-coloured fruits, such as pears or applesauce, to almost any batter without changing its colour. Adding yellow-orange fruits, such as puréed peaches or apricots, can often add an appetizing yellowish crumb.

➤ You can use pears and apples nearly universally in baking because their taste is mild and unnoticeable. Apricots, prunes, and pineapple add a much stronger flavour. Bananas and peaches are somewhere in the middle, adding a little flavour, but never an overwhelming one. Here's a secret: If you don't have a food processor to use to purée your own fruit, use baby food. It is already puréed, has a mild flavour, and usually is made without sugar.

15. Beat egg whites until soft peaks form before incorporating them into baked goods. This will increase the volume and tenderness.

16. Make a simple fat-free "frosting" for cakes or bar cookies by sprinkling the tops lightly with powdered sugar.

17. Increase the fibre content and nutritional value of dishes by using whole-wheat flour for at least half of the all-purpose white flour amount. For cakes and other baked products that require a light texture, use whole-wheat pastry flour, available in some well-stocked supermarkets.

18. Vegetables can be fat replacements in other recipes, too. Try...

➤ Adding baby carrot purée, roasted red pepper purée, or mashed potatoes to your pasta sauce to replace olive oil

➤ Replacing some of the fat in nut breads or cakes, such as carrot cake or zucchini bread, with vegetable purées or juices, such as carrot juice or pumpkin purée

➤ Substituting puréed green peas for half the amount of mashed avocado in guacamole or other dips

➤ Replacing fat in soups, sauces, muffins, or cakes with mashed yams or sweet potatoes

➤ Using white potatoes to thicken lower fat milks in cream soups and bisques

➤ Substituting a layer of vegetables in your favourite lasagna to replace meat or sausage

➤ Topping your pizza with vegetables instead of meat

Source: ADA. "Skim The Fat: A Practical and Up-to-Date Food Guide," 1995.

Top-10 List for Substitutions

Try some of these substitutions in your favourite recipes. They can help to reduce the fat while maintaining flavour.

1. Use low-fat plain yogurt instead of sour cream.
2. Use two egg whites instead of one whole egg.
3. Use 1% milk instead of whole milk.
4. Use half the fat that a recipe calls for.
5. Use 3 tablespoons (45 mL) cocoa powder and 1 tablespoon (15 mL) oil instead of baking chocolate.
6. Use evaporated skim milk instead of cream.
7. Use fruit purées, fruit juices, or buttermilk to replace fat in a recipe.
8. Use low-fat yogurt or reduced-fat mayonnaise instead of regular mayonnaise.
9. Use reduced-calorie margarine instead of regular margarine.
10. Use low-fat ricotta cheese or 1% cottage cheese instead of whole-milk cream cheese or ricotta cheese.

Breakfast: Two Creative Morning Recipes

Vanilla French Toast with Fresh Fruit

Serves three

2 egg whites (or egg substitutes)

1/3 cup (75 mL) 1% milk

1/2 tsp (2 mL) vanilla extract

2 tsp (10 mL) margarine

6 slices of whole grain bread

1 cup (250 mL) low-fat vanilla-flavoured yogurt

1 cup (250 mL) fresh blueberries, strawberries, and banana, mixed

Beat the egg whites, milk, and vanilla in a bowl. Melt the margarine in a skillet over medium heat. Dip both sides of the bread evenly in the egg batter. Next, brown each side of the bread in the hot skillet. Arrange the finished French toast on a plate (2 full slices or 4 halves per serving); top with a scoop of vanilla yogurt and fresh fruit. If you really miss your maple syrup, drizzle a little over top!

Nutrient Analysis for One Serving
Calories: 231
Total fat: 4 grams
Fibre: 7 grams
Protein: 13 grams
Sodium: 467 mg
Cholesterol: 1 mg

From the kitchen of Leslie Beck

Mexican-Style Egg-White Omelet

Serves two

8 egg whites

4 Tbs (50 mL) 1% milk

Pepper

1/2 cup (125 mL) sliced mushrooms

1/2 cup (125 mL) sliced green onions

2 Tbs (25 mL) water

Nonstick vegetable spray

1/4 cup (50 mL) grated part-skim cheddar cheese

1/3 cup (75 mL) medium salsa

Mix the egg whites together with the milk and some pepper; set aside. Place the mushrooms, green onions, and water in a separate dish. Cover and microwave the vegetables for approximately 2 minutes on high (depending upon how soft you like your veggies). Drain vegetables, and mix in the eggs. Apply nonstick spray to a large skillet, and cook the entire concoction over medium-high heat. When the eggs begin to set, sprinkle on the shredded cheese and allow it to melt. Drop spoonfuls of salsa over the omelet. When the omelet appears cooked but moist, fold over one side and gently lift onto plate. Round off the meal with some corn bread and you're set.

Nutrient Analysis for One Serving (1/2 large omelet)

Calories: 161
Total fat: 1 gram
Fibre: 2 grams
Protein: 26 grams
Sodium: 445 mg
Cholesterol: 1 mg

From the kitchen of Leslie Beck

Lunch: Not the Same Old Sandwich Again!

Chicken and Bean Salad

Makes 4 cups (1 L)

1 can (14 oz/398 mL) kidney beans, rinsed and drained

1 cup (250 mL) corn kernels, canned or frozen

1 cup (250 mL) cubed cooked chicken

3/4 cup (175 mL) diced red bell pepper

2 green onions, chopped

1/4 cup (50 mL) red wine vinegar

2 Tbs (25 mL) vegetable oil

1/2 tsp (2 mL) minced garlic

1/4 tsp (1 mL) salt

1/4 tsp (1 mL) black pepper

1/4–1/2 tsp (1–2 mL) hot pepper sauce (optional)

In a medium bowl, combine beans, corn, chicken, peppers, onions, vinegar, oil, garlic, salt, pepper, and hot pepper sauce. Toss gently until combined. Chill before serving.

<u>Nutrient Analysis for One Serving</u>
Calories: 245
Fat: 8.3 grams
Protein: 19 grams
Fibre: 7.2 grams
Sodium: 400 mg

By Lynn Homer, RD (Calgary, AB), in Great Food Fast, *Robert Rose Inc., 2000. Reprinted with permission.*

Tuna Salad Melt

Serves four

2 cans (6 oz/170 g) water-packed tuna, drained

$^1/_4$ cup (50 mL) finely chopped celery

$^1/_4$ cup (50 mL) finely chopped sweet pickle or sweet relish

$^1/_4$ cup (50 mL) finely chopped red or green bell pepper (optional)

$^1/_4$ cup (50 mL) light mayonnaise

2 Tbs (25 mL) low-fat plain yogurt

1 Tbs (15 mL) lemon juice or pickle juice

1 French stick or baguette

$^1/_2$ cup (125 mL) grated cheddar cheese

In a bowl, stir together tuna, celery, pickle, red pepper, mayonnaise, yogurt, and lemon juice. Blend well.

Slice French stick in half lengthwise. Cut each half into 4 equal portions, making 8 pieces; place on baking sheet. Toast under broiler for 1–2 minutes or until golden. Remove from broiler; spread tuna mixture evenly over each piece. Sprinkle with cheese. Broil for 2–3 minutes or until cheese is melted and golden.

<u>Nutrient Analysis for One Serving</u>
Calories: 208
Fat: 6.1 grams
Fibre: 0.6 grams
Protein: 14 grams
Sodium: 477 mg

By Bev Callaghan, RD, in Great Food Fast, *Robert Rose Inc., 2000. Reprinted with permission.*

Dinner: Recipes to "Wow" Your Taste Buds

Penne with Mushroom and Spicy Tomato Sauce

Serves four

8 oz (250 g) penne

1 Tbs (15 mL) olive oil

3 cups (750 mL) sliced mushrooms

1/2 cup (125 mL) sliced onions

1/4 cup (50 mL) red wine

3 cups (750 mL) homemade or commercially prepared tomato sauce

1/2 tsp (2 mL) hot pepper sauce

2 Tbs (25 mL) chopped fresh parsley

1/4 cup (50 mL) grated Parmesan cheese

In a large pot of boiling water, cook pasta until tender but firm; drain.

In a large nonstick skillet, heat oil over medium-high heat. Add mushrooms and onions and cook for 6–8 minutes or until softened and moisture has evaporated. Add wine and cook, stirring, until evaporated.

Stir in tomato sauce and hot pepper sauce; bring to a boil. Reduce heat and simmer for 1–2 minutes. Stir in parsley. Serve over pasta, sprinkled with Parmesan cheese.

Nutrient Analysis for One Serving
Calories: 382
Fat: 10 grams
Fibre: 6.8 grams
Protein: 13.7 grams
Sodium: 297 mg

By Laurie A. Wadsworth, PDt (Antigonish, NS), in Great Food Fast, *Robert Rose Inc., 2000. Reprinted with permission.*

Baked Chicken Parmesan

Serves four

2 tsp (10 mL) vegetable oil

4 boneless, skinless chicken breasts

1 cup (250 mL) diced zucchini

1/2 cup (125 mL) sliced onions

1 1/2 cups (375 mL) homemade or commercially prepared tomato sauce

1 tsp (5 mL) dried basil or Italian seasoning

1 cup (250 mL) grated partly skimmed mozzarella

1/2 cup (125 mL) Parmesan cheese

In a large nonstick skillet, heat 1 tsp (5 mL) of the oil over medium-high heat. Add chicken breasts and sear for 1–2 minutes per side until golden brown. Transfer to baking dish.

Heat remaining oil in skillet. Add zucchini and onions; sauté for 3–5 minutes or until lightly browned. Remove from pan and place on top of chicken.

Preheat oven to 350°F (180°C). In a small bowl, blend together tomato sauce and basil; pour over chicken and vegetables. Sprinkle with mozzarella and Parmesan cheese. Bake in preheated oven for 25 to 30 minutes or until juices run clear when chicken is pierced with a fork.

Nutrient Analysis for One Serving
Calories: 372
Fat: 14.7 grams
Fibre: 2.4 grams
Protein: 47 grams
Sodium: 542 mg

By Bev Callaghan, RD, in Great Food Fast, *Robert Rose Inc., 2000. Reprinted with permission.*

Skillet Pork Chops with Sweet Potatoes and Couscous

Serves four

2 tsp (10 mL) vegetable oil

4 boneless pork loin chops, trimmed and patted dry (about 1 lb/500 g)

$^1/_2$ cup (125 mL) chopped onions

$^1/_2$ cup (125 mL) chopped celery or fennel

2 cups (500 mL) diced sweet potatoes

1 chicken bouillon cube dissolved in 1 cup (250 mL) water

$^1/_2$–1 tsp (2–5 mL) crumbled dried rosemary

$^3/_4$ cup (175 mL) orange juice or apple juice

1 cup (250 mL) quick-cooking couscous

Black pepper

In a large skillet, heat 1 tsp (5 mL) of the oil over a medium-high heat. Add pork chops and cook, turning once, for 7–8 minutes, or until slightly pink at centre and juices run clear when pierced with a fork. Transfer pork to a plate and keep warm.

Add remaining oil to a skillet. Add onions and celery; cook for 3 minutes. Add sweet potatoes, bouillon mixture, and rosemary; bring to a boil. Reduce heat and simmer, covered, for 7–8 minutes, or until potatoes are barely tender.

Stir in orange juice and couscous. Return pork to skillet and simmer, covered, for 2 minutes. Remove pan from heat and let stand for 3 minutes. Fluff couscous with fork. Season to taste with pepper.

Nutrient Analysis for One Serving
Calories: 462
Fat: 9.4 grams
Fibre: 4.3 grams
Protein: 32.7 grams
Sodium: 397 mg

By Bev Callaghan, RD, in Great Food Fast, *Robert Rose Inc., 2000. Reprinted with permission.*

Sensational Side Dishes

Honey Glazed Carrots

Serves six

1 lb (500 g) carrots	2 tsp (10 mL) butter or soft margarine
1 Tbs (15 mL) liquid honey or brown sugar	1/2 tsp (2 mL) ground ginger
1 Tbs (15 mL) orange juice	1/2 tsp (2 mL) grated orange zest (optional)

In a medium saucepan over high heat, boil carrots until tender-crisp; drain. Add honey, orange juice, butter, ginger, and, if using, orange zest. Quickly stir for 2–3 minutes or until glaze forms.

Nutrient Analysis for One Serving
Calories: 77
Fat: 2.1 grams
Fibre: 2.5 grams
Protein: 1.1 grams
Sodium: 81 mg

By Lynn Roblin, RD, in Great Food Fast, *Robert Rose Inc., 2000. Reprinted with permission.*

Sautéed Spinach with Pine Nuts

Serves four

2 tsp (10 mL) olive oil	1 tsp (5 mL) minced garlic
1/4 cup (50 mL) pine nuts	1 tsp (5 mL) lemon juice
1 package (10 oz/300 g) fresh spinach trimmed of tough stalks	1/8 tsp (0.5 mL) nutmeg
	Black pepper

In a large nonstick skillet, heat 1 tsp (5 mL) of the oil over medium heat. Add pine nuts and cook, stirring constantly, for 2–3 minutes or until golden. Remove pine nuts from pan and set aside.

Add remaining oil to pan. Add spinach in several bunches (it will cook down quickly). Stirring constantly, add garlic and cook for 1–2 minutes. Stir in lemon juice and nutmeg. Season to taste with pepper. Add reserved pine nuts. Cook until heated through.

Nutrient Analysis for One Serving
Calories: 90
Fat: 7.6 grams
Fibre: 3.3 grams
Protein: 4.5 grams
Sodium: 48 mg

By Bev Callaghan, RD in Great Food Fast, *Robert Rose Inc., 2000. Reprinted with permission.*

Chunky Vegetable Lentil Soup

Makes 6 cups (1.5 L)

2 cups (500 mL) water

1 vegetable bouillon cube

1 cup (250 mL) chopped carrots

1 can (28 oz/796 mL) diced tomatoes

1 can (19 oz/540 mL) lentils, rinsed
and drained

2 tsp (10 mL) minced garlic

1 tsp (5 mL) dried basil

$^1/_2$ tsp (2 mL) ground thyme

$^1/_2$ tsp (2 mL) cumin

In a large saucepan, bring water to a boil. Add vegetable bouillon cube; stir until dissolved.

Add carrots; reduce heat to medium and cook, covered, for 10 minutes.

Add tomatoes, lentils, garlic, basil, thyme, and cumin; reduce heat to medium-low and cook, stirring often, for 10 minutes or until carrots are tender.

<u>Nutrient Analysis for One Serving</u>
Calories: 118
Fat: 0.7 grams
Fibre: 4.8 grams
Protein: 7.7 grams
Sodium: 541 mg

By Lynn Roblin, RD, in Great Food Fast, *Robert Rose Inc., 2000. Reprinted with permission.*

Decadent Desserts

Awesome Pineapple Cake

Cake

2 cups (500 mL) all-purpose flour

$1^1/_2$ cups (375 mL) granulated sugar

1 cup (250 mL) finely chopped pecans

1 tsp (5 mL) baking soda

1 can (19 oz/540 mL) crushed
pineapple with juice

2 eggs, beaten

1 tsp (5 mL) vanilla

Icing

2 Tbs (25 mL) butter, softened

1 4-oz (125 g) package light cream
cheese, softened

$1^1/_4$ cups (300 mL) icing sugar

1 tsp (5 mL) vanilla

Preheat oven to 350°F (180°C). Grease a 13 x 9-inch (3 L) baking pan with nonstick spray.

Cake: In a large bowl, combine flour, sugar, pecans, and baking soda. In another bowl, blend together pineapple, eggs, and vanilla. Make a well in the centre of the dry ingredients and pour in pineapple mixture; stir gently until combined.

Pour batter into prepared pan and bake in preheated oven for 40–45 minutes or until cake tester inserted into the centre comes out clean. Set aside to cool.

Icing: In a bowl, blend together butter and cream cheese until smooth. Beat in icing sugar and vanilla. Spread icing over cooled cake.

<u>Nutrient Analysis for One Serving</u>
Calories: 384
Fat: 11.7 grams
Fibre: 1.7 grams
Protein: 4.9 grams
Sodium: 175 mg

By Zita Bersenas-Cers, RD (Hamilton, ON), in Great Food Fast, *Robert Rose Inc., 2000. Reprinted with permission.*

Angel-Devil Smoothie

Serves four

2 cups (500 mL) nonfat plain yogurt

2 chocolate nonfat brownies, broken into small pieces (e.g., Snackwell's)

2 cups (500 mL) frozen sliced strawberries

1/4 cup (50 mL) skim milk

Combine all ingredients in blender or food processor. Pulse until all is puréed fine. Serve immediately.

<u>Nutrient Analysis for One Serving</u>
Calories: 140
Fat: 0 grams
Fibre: 2 grams
Protein: 8 grams
Sodium: 135 mg

Copyright Food for Health *newsletter, 1996. Reprinted with permission.*

Banana–Health Split

Serves one

1 banana, peeled
$^1/_2$ cup (125 mL) vanilla low-fat frozen yogurt
2 Tbs (25 mL) granola cereal (low-fat)

Split the banana lengthwise down the middle, and line up the two pieces on either side of an ice cream dish. Scoop frozen yogurt in the middle and sprinkle granola on top. You've now got a guilt-free banana split!

<u>Nutrient Analysis for One Serving</u>
Calories: 243
Fat: 1 gram
Fibre: 2 grams
Protein: 5 grams
Sodium: 65 mg

From the kitchen of Pam and Dan Schloss

Overrated–Undercooked

Be careful when cutting back on the amount of sugar in cakes, cookies, or other baked goods. Many times, reducing the sugar will affect the texture or the volume.

Start a Cookbook Library

Check with the following resources to begin your own collection of cookbooks. You can find healthy recipes in the following books (all are available at your local bookstore):

Great Food Fast: Brought to You by the Dietitians of Canada
Robert Rose Inc., 2000

Healthy Pleasures: Great Tastes from Canadian Dietitians and Chefs
Macmillan Canada, 1995

Sensationally Light Pasta & Grains
by Rose Reisman
Penguin Books Canada, 1999

Anne Lindsay's New Light Cooking
by Anne Lindsay
Ballantine Books, 1998

More HeartSmart Cooking with Bonnie Stern
by Bonnie Stern
Heart and Stroke Foundation of Canada, 1997

Simply HeartSmart Cooking
by Bonnie Stern
Random House Toronto, 1994

LooneySpoons: Low Fat Food Made Fun
by Janet and Greta Podleski
Garnet Publishing, 1996

Cooking Light Five Star Recipes
Oxmour House Inc., 1996

Great Taste—Low Fat
(A series of low-fat cookbooks)
Time Life Books, Time Life Inc.
1-800-621-7026

Everyday Cooking with Dr. Dean Ornish
by Dean Ornish, MD
HarperCollins Publishers

> ### The Least You Need to Know
>
> ➤ Simple ingredient substitutions can turn your favourite recipes into healthy, low-fat dishes.
>
> ➤ Stick with the healthier, lower fat cooking techniques such as steaming, poaching, stir-frying, broiling, grilling, microwaving, baking, and roasting. Jazz up the flavour with non-caloric spices and seasonings.
>
> ➤ Use puréed, cooked veggies instead of cream, butter, and egg yolks to thicken soups and sauces. For baked products, add puréed fruit instead of butter, lard, and other oils. When a recipe calls for a large amount of sugar, scale it down by 25 percent.

Chapter 12

Restaurant Survival Guide

In This Chapter

➤ Dining out healthfully

➤ Becoming a menu detective

➤ Best bets in ethnic cuisine

Too tired to cook, or just want to get out and socialize? Join the crowd! According to the Canadian Restaurant and Foodservice Association, the average Canadian spends $1,143 per year on food eaten away from home. Once considered a special occasion, eating out has become an everyday happening—and the food-service industry is growing by leaps and bounds. This chapter shows you that, along with convenience and atmosphere, restaurants can also provide healthy food. You just need to practise some defensive dining.

Common Restaurant Faux Pas

First, the problem of overeating. Are you the type who needs to loosen your belt buckle a couple of notches after each course? Keep in mind that this is *not* the last meal of your life, and there's no need to lick your plate clean even though your stomach is ready to explode. When you feel comfortably full, either ask the server to take away your plate, or simply pack up the leftovers in a doggie bag and enjoy them the following day.

What about the actual food choices? Making healthy food choices requires planning, nutrition know-how, and compromise: *planning* during the day so you can budget your fat and calories; *nutrition know-how* so you can order the healthier, lower fat items from your favourite ethnic cuisines; and the willingness to *compromise* between the foods you should be eating and the not-so-terrific foods you love to indulge in.

Fortunately, due to the increasing emphasis on health, most places, from fast-food joints to fancy establishments, are making an effort to prepare and offer at least a few healthy alternatives. Quite often, you will even notice a "Spa Cuisine" section on the regular menu listing nutrition information for the lower fat entrées. For the restaurants that don't provide this information, don't be shy or embarrassed: Speak up and ask for special requests such as salad dressing or sauce to be on the side, less oil and salt to be used during food preparation, and a baked potato or side salad to be substituted for french fries. Remember, good food does not have to come with the price tag of cellulite.

Become a Dining Detective

Go ahead and take on any type of restaurant. Ask yourself (and the server) the following five key questions before ordering something from the menu:

1. **How is the food prepared?** The same methods I advised for your own personal recipes also apply to foods prepared in restaurants. Scout out foods, whether entrées or side dishes, that are prepared by grilling, baking, poaching, roasting, boiling, blackening, steaming, broiling, or "lightly" stir-frying. If the menu doesn't indicate the cooking technique, ask your server. Don't assume that a food is not fried unless the menu clearly says it isn't.

2. **Are the cuts of meat lean?** Stick with the leaner cuts of meat. For instance, loin, round, flank, shoulder, leg, and extra-lean ground beef are the preferred choices when ordering red meat. Chicken and turkey breast are two of the leanest choices to make, and of course, all fish and seafood can be terrific when prepared in a healthful manner. When you do order steak, ask whether the chef melts butter on top before cooking it. Believe it or not, some establishments do this to make the meat seem more tender.

3. **What kind of sauces come with your meal?** Ask about the ingredients used for sauces. Generally, avoid hollandaise, butter, cheese, and cream sauces that come slathered on your meal. If you're not sure about a sauce, or it sounds delicious and hard to pass up, ask to have it on the side and enjoy it in smaller amounts.

4. **Are the ingredients loaded with sodium?** If you're on a sodium-restricted diet for medical reasons, it's especially important to avoid entrées and side dishes that are loaded with salt. Stay away from meats and fish that are smoked, cured, pickled, or canned. Also avoid sauces, seasonings, and marinades that use soy sauce, teriyaki sauce, dried stock, MSG, or plain old table salt during preparation.

5. **How can you balance out your meal?** If you order a pasta entrée, pass up the bread. If you know that you like to splurge on dessert, order lean grilled fish for your main dish with a lot of vegetables. If the breadbasket is your thing, skip the side starch that comes with your main meal and enjoy a few slices of fresh bread instead. If you like to use up calories on a few glasses of wine, skip the bread and get fresh fruit for dessert.

Q & A

Can you ever just "go whole hog" and order whatever you want without worrying about all the unhealthy ingredients?

Sure you can, but save it for occasional splurges–not everyday habit. In fact, some things are so obscenely scrumptious that if you didn't periodically indulge, I'd think you were too good to be true!

Ethnic Cuisine: the Good, the Not-So-Great, and the Downright Bad

Take a quick trip around the world, and check out the best bets in French, Italian, Chinese, Japanese, Mexican, Indian, and North American cookery. Be adventurous and excite your palate with exotic new flavours. *Bon appétit!*

Chinese Food

Loaded with vegetables, rice, and noodles, the typical Chinese cuisine available in North America offers an assortment of healthy selections. Because most Chinese cooking is done in a wok (stir-fried), varying amounts of peanut oil are used. The good news is that peanut oil is unsaturated and won't clog up your arteries. The bad news is that excessive amounts of *any* oil can add a lot of fat calories. As you can imagine, some of the dishes have *startling* numbers.

If your thighs can't afford those extra fat calories, avoid anything fried. Try one of the steamed versions, or carefully drain off some of the fat in a stir-fried entrée by taking your portion from the serving plate drenched in sauce and transferring it to your dish with rice. Another idea, if you're dining with a friend, is to order one dish in sauce and a second steamed vegetable dish. Mix the two together, and you'll have half the sauce and double the vegetables.

Another problem with Chinese food can be sodium because a lot of the sauces are high in salt. If you're on a salt-restricted diet, you should probably stick with the plain steamed dishes.

Lower Fat Foods	Higher Fat Foods
Hot and sour soup	Egg drop soup
Won ton soup	Egg rolls
Steamed dumplings (vegetable, chicken, and seafood)	Fried dumplings
	Fried won tons
Stir-fried or *steamed* chicken and vegetables	Fried rice
	Cold noodles with sesame sauce
Stir-fried or *steamed* beef and vegetables	Moo-shu pork
	Sweet and sour pork
Stir-fried or *steamed* seafood and vegetables	Fried chicken and seafood dishes
	Seafood with lobster sauce
Stir-fried or *steamed* tofu and vegetables	Spareribs
Steamed whole fish	
Sesame Chicken	
General Tsao Chicken	
Moo-shu vegetables (with pancake rollups)	
Steamed brown and white rice	
Fortune cookies	
Lychee nuts	
Orange and pineapple slices	
Low-sodium soy sauce (if available)	
Duck sauce and plum sauce	

French Food

Many positive changes (nutritionally speaking) have occurred in French cuisine during the 20th century, from classic *haute* cuisine that generally uses heavier cream sauces to *nouvelle* cuisine that uses a lighter and healthier approach to food preparation.

Lower Fat Foods	Higher Fat Foods
Steamed mussels	Appetizers with olives, anchovies, or capers
Consommé	Quiche
Endive and watercress salads	French onion soup (with cheese)
Nicoise salads	Cream-based soups
Poached fish	Pâté
Steamed fish	Fondue
Lightly sautéed vegetables	Crêpes
Bouillabaisse	Brioche
Chicken in wine sauce	Duck or goose with skin

Lower Fat Foods	Higher Fat Foods
French bread and baguettes	Bérnaise sauce
Flambéed cherries	Hollandaise sauce
Peaches in wine	Béchamel sauce
Fresh and poached fruit	Mornay sauce
Fruit sorbet	Anything with the word "cream" or "au gratin"
Wine in moderation	Chocolate mousse
	Crème caramel
	Croissants
	Pastries and éclairs

Indian Food

As with most ethnic cuisines, there are pros and cons to Indian cookery. Beginning with the pros, Indian cuisine emphasizes foods high in carbohydrates, such as basmati rice, breads, lentils, chickpeas, and vegetables, all accented with an array of spices. The most common veggies are spinach, cabbage, peas, onions, eggplant, potatoes, tomatoes, and green peppers. The con is that fat can easily find its way into many of the entrées, breads, and vegetable side dishes.

Scrutinize the menu and watch out for the word *ghee*, which is the clarified butter used frequently in Indian cooking. Other oils that are used for sautéing and frying are sesame oil and coconut oil. Although sesame oil is unsaturated, it's quite the contrary for coconut oil—arteries beware! If salt is an issue, forgo the soups, and ask the waiter to please prepare your meal without any added salt.

Lower Fat Foods	Higher Fat Foods
Tamatar salat	Anything made with ghee (clarified butter)
Mulligatawny soup (lentil, veggies, and spices)	Coconut soups
	Samosas (fried vegetable turnover)
Chicken or beef tikka	Korma (meat with rich yogurt cream sauce)
Tandoori chicken, beef, or fish	Curries made with coconut milk or cream
Chicken, beef, and fish saaq (with spinach)	Pakora (fried dough with veggies)
	Saaq paneer (spinach with cream sauce)
Chicken, beef, and fish vindaloo (with potatoes and spices)	Creamy rice dishes
	Fried breads
Shish kabob	Honeyed pastries
Gobhi matar tamatar (cauliflower with peas and tomatoes)	

Lower Fat Foods	Higher Fat Foods
Matar pulao (rice pilaf with peas)	
Steamed rice	
Papadum or papad (crispy, thin lentil wafers)	
Coriander, tamarind, and yogurt-based sauces	
Chapati (thin, dry whole-wheat bread)	
Naan (leavened, baked bread)	
Kulcha (leavened, baked bread)	
Mango, mint, and onion chutney	

Italian Food

Among my friends and family, Italian seems to be the one type of food that we can always agree on. (It's amazing how quickly you can get into the mood.) Unfortunately, as with every other cuisine, if you take one wrong turn on the menu, you're headed for a nutritional no-no. For instance, pasta can be a terrific meal if it is ordered with the right kind of sauce; stick with meatless marinara, red clam, pomodora, or white wine sauce, or a light olive oil. On the other hand, a pasta entrée swimming in one of those cream sauces is a dieter's demise. Also, watch out for super-cheesy entrées such as stuffed shells, manicotti, lasagna, and parmigiana. Of course, every once in a while, we are all entitled to indulge. Just make sure the rest of your day was pretty low-fat because some of these dishes can pack away the fat grams.

Lower Fat Foods	Higher Fat Foods
Roasted peppers	Fried calamari and fried mozzarella
Mussels marinara	Garlic bread
Steamed clams	Caesar salads
Grilled calamari	Sausage and meatball heros
Minestrone soup	Calzones and pizza with pepperoni and sausage
Pasta with meatless marinara sauce	
Pasta primavera (not creamy)	Antipasto salad with high-fat meats and cheese
Pasta with red and white clam sauce	
Pasta with marsala	Cheese- or meat-filled ravioli and manicotti
Chicken breast with red sauce	Meat lasagna and cheesy vegetarian lasagna
Chicken cacciatore	Cannelloni and baked ziti
Shrimp, chicken, or veal in wine sauce	Chicken, veal, or eggplant parmigiana
Chicken and veal piccatta	Fettuccine alfredo and pasta carbonara
Pizza with fresh vegetable toppings	Shrimp scampi
Lightly marinated mushrooms	Chicken or veal scaloppini
Fresh Italian bread	Cannoli, spumoni, and tartufo

136

Lower Fat Foods	Higher Fat Foods
Fresh fruit or sorbet	
Italian ices	
Skim milk cappuccino	
Wine in moderation	

Japanese Food

The Japanese have perfected low-fat cooking with food-preparation methods that require little or no oil. Highlighting rice, vegetables, soybean-based foods, and small quantities of fish, chicken, and meat, these meals are artistic, healthy, and, best of all, delicious. What's more, once you master the art of using chopsticks, Japanese dining can be a lot of fun. The one drawback is the high-sodium marinades and traditional sauces, which include soy and teriyaki. Ask your waiter whether low-sodium soy sauce is available, and if it isn't, dilute the regular sauce with some water.

Lower Fat Foods	Higher Fat Foods
Miso soup (soybean-paste soup with tofu and scallions)	Vegetable tempura (battered and fried veggies)
Steamed vegetables	Shrimp tempura
Fish and vegetable sushi	Eel and avocado rolls
Sashimi (raw fish served with wasabi and dipping sauce)	Tonkatsu (breaded pork cutlet)
Hijiki (cooked seaweed)	Fried dumplings
Oshitashi (boiled spinach with soy sauce)	Fried bean curd
Yaki-udon	Oyako domburi (chicken omelet over rice)
Yakitori (skewers of chicken)	Chawan mush (chicken and shrimp in egg custard)
Su-udon	Yo kan (sweet bean cake)
Sukiyaki	
Sushi and sashimi (pieces and rolls)	
Nabemono (a variety of casseroles)	
Yosenabe (seafood and veggies in broth)	
Miso-nabe	
Shabu-shabu (sliced beef, vegetables, and noodles)	
Sumashi wan (broth with tofu and shrimp)	
Chicken, fish, or beef teriyaki	
Steamed rice	

Mexican Food

If your taste buds cry out for hot and spicy, Mexican food is probably high on your list of favourites. Unfortunately, some typical dishes on a Mexican menu can send you straight to nutrition jail. On a positive note, Mexican food can be healthy, especially because many dishes are high in complex carbohydrate and fibre; you just need to manage the menu. For example, we all know those fried tortilla chips can be addictive. If you typically gobble down three baskets before your food even arrives, get them off the table. Stick with cheeseless entrées that include beans, rice, and grilled chicken or fish, and use plenty of salsa in place of high-fat sour cream and guacamole. (Although guacamole contains unsaturated fat, there's still a lot of it.)

Lower Fat Foods	Higher Fat Foods
Gazpacho	Tortilla chips
Corn tortillas with salsa	Nachos with cheese
Ceviche (raw fish cooked in lime or lemon juice)	Chorizo (sausage)
	Carnitas (fried beef)
Chicken fajitas	Refried beans
Enchiladas	Quesadillas with cheese
Camarones de hacha (shrimp sautéed in tomato coriander sauce)	Beef tacos
	Burritos with cheese
Arroz con pollo (chicken breast with rice)	Beef and cheese enchilada
	Chimichangas
Cheeseless burritos	Sour cream and guacamole
Grilled fish or chicken breast	Sopapillas (fried dough with sugar)
Frijoles a la charra	Frozen margaritas and piña coladas
Borracho beans and rice	
Soft chicken taco	
Chicken tostada	
Salsa, pico de gallo and cilantro	
Jalapeño peppers	

North American Food

North American–style restaurants borrow an assortment of ethnic dishes from around the world. Of course, we *are* responsible for salad bars, steak and potatoes, chicken and ribs, a bunch of sandwiches, and good ol' American apple pie, but the typical North American menu could represent the United Nations.

For example, you can usually expect to find chicken teriyaki from Japan, a stir-fried dish from China, chicken fajitas from Mexico, and a pasta dish from Italy on the spread. The nice part about such a comprehensive menu is that it offers something for everyone

Overrated–Undercooked

Don't let the words "salad bar" fool you. There are just as many high-fat pickings displayed on the buffet as there are low-fat ones. Survey the offerings and load your plate with fresh vegetables, beans, whole grains, and low-fat dressings. On the flip side, watch out for the high-fat mayonnaise traps (such as macaroni, tuna, egg, seafood, and chicken salads), and take it easy on the creamy dressings, bacon bits, high-fat cheeses, olives, nuts, and seeds.

(even finicky kids). Placing heavy emphasis on appetizers, salads, and sandwiches, North American food can certainly swing both ways. When you're in the mood for a sandwich, stick with the unadulterated versions such as turkey, roast beef, and chicken breast. Beware of breads and buns that are pre-buttered before they reach your table (such as the buttery grilled cheese sandwich). Ask your waiter to substitute a side salad for those greasy french fries, and stay clear of large salad entrées that pack in more fat than you want to know about. (Read the descriptions and go easy on bacon, avocado, shredded cheese, olives, and dressings.) For standard entrées, look for the usual green-light words (grilled, broiled, and blackened); you know the routine by now.

Lower Fat Foods	Higher Fat Foods
Shrimp/seafood cocktails	Creamy soups
Tossed salads with light vinaigrette	Caesar salads
Broth and vegetable-based soup	Salads with avocado, bacon, and
Turkey, roast beef, and	creamy dressings
grilled chicken sandwiches	Buffalo/chicken wings
Broiled, blackened, and grilled	Fried zucchini and mushrooms
fish and chicken	Cheeseburgers
Plain hamburgers, turkey burgers,	Grilled cheese sandwiches
and veggie burgers	Philadelphia cheese steaks
Grilled chicken on salad	Rueben sandwiches and tuna melts
Grilled vegetables over rice	Tuna salad, egg salad, and chicken salad
Chicken kabobs and rice	Fried chicken or fish
Baked potatoes with Dijon mustard,	Hot dogs
ketchup, marinara, salsa, or small	French fries and potato salad
amount of butter	Fruit pies, cookies, cakes, and
Pasta with tomato-based sauce	ice cream sundaes

Lower Fat Foods	Higher Fat Foods
Steamed or lightly sautéed vegetables	
Frozen yogurt, fruit ice or sherbet	
Fresh fruit	
Angel-food cake	

Fast Food

The restaurants might lack ambiance, but fast food is certainly one hopping business! It's quick, convenient, and cheap. The nice thing about fast food today is that most places offer an assortment of healthy alternatives due to the growing number of nutrition-conscious customers. Try your best to keep things simple. Generally, the items with complicated names are laden with high-fat meats and "special sauces." For example, the Bacon Double Cheeseburger Deluxe at Burger King has a whopping 39 grams of fat with 16 grams from saturated fat. Be sure to also skip the fried chicken and all sandwiches smothered with cheese. Also, don't ever assume that fish automatically gets a nutrition gold medal. Did you know that McDonald's Filet-O-Fish (breaded and fried) contains 18 grams of fat, compared to the plain hamburger, which has only 9 grams? Stick with the healthier choices to make the best of your fast-food outings.

Lower Fat Foods	Higher Fat Foods
Bagel with jam	Biscuits and Danish
Hot cakes (no butter)	Egg sandwiches with sausage or bacon
Grilled chicken sandwiches	Cheeseburgers
Plain hamburgers	Jumbo burger combinations
Turkey burgers	Fried chicken sandwiches and
Veggie burgers	fried chicken nuggets
Vegetable pizza	Fried fish fillets
Vegetable salads with calorie-reduced	Pepperoni or sausage pizza
dressings, or plain baked potato	French fries
Chunky chicken salads	Baked potatoes with butter,
Turkey sandwiches (no mayo)	sour cream, or cheese
Lean roast-beef sandwiches (no mayo)	Nachos with cheese
Onion rings and fried vegetables	Apple pie and milkshakes
Chicken fajitas	
Mashed potatoes	
Baked potatoes with vegetables,	
salsa, ketchup, or vegetarian chili	
Grilled or steamed veggies	
Fruit salads and fresh fruit	

Lower Fat Foods	Higher Fat Foods
Frozen yogurt cones	
Juice or low-fat milk	
Ketchup, mustard, barbecue, and honey mustard sauce	

Your best bets in fast food are these:

➤ At McDonald's, try the McChicken Wrap, a side salad with calorie-reduced vinaigrette, and a bottle of water.

➤ At Pizza Hut, try the Edge Pizza (thin crust) with vegetable toppings, a side salad with calorie-reduced dressing, and a tall glass of water.

➤ At Wendy's, try the Grilled Chicken Sandwich on a multigrain bun, or a baked potato with plain broccoli (or chili), and a salad tossed with calorie-reduced dressing. Wash it down with some water or juice.

➤ At Mr. Sub, try the Grilled Chicken Wrap (whole-wheat), no cheese, with veggies and barbecue sauce. Order a bottle of water or unsweetened fruit juice.

➤ At Harvey's, try the Veggie Burger and a salad tossed with calorie-reduced dressing. Have water or unsweetened juice with your meal.

➤ At Swiss Chalet, order a Quarter Chicken Breast (no skin) with a baked potato and a side salad tossed with calorie-reduced dressing. If you're really hungry, start with a chicken soup. And yes, go ahead and enjoy the barbecue sauce—it's low in fat!

Going Out for Breakfast or Brunch?

Master the following do's and don'ts.

Do order pancakes and waffles with plenty of fresh fruit and just a touch of syrup. Choose egg-white omelets stuffed with various veggies, peameal bacon, unsweetened cereals with skim or 1% milk, and fresh fruit. Other healthy alternatives are hot oatmeal, cream of wheat and rice (made with low-fat milk), English muffins, bagels, and whole grain breads with some jam and low-fat yogurt. Opt for some fresh unsweetened juice or low-fat milk to drink.

Don't make it a habit to start your day with higher fat fare, such as scrambled eggs, bacon, sausage, hash browns, cheese omelets, biscuits, croissants, bagels with butter, large cake-like muffins, donuts, pancakes and waffles smothered in butter and syrup, deep-fried French toast, or steak and eggs.

The Least You Need to Know

➤ Once considered a luxury, dining out has become commonplace for most all Canadians today.

➤ Remember that "eating out" does not mean "pigging out." Don't allow yourself to overeat just because you are in a restaurant. Eat slowly and selectively, and stop when you are comfortably full.

➤ With the proper planning, nutrition know-how, and willingness to compromise, you can fit almost any ethnic restaurant into a healthy low-fat eating plan.

➤ Become a dining detective and examine the menu carefully. Look for lean cuts of meat, poultry, and fish that have been prepared using low-fat cooking methods. Ask your server about the type of sauce that accompanies your meal. If salt is an issue, watch out for high-sodium marinades.

➤ Always remember: You're the paying customer. Don't be shy to order it *your* way.

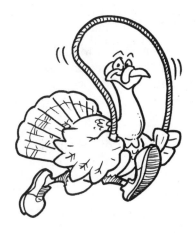

Chapter 13

Trimming Down the Holidays

In This Chapter

➤ Cutting fat and calories out of your holiday season

➤ Healthy menu alternatives for each major holiday

➤ Some great-tasting recipes

We all love holidays. There are family, friends, gifts, days off from work, and more delicious treats than we know what to do with. Doesn't it seem like we can eat whatever we want—with no consequences in the morning?

Unfortunately, overindulging leaves most of us feeling heavy and sluggish—and guilty. And suddenly you don't fit into your pants. The fact is, holidays are hard when it comes to making smart food choices, but there are ways to help you keep making them.

Staying on Track During the Holidays

No matter how much you expect to eat at your relatives', stick with your regular meals. Skipping breakfast and barely eating lunch will only make you more ravenous and prone to overeating at a holiday party. Just because your holiday agenda involves sitting around, telling stories, and eating doesn't mean you have to stop your regular exercise routine. The more active you are during the holiday season, the better you'll feel, and hence, you'll be more likely to feed your body in a healthy manner. What's more, exercise doesn't have to mean hitting a gym: You can do little things such as parking your car a little farther from your destination, taking the stairs instead of the elevator, or taking a quick walk around the block.

It's also important to be selective with your food choices. Survey the spread *before* you dive in and eat everything. Figure out what you really want, and then monitor everything else so you can balance it out. Don't deprive yourself! If you want a piece of cake, have some, but remember that quality is more important than quantity.

Follow these simple holiday menus to help cut your calorie and fat intakes down from one holiday to the next. Keep in mind that the nutritional information was based on real-life, *generous* holiday portions.

Easter

The spirit of Easter is all about new beginnings. It's the onset of spring; there are flowers blooming and birds returning. As the days get longer and the sunshine gets warmer, it's time to pull yourself out of those winter doldrums, peel off those big winter sweaters, and add some spring to your step...and your meal.

Your Easter meal doesn't have to be heavy and filling; it can be light and airy, like the holiday. Just revamp your traditional menu, and lose half the calories and one third of the fat; doing so will leave a little room for those wonderful chocolate bunnies.

Traditional Meal	**Nutrition Information**
Poached salmon with cucumber dill sauce	Calories: 1,532
Baked ham with pineapple, drenched in syrup	Total fat: 77 grams
Scalloped potatoes with cream and cheese	Saturated fat: 37 grams
Peas with black olives and hard-cooked eggs	Cholesterol: 366 mg
Bread and butter	Sodium: 1,381 mg
Vanilla ice cream	Dietary fibre: 9 grams
Easter candy	Protein: 69 grams

Healthier Meal	**Nutrition Information**
Poached salmon with honey mustard dill sauce	Calories: 867
Baked ham with fresh pineapple	Total fat: 27 grams
Wild rice salad with chopped dried fruit	Saturated fat: 7 grams
Asparagus with shallot vinaigrette	Cholesterol: 138 mg
Whole grain rolls	Sodium: 523 mg
Fruit sorbet	Dietary fibre: 11 grams
Chocolate fondue (small bowl of chocolate syrup or any other ice cream topping with strawberries, orange slices, and banana chunks for dipping)	Protein: 60 grams

Passover

One of the oldest and most continuously celebrated holidays, Passover commemorates the Jewish exodus from Egypt after years of suffering and slavery. It is the tradition of the Jewish people to remember their ancestors with a big meal! Well, with a few minor changes to the menu, you can still indulge in the Passover meal with all the taste, a lot less fat, and fewer calories. What's more, the extra fibre in the healthier version can help to move along that matzo meal!

Traditional Meal	**Nutrition Information**
Matzo ball soup	Calories: 2,086
Gefilte fish	Total fat: 101 grams
Brisket	Saturated fat: 35 grams
Roast chicken	Cholesterol: 734 mg
Potato kugel	Sodium: 1,768 mg
Chopped broccoli casserole	Dietary fibre: 17 grams
Tzimmis	Protein: 116 grams
Chocolate Passover cake	
Macaroons	

Healthier Meal	**Nutrition Information**
Matzo ball soup (substitute kosher olive oil for chicken fat and use seltzer instead of another liquid to get your matzo balls fluffy)	Calories: 1,575
	Total fat: 56 grams
	Saturated fat: 11 grams
Gefilte fish on green salad with lemon and olive-oil vinaigrette (use salmon instead of white fish; it's a great source of omega-3 fatty acids)	Cholesterol: 454 mg
	Sodium: 1,715 mg
	Dietary fibre: 27 grams
	Protein: 84 grams
Rock Cornish game hens stuffed with dried fruit and tomatoes	
Sweet potato and carrot tzimmis	
Artichokes stuffed with herbed matzo	
Large fruit salad	
Chocolate Passover cake	

Summer Long Weekends

Think fun-filled, pool or lakeside barbecues with your friends and family. It's about soaking up the sun and being comfortable in your body, not feeling bloated and so heavy that you'd rather cover up and stay inside. The best way to keep yourself looking good and feeling fine is to cut down on those heavy, high-fat foods and splurge on the fresh fruits and veggies that are in season. The traditional barbecue menu below has a whopping 2,099 calories and 116 grams of fat, but the healthier menu has 688 fewer calories and 40 percent of the fat—so you can say goodbye to that beer gut and greet some great abs without feeling the least bit deprived.

Traditional Meal	**Nutrition Information**
Grilled hamburgers and hot dogs on buns	Calories: 2,099
Cold fried chicken	Total fat: 116 grams
Potato salad	Saturated fat: 40 grams

Macaroni salad
Cole slaw
Potato chips
Brownies
Watermelon
Ice cream cones

Cholesterol: 381 mg
Sodium: 3,741 mg
Dietary fibre: 10 grams
Protein: 72 grams

Healthier Meal

Turkey or veggie burgers on buns
Grilled tuna, salmon, or chicken fillets
Pasta salad with tomato-basil vinaigrette
Grilled vegetables
Green or spinach salad
Baked potato chips
Low-fat brownies
Watermelon
Frozen fruit pops

Nutrition Information

Calories: 1,411
Total fat: 55 grams
Saturated fat: 10 grams
Cholesterol: 110 mg
Sodium: 1,640 mg
Dietary fibre: 14 grams
Protein: 47 grams

Thanksgiving

This holiday is supposed to be about giving thanks and feeling grateful for all the positive things in your life. But come on, we know we really focus on the delicious feast: mounds of turkey, rich gravy, starchy stuffing, cranberry sauce, four kinds of potatoes, veggies soaked in butter or oil, pumpkin pie, and going in for round two a few hours after your stomach finally settles. Then, there's all those leftovers: Thanksgiving eating goes on for days!

Keep your family traditions and indulge. If you make minor alterations in your meal, you'll feel a whole lot better in the morning—and maybe even have the energy to make it outside for a healthy walk amid the beautiful fall colours.

Traditional Meal

Roast turkey
Stuffing with onions and sausage
Yams with brown sugar
Green bean casserole
Creamed onions
Cranberry sauce
Vanilla ice cream or whipping cream
Pumpkin pie

Nutrition Information

Calories: 1,713
Total fat: 59 grams
Saturated fat: 21 grams
Cholesterol: 246 mg
Sodium: 2,904 mg
Dietary fibre: 13 grams
Protein: 79 grams

Healthier Meal

Roast turkey (no skin)
Cornbread stuffing with apples, celery,
   and cranberries
Baked yams
Mashed potatoes made with buttermilk
   and roasted garlic
Roasted vegetables (drizzled with olive oil)
Cranberry chutney
Cinnamon frozen yogurt
Pumpkin chiffon pie

Nutrition Information

Calories: 1,090
Total fat: 39 grams
Saturated fat: 9 grams
Cholesterol: 143 mg
Sodium: 1,238 mg
Dietary fibre: 18 grams
Protein: 72 grams

With Thanksgiving leftovers coming out of your ears, here are some creative ways to have seconds and thirds:

Ready-Made Menu

➤ Turkey and cranberry risotto

➤ Turkey and roasted vegetables stuffed in a pita

➤ Turkey and rice soup

Hanukkah

For the kids, the festival of lights is all about the presents, but for us adults, it seems to be all about the scrumptiously fried food (and, of course, about commemorating the Maccabean victory over Antiochus of Syria and how the Maccabees created a miracle and lit the menorah with a drop of oil that lasted for eight long nights). Today, we're a lot more nutritionally enlightened; we realize that fried foods aren't a good base for any meal, holiday or not. With a few minor adjustments to the traditional menu, you can take the healthy route, avoiding 645 calories and cutting your fat in half, and still have your potato latkes. (A Hanukkah without them would be sacrilegious, wouldn't it?)

Traditional Meal

Chicken soup
Brisket
Potato latkes
Applesauce
Green salad with vinaigrette
Jelly donuts
Hanukkah gelt

Nutrition Information

Calories: 2,038
Total fat: 105 grams
Saturated fat: 27 grams
Cholesterol: 520 mg
Sodium: 2,896 mg
Dietary fibre: 8 grams
Protein: 114 grams

147

Healthier Meal	Nutrition Information
Chicken soup	Calories: 1,393
Roast chicken breast, no skin	Total fat: 53 grams
Potato latkes	Saturated fat: 11 grams
Applesauce	Cholesterol: 322 milligrams
Green salad with vinaigrette	Sodium: 1,959 milligrams
Fresh fruit salad	Dietary fibre: 13 grams
Low-Fat Apple Streusel Pot Pie (see recipe)	Protein: 76 grams

Low-Fat Apple Streusel Pot Pie

Serves six
Calories/serving: 300

Honey	1 tsp (5 mL) ground cinnamon
Canola oil	1/2 tsp (2 mL) ground nutmeg
8 sheets phyllo dough	Lemon juice
8 cups (2 litres) sliced apple	Vanilla extract
1/2 cup (125 mL) golden raisins	Cornstarch
1/2 cup (125 mL) packed brown sugar	

Preheat oven to 350°F (180°C). In a small bowl, combine equal parts honey and canola oil. Remove 4 sheets of phyllo dough, not separating the leaves. Place on an even surface and cut 3 rounds of dough with a paring knife, following the outline of the bowl in which an individual serving will be served. Remove phyllo rounds to a nonstick sheet pan, and brush top with honey mixture. Repeat with remaining 4 sheets of phyllo dough. Place sheet pan in oven and bake for about 10 minutes. (Do not let rounds get too dark.) Remove from oven, gently flip, and brush dry side with honey mixture. Bake for 2 more minutes and remove from oven.

In a large bowl, combine apple, raisins, brown sugar, cinnamon, nutmeg, lemon juice, vanilla, and 1 Tbs (15 mL) oil. Mix well. Put in saucepan and cook over low heat, covered, for 20 minutes or until apples are soft.

Remove apples with slotted spoon and place in serving bowls. Whisk cornstarch into remaining liquid and bring to a boil. Add thickened liquid to apple mixture in bowls. Top with phyllo round and let cool before serving.

Christmas

With homemade Christmas cookies, creamy veggie dishes, and what always seems like 24 hours of nibbling, you'll be praying to open up boxes of oversized sweaters from under the tree. What better way to hide all the pounds we tend to pack on during the chilly season of decked halls and tons of parties? Well, you can still splurge on warm, rich comfort foods that are good for the soul, but if you lighten up your menu just a tad, you'll be indulging in yummy eats that are good for the arteries, too. See, it can still look a lot like Christmas with almost half the calories and 20 percent of the fat! Since the typical Christmas meal is pretty much identical to Thanksgiving fare, I've come up with an alternative festive dinner.

Traditional Meal

Oyster stew
Roast beef with gravy
Yorkshire pudding
Oven-roasted potatoes
Creamed spinach
Chocolate mousse
Christmas cookies

Nutrition Information

Calories: 1,915
Total fat: 122 grams
Saturated fat: 56 grams
Cholesterol: 717 milligrams
Sodium: 2,516 milligrams
Dietary fibre: 7 grams
Protein: 107 grams

Healthier Meal

Manhattan oyster chowder
Beef tenderloin with horseradish yogurt sauce
Potato and Caramelized Onion Gratin (see recipe)
French green beans, tied with leek bow
Chocolate angel-food cake
Vanilla frozen yogurt

Nutrition Information

Calories: 1,068
Total fat: 25 grams
Saturated fat: 6 grams
Cholesterol: 130 milligrams
Sodium: 1,620 milligrams
Dietary fibre: 10 grams
Protein: 66 grams

Potato and Caramelized Onion Gratin

Serves eight
Calories/serving: 134

1 Tbs (15 mL) canola oil

4 cups (1 L) sliced onion

1 Tbs (15 mL) balsamic vinegar

4–5 large russet potatoes

1 tsp (5 mL) mixed dried herbs

1 tsp (5 mL) table salt

3 Tbs (45 mL) chopped sun-dried tomatoes

$^3/_4$ cup (175 mL) reduced-fat chicken broth

Preheat oven to 350°F (180°C). In a large nonstick sauté pan, heat oil and add onions. Cook over medium heat, stirring frequently, for about 30 minutes or until onions are very soft and beginning to brown. Add balsamic vinegar and cook for another few minutes. Set aside.

Slice potatoes $^1/_4$-inch (6 mm) thick and put in a large bowl with herbs and salt. Do not rinse or soak potatoes in water.

In a casserole dish, sprinkle $^1/_3$ of the caramelized onions and $^1/_3$ of the sun-dried tomatoes on the bottom of the pan. Shingle $^1/_3$ of the potatoes on top; repeat this process two more times. Add chicken stock and cover with foil.

Bake for 1 hour, remove foil, and bake for 15 more minutes.

149

The holidays are about celebration and rejoicing—not overeating and gaining weight. Remember to exercise, eat something before going to a party, and eat smaller portions of the higher-fat entrées and desserts. Also, try some of my menu ideas and recipes at your next holiday gathering. You and your family will enjoy the tradition with a lot less fat and calories.

The Least You Need to Know

➤ Trim down your Easter meal by using honey mustard dill sauce on the poached salmon. Also, trade in white bread and butter for some fresh whole grain rolls.

➤ For Passover, forget brisket and go with some gourmet Rock Cornish game hens. You can also cut your saturated fat intake substantially by making your matzo ball soup with kosher olive oil instead of chicken fat. Sure, you can have potato latkes on Hannukah; just balance it out by serving roast breast of chicken instead of the brisket.

➤ At your summer long-weekend barbecues, say goodbye to higher fat burgers and hot dogs and hello to turkey and veggie burgers.

➤ Reduce the traditional Thanksgiving meal by switching from pumpkin pie to pumpkin chiffon pie—and using plain baked yams instead of mashed yams with brown sugar and butter.

➤ For Christmas, have beef tenderloin instead of roast beef with gravy—and lighten your dessert load by enjoying chocolate angel-food cake topped with vanilla frozen yogurt.

Part 3

The ABCs of Exercise

Exercise goes hand in hand with eating well. It can make you feel more energetic, enhance your mental outlook, increase your balance and coordination, help to prevent certain diseases, and make you look and feel terrific.

Part 3 provides you with the inspiration and know-how to get you moving and keep you moving. It's a crash course on becoming physically fit.

In the following chapters, I supply vital information on how to get started on an exercise program that's right for you. You'll hear the lowdown on strengthening your heart and lungs through aerobic exercise and get tips to buff your bodacious bod through proper weight-training techniques. In addition, you'll get the education you need to enter a gym with confidence and learn how to fuel your body properly —whether for casual exercise or competitive sport.

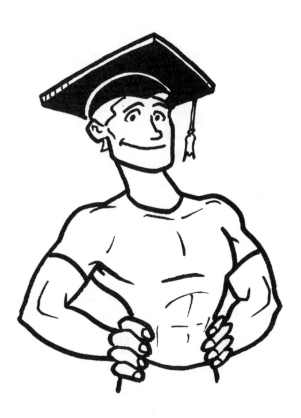

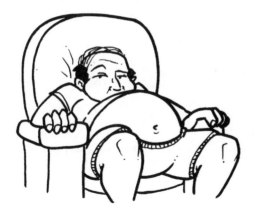

Chapter 14

Getting Physical

In This Chapter

➤ All the great stuff exercise can do for you

➤ How to properly warm up, cool down, and stretch

➤ All about aerobic exercise

➤ Getting started on a weight-training program

➤ Some great ideas for your personal workout plan

Throughout history, health professionals have promoted the notion that people who regularly exercise have better overall health, improved physical functioning, and increased longevity. Even as long ago as 400 B.C., one health professional, the Greek physician Hippocrates (known as "the father of medicine"), addressed exercise in one of his works when he wrote, "Eating alone will not keep a man well; he must also take exercise." Same thought, different century!

What is exercise, anyway? Exercise is formally defined as physical activity that is planned, structured, and repetitive and has the objective of improving or maintaining a level of physical fitness. Simply stated, *exercise whips your body into shape.* Put down the TV remote and say adios to the sofa; this chapter offers concrete guidelines and information on becoming physically active.

Of course, if you have any medical conditions, be sure to check with your physician before plunging full force into any type of exercise program.

Why Bother Exercising?

Simply put, exercise

- ➤ Makes you feel better physically
- ➤ Improves self-esteem and provides a more positive mental outlook
- ➤ Makes you look better and helps control your weight
- ➤ Increases your balance, coordination, and agility
- ➤ Helps prevent osteoporosis, cardiovascular disease, and non-insulin-dependent diabetes
- ➤ Makes you feel invigorated and more energetic
- ➤ Strengthens bones and muscle, giving you the functional strength for everyday living

Before you begin, there are some things to consider:

- ➤ **Have realistic expectations.** For all you beginners, don't expect to turn into Arnold Schwarzenegger or Cindy Crawford overnight. (The majority of us never will.) It's great to have a hero, but understand that people come in all shapes and sizes, and genetics plays a major role in your body makeup and proportion. Rule number 1: Exercise is about looking and feeling *your* best—not somebody else's best.

- ➤ **Set reasonable goals for yourself.** Plan reachable short-term goals each week that will not leave you overwhelmed or set you up for failure. An example of a reasonable goal is, "I will work out four days this week and eliminate all high-fat desserts."

  Not a reasonable goal: "I will work out two hours every day and lose 10 pounds in three weeks."

- ➤ **Work exercise conveniently into your day.** You know the story: Unless exercise sessions are planned during realistic time slots, your workouts aren't going to "work out." Take into consideration your schedule. Are you a morning person or a night owl? Some people are lucky enough to have leisurely lunch breaks and can sneak in a quick workout during their day.

- ➤ **Rise and shine.** Studies show that exercisers who work out in the morning are 50 percent more likely to stick with it. Basically, get it out of the way before the day wipes you out. If you have the capacity to endure a gruelling day at the office and then *shake, rattle, and roll* in the gym—more power to you.

- ➤ **Keep it short and sweet.** Most people have hectic lifestyles and cannot afford to dedicate hours each day to the gym. And they shouldn't! Each workout should be short and efficient. The *consistency* of regular physical activity is as important as duration and intensity. Without any of these three elements, exercise is simply not effective. Furthermore, people who get carried away usually wind up with injuries or exercise burnout.

What's an Appropriate Exercise Program?

An effective exercise program has three main parts: the before, the middle, and the after. The *before* includes a brief warm-up; the *middle*, or bulk of the workout, involves aerobic activity and weight training; and the *after* consists of a cool-down and stretch. Let's take a closer look at each.

Warming Up

A warm-up literally *warms up* the body. By increasing your internal temperature and preparing muscles for the activity ahead, a proper warm-up can help prevent injury to muscles, joints, and connective tissue. Further, a quick 5–10 minute warm-up will increase the blood flow to the primary muscle groups so that they are ready to go.

When you think of a warm-up, do you visualize yourself sitting in a straddle position on the floor, moaning loudly while reaching for your left toe (which feels like it's somewhere south of the equator)? You're not alone. But contrary to what most people think, a warm-up doesn't necessarily involve stretching exercises. Actually, 5–10 minutes of light aerobic activity (such as biking, rowing, walking, or even marching in place) is an effective warm-up. More specifically, warm up with a lighter version of the exercise you will be doing.

For instance, runners can start with a 5–10 minute brisk walk, and swimmers can warm up with a couple of easy, slow laps in the pool. Even take a 5–10 minute walk on a treadmill (and include arm circles) before hitting the weight room.

The Cardiovascular Workout: Challenge Your Heart and Lungs

What is aerobics? If you think that aerobics is just jumping around to loud music, dust off your sneaks; you're way behind the times. The term *aerobic* literally means "with air." Therefore, the exercises in which your muscles require an increased supply of air (more specifically, the *oxygen* within air) are termed aerobic. Aerobic activity is also known as cardiovascular activity (or *cardio*) because it most definitely challenges your heart and lungs. Think about this: When you jog, the large muscles of your lower body are continuously working over an extended period of time and therefore require more than their usual supply of oxygen. Because your heart and lungs are the key players in retrieving and circulating oxygen, they go into overdrive to increase oxygen delivery. Therefore, in addition to working out the large muscles, aerobic activity provides one heck of a workout for your heart and lungs.

> **Nutri-Speak**
>
> **Aerobics**, also known as *cardio*, involves exercises in which your muscles require an increased supply of oxygen.

Normally, aerobic exercise should last for 20–60 minutes, depending upon how much time you have and how fit you are. People who are fit can work longer and harder than those who are not, simply because they can handle the increased demand for oxygen. For all you beginners, don't let a few discouraging workouts get you down. Doing aerobics is like playing the piano; the more you practise, the better you get at it.

Walking briskly, biking, jogging, stair climbing, cross-country skiing, jumping rope, and, yes, aerobic dance are all examples of aerobic activity. Generally speaking, anything involving weights and machines or a fair amount of standing in place is *not* considered aerobic activity.

What can aerobics do for you? It can

➤ Burn calories and help with weight management (most people are happy to hear that one)

➤ Improve the functioning of your heart and lungs, therefore making you less likely to suffer from serious problems involving these key organs

➤ Improve your circulation

➤ Improve your sleep patterns

➤ Improve your state of mind

➤ If intense, can release endorphins, in other words, the "natural" or "runner's high"—legal in all provinces, with no nasty side effects the day after

How Long, How Much, How Hard?

The Canadian Society for Exercise Physiology set the following guidelines:

➤ **How long:** 20–60 minutes of aerobic activity per session

➤ **How much:** 3–5 times per week (if you're new to exercise, start with 3 times per week and build from there)

➤ **How hard:** Low-to-moderate intensity, that is, at 60–90 percent of your maximum heart rate

Beginners should start with a modest game plan. In fact, beginners need to shoot for 40 percent of their maximum heart rate and work up from there. As you improve, you can do more activity by going longer, harder, or more frequently. But keep in mind that you should increase the length, frequency, and intensity only one at a time. Increasing all three at once is the perfect recipe for injuries and exercise burnout.

Cooling Down

The goal of a cool-down is to gradually stop the activity, allowing your heart rate, blood pressure, and body temperature to slowly return to normal. Think about how rapidly your heart is pounding and blood is pumping following an intense bout of exercise—*not* a good time to hit the shower. In fact, stopping an intense workout abruptly is a sure way to get dizzy and feel terrible after a workout. Furthermore, cooling down properly can help prevent serious health risks for older or out-of-shape participants. Take an extra 5–10 minutes and slowly reduce the intensity of the exercise you've been doing. Your body will thank you.

Stretching

Stretching is definitely important for maintaining and increasing flexibility, which in turn makes it easier for you to move around. The best time to stretch is when your body is warm, either after you have done a light aerobic warm-up *or*, even better, at the end of your workout following a cool-down period. Proper stretching allows the muscles to relax and lengthen, and it can even help alleviate some built-up body tension. What's more, it *might* also aid in the removal of waste products, such as lactic acid, from your body. This can prevent injury and improve muscle tone.

Here are some general stretching guidelines:

➤ Always get your blood pumping and body warmed up before you stretch.

➤ Stretch *all* your major muscle groups (not just the ones you think were used).

➤ Hold each stretch for at least 15 seconds; never bounce. You can still feel a good stretch with slightly bent knees.

➤ Stretch only to the point of mild tension, not to the point of agonizing pain!

➤ Ask a qualified personal trainer to show you the correct stretching techniques; there's a lot more to it than touching your toes.

Are You Working Hard Enough?

Let's check it out. A couple of easy ways to tell whether you are working hard enough during an aerobic workout are taking your heart rate (the number of times your heart beats per minute) and the talk test.

Follow this mathematical equation to check whether you are working in your training heart rate zone (also called the target heart rate zone). Generally, your training heart rate falls between 60 and 90 percent of your *maximum heart rate* (the maximum number of times your heart can beat in 1 minute). Although this formula only provides an estimate, it's a great indication of whether you are working too hard or not hard enough:

Training heart rate formula: (220 − your age) × .60 or .90

Let's break it up and take it step by step:

Step 1   Calculate your estimated maximum heart rate (220 − your age).

Step 2   Multiply your maximum heart rate × .60 for the lower end of your target range.

Step 3   Multiply your maximum heart rate × .90 for the upper end of your target range.

157

Here's the training zone for a 35-year-old man:

(220 − 35) × .60 = 111 Lower end of target range

(220 − 35) × .90 = 167 Upper end of target range

Therefore, his target heart rate zone would range between 111 and 167 beats per minute. This means if his heart rate is lower than 111, he needs to step on the accelerator, and if it's more than 167, he needs to ease up slightly.

Test Your Heart Rate and Your Math Skills

Now that you know the math, take some time during your workout and try using the formula. Place two fingers (your pointer and middle finger) on the inside of your wrist (just to the thumb side of the large cords you feel) *or* on your neck (below and off to the side of your chin). If you can't find your pulse, ask for assistance. (Don't worry, you're alive.) Once you locate your pulse, look at the second hand of your watch or a clock and count the beats in 15 seconds; then, multiply that number by 4. That's your working heart rate. Just make sure it falls within the range you've calculated as your training zone—not slower, not faster.

Try the "Talk" Test

Here's a *much* easier way to tell whether you're working at an appropriate level. Can you comfortably carry on a conversation while exercising? If the answer is yes, you're doing fine. If you're so out of breath that you can't say, "Yippee! I'm rich," when someone announces you've won the lottery, you need to slow down. On the other hand, if you can belt out the chorus to "YMCA" by the Village People, you'd better step it up. In the final analysis, you should feel like you're working, but not to the point of a cardiac explosion.

Nutri-Speak

Hypertrophy is an increase in muscle size.

Hit the Weights and "Pump Some Iron"

Let's clear something up: Weight training is *not* the same as body building. Weight training is about improving muscle strength and muscle tone. For men, who have naturally higher levels of testosterone than women, weight training usually does mean an increase in muscle size, or *hypertrophy*. On the other hand, women tend to increase muscle tone without significantly increasing muscle size. Typically, muscle conditioning uses dumbbells and barbells (called free weights) and various types of weight machines (usually referred to by brand names such as Cybex and Nautilus).

What can weight training do for you?

➤ Stronger muscles can improve your posture and help keep your body in balance.

➤ Stronger muscles can prevent injuries.

➤ Weight training helps to tone, lift, firm, and shape your body.

➤ Stronger muscles can help you do your everyday activities such as lugging shopping bags, moving furniture, lifting kids and strollers, and so on.

➤ Weight training can help prevent osteoporosis.

➤ Weight training can help *reshape* problem areas such as your sagging arms and your butt. Unfortunately, there is no such thing as "spot reducing"—zapping off fat from specific body parts. But don't fret because the combination of a low-fat diet and aerobic activity burns *total fat* from all over your body, and chances are the fat will eventually come off your personal problem spots.

➤ Weight training can increase your lean body mass and therefore increase your metabolism.

Your Weekly Weight-Training Routine

Your weekly schedule is just as important as the exercises themselves. Set aside time for two to three muscle-conditioning workouts per week, targeting all of your major muscle groups. A major warning here is to *not* work the same muscles on consecutive days. Leave a day of rest in between to allow all those important biological changes to take place. In fact, *resting is just as important as the workout itself*. For instance, if you'd like to work all of your muscle groups on the same day, an effective schedule is a workout on Monday, Thursday, and Saturday.

Another option is doing *split routines*. In this case, you can lift more often simply because you split up the muscles being worked over the week. In other words, train your upper body one day and your lower body the next. For those truly gung-ho types, train your chest, triceps, and shoulders on one day and your legs, back, and biceps on the next. Go ahead and plug in your abdominal exercises whichever day you like. Chest and triceps are involved in pushing-type activities, and your back and biceps are involved in pulling activities; therefore, they should be worked in pairs if you want to split up the upper-body workouts. One reason people prefer a split-routine workout is that they can devote more energy to the muscles worked on a particular day.

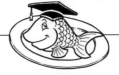

Food for Thought

When training with weights, your three sets should be 6–15 repetitions at 70–90 percent of the maximum weight you can lift.

Cardio and Weight Training: the Perfect Combination

Some people ask, Which is more important, cardio or weight work? The answer is both. You need the combination of aerobic and weight training for overall fitness. As one of my clients once said, "Weights make it hard; cardio gets rid of the lard."

Q & A

Cardio or muscle conditioning: Which comes first?

If you want to do cardio and weights on the same day, that's fine. It's also fine to alternate days, whichever you fancy. There is not, as of yet, a definite rule about which you should do first—merely follow your personal preference. Some people like to be good and sweaty before they hit the weights, whereas others prefer to get the weight training out of the way and then loosen up with cardio afterwards. The choice is yours.

Top-Five Exercise Myths

This list will help debunk the common misconceptions floating around the gym. Read on and learn the whole truth.

1. **No pain, no gain.** False! It is true that both weight training and cardiovascular exercise usually involve *some* type of minor discomfort, such as feelings of slight burning or fatigue and moderate to heavy breathing. However, pain is entirely different. If you feel pain when you work out (particularly joint pain), you're doing something wrong. Stop exercising immediately, and get checked by your physician. Pushing through agony can lead to serious trouble. If you check out okay, seek the assistance of a qualified personal trainer; something is probably wrong with your exercise program or technique.

2. **Eating lots of protein builds muscle.** We already went over this one in the protein chapter, but allow me to drive the point home. The increase in muscle size, known as hypertrophy, has nothing to do with eating excessive protein. Muscles get bigger when you overload them via weight training—*not* by eating kilos of tuna. If you are trying to gain muscle mass, you need to hit the weights *and* take in more calories coming from protein and carbohydrate. Consult a dietitian to find out how much extra you need to eat—it's probably less than you think.

3. **Weight training will give you bulky muscles.** After reading that weight training causes muscles to increase in size, it's no wonder some women are hesitant to lift weights. Fear not: Your lower testosterone levels cause increases in strength and tone without all that increase in size. Incidentally, even men have to have a genetic predisposition to getting bigger. Some guys can cut and bulk quickly, whereas others work their tails off without much visible result. Stick with a moderate weight-training program, and you'll be fine.

4. **You only burn fat working cardio at a slower pace.** This myth got a lot of play back in the 1980s, with exercise classes actually slowing down the pace to "burn more fat." In terms of weight loss, that's just not the case. The crucial factor for losing weight is *the total number of calories burned*, and it doesn't matter whether it comes from carbs, protein, or fat. For instance, a 130-pound (59 kg) woman doing a high-intensity workout (such as jogging) for 30 minutes will burn approximately 350 calories; that same woman will burn only 140 calories doing a low-intensity workout (such as walking).

   What if you're just starting out and can't sustain a fast pace for more than 5 to 10 minutes? In that case, you're certainly better off doing something at a slower pace for a longer period of time. Again, the reason is that you'll burn more total calories in the end.

5. **Sit-ups can burn fat off your waist.** Not a chance! Remember, there is no such thing as spot reducing or burning the fat off a particular body part. Fat comes off the body as a whole (through aerobic activity and proper nutrition) and, unfortunately, not always from the places you want it to come from first (as happens in the case of "the incredible shrinking bra"). You can buy every tummy-tucker and blubber-blaster on the market. Abdominal-toning exercises strengthen *only* the tissue underneath; they don't zap off that mid-section fat (contrary to what the ads might say). Look on the bright side: Below all the flab, you probably have some dynamite muscles—something to look forward to when you lose that outer layer.

How to Get Started: Your Personal Plan of Attack

Before embarking on an exercise program, figure out what type of plan will best fit your personality and schedule. Take a paper and pen and answer the following questions:

1. What type of activities do you enjoy doing?

2. What are your time restraints?

3. Are you a morning person or a night owl?

4. Do you like to work out alone or with people?

5. Do you prefer to exercise indoors or outdoors?

6. What's the weather like in your neck of the woods?

7. Do you want to travel to a facility, or does the privacy of your own home sound more appealing?

8. What is within your budget?

A Million Things You Can Do to Stay in Shape

Now that you've answered the previous questions, you should have a pretty good idea of your personal preferences and limitations. Read through the possible exercise options and determine which ones are feasible. Be sure to focus on both categories: aerobic (3–5 times per week) and muscle conditioning (2–3 times per week). Remember, nothing is set in stone; mix and match often to avoid getting bored or burnt out.

Suggestions for Aerobics

Activity	Where You Can Do It
Walking	Outside or treadmill (at gym or home)
Running	Outside or treadmill (at gym or home)
Biking	Outside or stationary bike (at gym or home)
Swimming	Outside or indoor pool
Skating	Outside or indoor rink
Stair climbing	Indoor staircase or stair-climbing machine (at gym or home)
Cross-country skiing	Outside or machine (at gym or home)
Rowing	Outside or rowing machine (at gym or home)
Aerobic classes	At the gym or home (using videos):
	Low-impact
	Multi-impact
	Step
	Spinning
	Jazz
	Tap
	Funk
	Hip-hop
	Boxing
	Tai Boe

Suggestions for Muscle Conditioning

Activity	Where You Can Do It
Body sculpting	Classes at the gym or videos at home
Circuit/interval workouts	Classes at the gym or videos at home
Weight training	Gym or home equipment
Weight machines	Gym or home equipment
Free weights	Gym or home equipment

When Formal Exercise Is Just Not Your Thing!

Not into planned sweat? Only read this far to humour yourself? Well, you're not hopeless yet; you can still cash in on some of the benefits of exercise. In fact, everyday activities can also benefit your health substantially, even if they are done *intermittently* throughout the day. For example, take the stairs instead of the elevator (you live on the 25th floor—great!), walk short distances instead of driving the car, join your kids in a game of tag, do some gardening, rake the leaves, shovel the snow—and let's not forget how physical housecleaning can be. Whatever your style, formal exercise *or* increasing plain old daily activity, make your life a healthy and active one.

Take a look at the number of calories you can burn doing everyday chores:

Overrated-Undercooked

Pushing your body more often than the experts recommend (unless you are in an athletic training program) can and usually *does* lead to injuries from over-used muscles, tendons, and joints. What's more, *varying* the intensity and duration of your exercise is important to prevent overtraining. For example, some days you should work hard and long, but on other days, make it short and sweet. Pay attention to the cues your body gives you and make exercise an enjoyable part of your life.

Activity	130-lb (59 kg) Person	183-lb (83 kg) Person
Car washing	123	171
Housecleaning	111	153
Raking leaves	96	135
Shovelling snow	150	213
Wallpapering	84	120
Weeding	96	135
Window cleaning	105	147

Whether you are 18, 50, or 70 years old, invest the time in becoming more physically active. Regular exercise will help you feel your best and keep you fit—while increasing bone strength, reducing your risk of disease, and helping to maintain an ideal body weight. Keep in mind that the perfect complement to fuelling your body properly is moving your body.

The Least You Need to Know

➤ Exercise reduces your risk for certain diseases, helps you control your weight, provides you with strength and vigour for everyday activities, and makes you feel great both mentally and physically.

➤ The important parts of an exercise program include the warm-up, aerobic activity and weight training, cool-down, and total-body stretch.

➤ Aerobic exercise (also known as cardio) is any continuous activity that requires increased oxygen and therefore challenges your heart and lungs.

➤ How long, how much, and how hard should you do aerobic activity? The experts recommend 3–5 days each week for 20–60 minute sessions at a low to moderate intensity.

➤ Don't forget about your muscles! A proper weight-training program 2–3 times per week can increase your strength, reduce the risk of osteoporosis, enhance your posture, and help reshape your body.

➤ Select activities that complement your personality and time schedule, and vary your routine often to avoid exercise burnout.

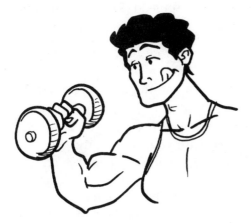

Chapter 15

The Gym Scene

In This Chapter

➤ Acquainting yourself with the health-club scene

➤ Translating gym jargon into English

➤ Popular exercise equipment for cardio and weight training

➤ Some exercises to work your muscles

Now that your body is ready and eager to go, you might want to join a local health club. Be sure to prepare yourself for more than a physical experience: When you encounter the language barrier, high-tech equipment, and people with enormous biceps, you may find that going to the gym feels like travelling to a foreign land or outer space. But don't be intimidated. The gym scene can be terrific. Where else can you have such a tremendous variety of workout choices? There's always someone available for instruction, encouragement, and motivation. Check out the health clubs in your area, but browse through the basics in this chapter before hitting the locker room.

Gym Jargon 101

Here's the gym terminology you'll need to hang with the muscle-heads; it's sure to make your conversations with the locals a bit easier:

➤ **Reps**—Short for repetitions, meaning the number of times you do an exercise. Usually 6–15 reps make a set.

➤ **Sets**—A group of repetitions. Usually you do 1–3 sets per exercise. (A man working on bicep curls might do 3 sets of 10 reps. This translates to 3 full rounds of 10 bicep curls each.)

➤ **"He's/she's ripped"**—A major compliment about someone's defined physique.

➤ **"You've really got great definition in your..."**—A tired but effective gym come-on. Gym slang for "Wow."

➤ **Being cut**—Having well-defined muscles.

➤ **Being pumped**—Experiencing a temporary increase in the size of a muscle due to increased blood flow during exercise.

➤ **"Can I work in?"**—Someone wants to use the weight machine you are using, and she is asking whether she can alternate sets with you. Because the gym is usually crowded, it's normal practice to share equipment. For example, you do a set of 8 reps, then someone else changes the weight to do a set, then you do another set, and so on. This only makes sense when you have a bunch more to go. If you have only one more set left, reply, "This is my last set"—gym slang for "Hold your horses, I'm almost done."

➤ **"How many more sets do you have here?"**—Someone is getting antsy to use the weight machine and doesn't particularly want to "work in" with you. This is a polite way of saying, "Are you planning on staying here all day? Perhaps I could order you a cappuccino."

➤ **"Can I get a spot?"**—Basically, someone is asking you to help him do an exercise with an amount of weight he is nervous about. Politely pass on this one if you don't know how to spot the exercise. Things could get ugly if a bad spot ruins his set (or worse, the weight falls on him).

➤ **Juice**—Slang for steroids. If muscle-heads are said to be "juicing," you can be sure they're not talking about juicing fresh fruits and vegetables.

A Tour of the Equipment

Health clubs are loaded with amazing machinery. With all the high-tech, futuristic equipment that's available, it can almost feel like you're on *The Jetsons*. ("Hey Jane, how long you been on that Stairmaster?") Take advantage and try them all. Don't get stuck in that "same machine day-in day-out" routine. Swap around from week to week and keep your workouts interesting and fun.

Get to Know the Aerobic Contraptions

All cardiovascular exercise equipment is designed to get large muscles pumping in a rhythmic fashion—to increase the heart rate and blood pressure and burn calories. What's the best piece of cardio equipment? The answer: any machine you'll use. Pop some great tunes in your Walkman, read the paper, or watch TV (*Canada AM, Oprah, The Young and the Restless*—whatever grabs you), and you'll be surprised how quickly the time flies when you're using exercising machines such as these:

➤ **Treadmills**—Cardiovascular equipment that presents light to moderate impact to your joints, depending on whether you're walking or running. Walking on a flat grade is a good starting place for beginning exercisers. As your fitness and confidence builds, you can fool around with increasing the incline and speed.

➤ **Stairclimbers**—Cardiovascular equipment that provides a challenging workout with some potential stress to your knees and lower back. (Listen carefully to your body.) This is a more advanced piece of machinery because of the importance of technique, and, therefore, you need a base level of stamina and strength to use this machine, even on lower levels.

➤ **Stationary bikes**—These come in two types—the upright bike (which you ride like a regular outdoors bicycle) and the recumbent bike (which you ride with your legs out in front of you while sitting in a high bucket seat that gives support to your lower back). Because these bikes involve a non-weight-bearing activity, both types provide an aerobic workout that gives your joints a break. Make sure the tension isn't too high and the seat isn't too low. If you're a beginner, ask a certified personal trainer to help you get into the proper position. When you're ready to pump up the intensity, increase your speed before increasing the tension.

➤ **Cross conditioners/cross-country ski machines**—Great aerobic exercise machines that use the entire body and burn tons of calories without any jarring impact. These are also good for quick warm-ups because they get the whole body going. There is, however, one catch: Learning the movement can be tricky for some people, and let's just say the term "poetry in motion" takes on a whole new meaning.

➤ **Rowing machines**—These are another good way to get a total-body workout (and warm-up) without any impact. Be sure to get some pointers on technique; there's an easy way and the *right* way to use them. Obviously, the right way requires more energy, concentration, and muscular effort.

> *Moo!*

Overrated-Undercooked

Do something too much, too hard, or too often, and sooner or later it'll get stale. Don't be afraid to vary your activities and change your program. In fact, I encourage it. Try inline skating instead of using the treadmill. Use weight machines instead of free weights. Attend an exercise class instead of riding the Life Cycle. Hey, if you want to dance around stark naked, go for it (just do it at home and close the window shades).

Become Familiar with the Weight-Training Tools

Weight-training equipment can be very high-tech (multimuscle machinery) or very low-tech (a pair of dumbbells and a box). Don't be fooled into thinking that something more complicated means a better workout. That's not the case at all:

➤ **Weight-training machines**—In general, machines are a good starting point for beginners. They remove a lot of the guesswork; you just move from machine to machine. (Adjust your seat, stick in a pin, and you're ready for action.) Different types of machines have either weight stacks with pulleys and cords (such as Universal and Cybex), metal rod systems (such as Cybex and Med-X), cams and chains (such as Nautilus), or air pumps (such as Kaiser). Just name the nut and bolt, and there's a machine out there that has it. Test them all and find the one you're most comfortable with.

➤ **Free weights**—These, on the other hand, require a fair amount of coordination, strength, and skill because they depend on your balance and body control. Although weight training with barbells and dumbbells (free weights) might seem significantly harder at first, some people claim free weights yield greater gains than machines. When embarking on a free-weight program, consult a certified personal trainer for tips on proper form and technique. Bad habits lead to bad injuries.

Q & A

Do I really need to buy all of the belts, wraps, and straps associated with weight training?

No. In fact, the only peripheral equipment you might need is a pair of gloves to help protect against calluses.

Learn Your Muscles and "Buff That Bod"

This section provides a quick rundown on the major muscles that conscientious gym folks tend to work out. Of course, your body is packed with hundreds more. Browse through the list, and become familiar with your muscles *and* the exercises that work them out. Be sure to ask a qualified trainer to show you the correct form and technique for each and every exercise.

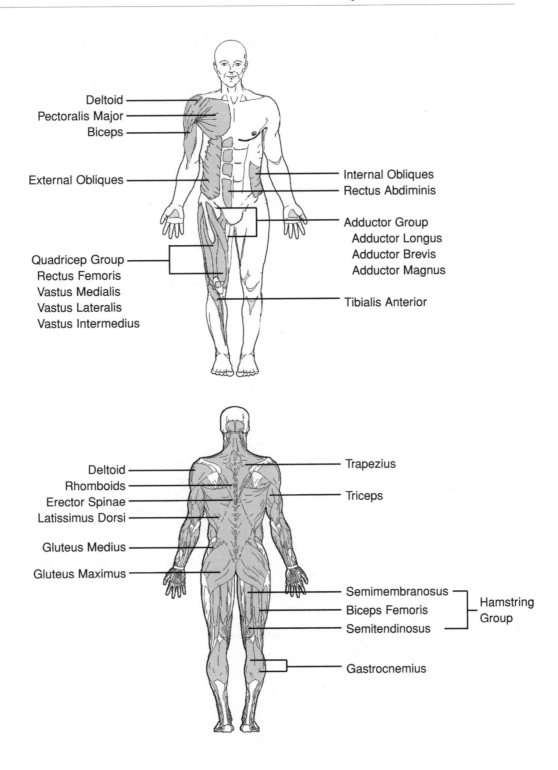

Deltoid
Pectoralis Major
Biceps

External Obliques

Internal Obliques
Rectus Abdiminis

Adductor Group
Adductor Longus
Adductor Brevis
Adductor Magnus

Quadricep Group
Rectus Femoris
Vastus Medialis
Vastus Lateralis
Vastus Intermedius

Tibialis Anterior

Deltoid
Rhomboids
Erector Spinae
Latissimus Dorsi

Trapezius

Triceps

Gluteus Medius

Gluteus Maximus

Semimembranosus
Biceps Femoris
Semitendinosus

Hamstring
Group

Gastrocnemius

Gym Slang	Muscle Group	Exercises That Work 'Em
Traps	Trapezius	Upper traps: shoulder shrugs Mid traps: reverse flys, seated rows Lower traps: dips
Delts	Deltoids	Anterior delts: frontal raises Medial delts: lateral raises Posterior delts: reverse flys
Midback	Rhomboids Mid trapezius	Seated rows Reverse flys
Pecs	Pectoralis major	Dumbbell bench press Dumbbell flys Push-ups Dips
Lats	Latissimus dorsi	Lat pulldowns Seated row pulley rowing
Lower back	Erector spinae	Lower back lifts (on a mat) Opposite arm/leg lifts on all fours
Bis	Biceps	Bicep curls Supination curls with dumbbells
Tris	Triceps	Tricep dips Tricep pulldowns
Abs	Abdominal group: *internal obliques* *external obliques* *rectus abdominis*	Stomach crunches Oblique twist Side crunches
Butt	Gluteus maximus	Leg press/squats Hip extension (with a low pulley cable)
Outer hips	Abductor group: *gluteus medius* *gluteus minimus*	Abductor machine Side leg lifts (with a low pulley cable)
Inner thighs	Adductor group: *adductor longus* *adductor brevis* *adductor magnus*	Adductor machine Inward leg lifts (with a low pulley cable)
Quads	Quadricep group: *rectus femoris* *vastus medialis* *vastus lateralis* *vastus intermedius*	Leg press Leg extension (also includes squats, lunges, and step-ups with dumbbells)
Hams	Hamstring group: *biceps femoris* *semitendinosus* *semimembranosus*	Leg press Leg curl

Gym Slang	Muscle Group	Exercises That Work 'Em
Calves	Gastrocnemius Soleus	Heel raises straight leg Toe presses straight leg Heel raises bent leg Toe presses bent leg
Shins	Tibialis anterior	Toe taps Toe backs

Do You Need a Personal Trainer?

Some people decide to hire a personal trainer to help them get into shape. Although some exercisers require a personal trainer only for a single "show you the ropes" session, others enjoy continual weekly appointments that help keep them focused and motivated. If you decide to work with a trainer, be selective about whom you hire because the unfortunate truth is that *anyone* can call herself or himself a personal trainer.

Consider hiring a personal trainer if you fall into any of the following categories:

➤ You are completely out of shape and haven't the slightest idea how to begin an exercise program. A trainer can acquaint you with all of the up-to-date exercise techniques and aerobic and weight machinery available.

➤ You are in a *huge* exercise rut and have been doing the same old routine for as long as you can remember. A trainer can show you variations on your day-to-day workout and make exercising more efficient and effective.

➤ You just plain lack the oomph to exercise on your own. A trainer can push and motivate you to whip your butt into shape.

➤ You want to take your workouts to a higher level; you'd like to try a half marathon or triathlon and need an expert to map out a sound training program.

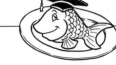

Food for Thought

Studies report that arthritis sufferers who regularly participate in strength training and stretching programs can greatly improve their balance, speed, and ability to walk, as well as reduce joint pain and fatigue. Check it out with your doctor first to be sure there's not too much joint inflammation.

Find out what local programs are offered by your provincial arthritis society. Call 1–800–321–1433 or visit the Arthritis Canada Web site at www.arthritis.ca for more information about exercise.

Seek out somebody with a bachelor of science degree (B.Sc.) (or better yet, a masters degree) in exercise physiology, physical education, or kinesiology. You can also look for a *certified* fitness trainer, which means he or she has studied for and passed a comprehensive training exam. Some of the most reputable organizations that provide certifications, include

➤ PFLC (Professional Fitness and Lifestyle Consultant) certificate

➤ CSEP (Canadian Society for Exercise Physiology)

➤ CPTN (Canadian Personal Trainers' Network)

➤ CATA (Canadian Athletic Therapists' Association)

➤ Your provincial kinesiology association

Other comprehensive fitness certification programs are offered at various universities. Most offer a variety of certification programs (aerobic instructor, yoga, and so on). Make sure your trainer is specifically certified in *personal training* or *fitness instruction* and that his or her certification is up to date.

Interview a trainer to be sure you feel comfortable with his or her workout philosophy, personality, and fee scale before you actually set up an appointment for training. Rates vary tremendously, anywhere from $25 to $85 per workout. They can even cost more than $100 if you're looking for a "trainer to the stars."

The Least You Need to Know

➤ Joining a local gym can be invaluable to your pursuit of a fit, healthy body. Take advantage of the variety of workout choices and the qualified staff of trainers who can instruct, motivate, and encourage you.

➤ Some of the popular aerobic equipment commonly found in most gyms includes treadmills, bikes, stairclimbers, rowing machines, and cross-country ski machines. Weight-training equipment generally involves either multipurpose machinery (Cybex, Nautilus) or free weights (barbells and dumbbells).

➤ Because bad form and technique can lead to injuries, seek the assistance of a certified personal trainer before embarking on any type of program.

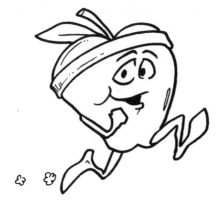

Chapter 16

Sports Nutrition

In This Chapter

➤ Superfuelling your body with carbohydrates

➤ Where to find high-carbohydrate foods

➤ Increased protein requirements for athletes

➤ What to eat before, during, and after exercise

If you've read this far, you know the basics of sports nutrition. Contrary to what some people think, there isn't any magic ingredient that helps optimize exercise and training (such as instant-muscle shake concoctions or endurance potions). In fact, the same healthy eating guidelines you read about in the earlier chapters also apply to competitive sport and casual exercise. You know the story: high on the carbs, low on the fat, and moderate in the amount of protein. You might just need to increase the total number of calories you take in to compensate for the amount you're now burning with all that activity.

Just because you're familiar with *Canada's Food Guide to Healthy Eating*, don't stop there: This chapter clues you in to a lot more sport-specific nutrition. Stay tuned for a mouthful of information that can help enhance your athletic performance and secure that competitive edge.

Carbohydrates: Fuel of Choice

Carbohydrate is the high-octane fuel for exercise and should provide at least 55 percent of an athlete's total daily calories. Let's get a bit more technical: You should consume approximately 3.0–4.5 grams of carbohydrate per pound of body weight (for all you metric buffs, that's 6.6–9.9 g/kg). Where do you fit in? If your sport is pretty low-key—not a lot of nonstop running around—your intake should be at the lower level of this range. On the other hand, if you participate in a super-endurance sport that involves hours of heavy training each day, your intake should be up near the higher level of this range.

What does this mean, anyway?

Math time—grab a calculator. Take your weight in pounds (kg) and multiply it by 3.0 grams (6.6 g) if you participate in moderate intensity sports and by 4.5 grams (9.9 g) in you participate in strenuous endurance training. Obviously, these are two extremes; most exercisers and athletes fall in the middle. In fact, give yourself a range; play around and see where your body feels most vigorous.

For example: Here's the carbohydrate requirement for a 150-pound (68 kg) *elite* runner training several hours each day (note that the metric totals are slightly different due to rounding):

150 pounds × 4.5 grams = 675 grams of carbohydrate

(68 kilograms × 9.9 g = 673 grams of carbohydrate)

Because 1 gram of carbohydrate = 4 calories, we can now convert 675 (673) carb grams into carb calories by using the following equations:

675 × 4 = 2,700 carbohydrate calories

(673 × 4 = 2,692 carbohydrate calories)

Now let's look at a typical 150-pound (68 kg) health-club member, working out at a moderate intensity (approximately 45 minutes), 4–5 days a week:

150 pounds × 3.0 grams = 450 grams of carbohydrate

(68 kilograms × 6.6 grams = 449 grams of carbohydrate)

Now convert into carb calories:

450 × 4 = 1,800 carbohydrate calories

(449 × 4 = 1,796 carbohydrate calories)

As you can see, a more intense endurance exercise program will demand more carbohydrate. But keep in mind that the proportion of carbs, protein, and fat pretty much remains the same as that described in the previous chapters (about 55% carbs, 15% protein, and less than 30% fat) because in the end, you're taking in more of everything.

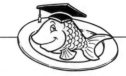

Food for Thought

Without question, carbohydrate-rich foods are the fuel of choice for athletes. Carbs provide the muscles with ongoing energy in the form of glucose and help maintain prolonged endurance and optimal performance.

Develop Your Own High-Carb Diet

Need to boost your carbs? Take a look at the variety of foods you can choose from, and watch how fast you can rack up the grams.

The Starchy Carbs

Generally speaking, breads, grains, and other starchy foods contain approximately 15 grams (give or take a few) of carbohydrate per serving (1 slice bread, $^1/_2$ cup/125 mL pasta, 1 serving of cereal). These foods receive top billing for endurance athletes simply because it's easy to eat multiple servings in one sitting. For instance, a pasta entrée can easily total five grain food servings, and because one pasta serving contains about 20 grams of carb, five servings supplies a whopping 100 grams of carbohydrate. Clearly, this is the reason why marathon runners pack in the pasta before they run long distances.

Fruits

Next up are fruits, which also provide about the same amount—15 grams—of carbohydrate per serving (1 medium fresh fruit, 1 cup/250 mL berries or chopped melon, $^1/_2$ cup/125 mL fruit juice). Why are they second? Athletes looking to load up on carbs can eat 10+ servings of grain more comfortably than 10+ servings of fruit. Remember, fruit has a lot of fibre and tends to fill you up more quickly. (You might be "bursting with fruit flavour" in more ways than one!) Incorporate a lot of fresh fruit into your regimen, but don't skimp on the grains and rely solely on fruit. You'll probably get a stomachache and more than likely *toot* your way to the finish line.

Milk Products

Milk products contain about 12 grams of carbohydrate per serving (1 cup/250 mL milk or yogurt) and can certainly boost your total carbs, together with the starchy foods, fruits, and vegetables. What's more, milk pumps you with calcium, a key ingredient for maintaining strong, athletic bones.

Vegetables

Vegetables provide approximately 5 grams of carbohydrate per serving (1 cup/250 mL raw or $^1/_2$ cup/125 mL cooked) and are certainly packed with vitamins and minerals. Although veggies alone can't supply enough concentrated carbohydrate for increased requirements, they can sure spruce up your meals and add tremendous amounts of nutrition to your table.

Common High-Carb Foods	Carbohydrate Grams
Medium bagel	45
2 slices whole-wheat bread	23
1 cup (250 mL) oatmeal	25
1 cup (250 mL) cereal (ready to eat)	16
10 crackers	21
1 cup (250 mL) cooked pasta	40
1 cup (250 mL) cooked rice	35
Granola bar	16
1 ounce (30 g) pretzels	21
2 fig cookies	23
1 PowerBar	42
1 banana	27
Glass of orange juice (8 oz/250 mL)	26
1 medium baked potato	51
$^1/_2$ cup (125 mL) peas	11
$^1/_2$ cup (125 mL) corn	17
1 cup (250 mL) low-fat milk	12
$^3/_4$ cup (175 mL) low-fat yogurt (plain)	13
$^3/_4$ cup (175 mL) low-fat yogurt (fruit)	34
1 cup (250 mL) brown beans in tomato sauce	51

Note that the carbohydrate grams are calculated for serving sizes that are *commonly eaten*, not the standard *single* serving sizes frequently listed throughout this book and in Canada's Food Guide.

Food for Thought

You can take in more than 100 grams of carbohydrate by eating 4 bananas, or $2^1/_2$ power bars, or 3 cups (750 mL) of pasta, or 6 medium pancakes, or $2^1/_2$ cups (625 mL) of Raisin Bran cereal, or 2 medium baked potatoes, or 8 fig cookies and a glass of milk.

All About Muscle Glycogen

Muscle glycogen is stored carbohydrate in your muscle. Imagine this: After you eat and digest a meal, the amount of carbohydrate that you need immediately will get used as fuel, but the rest (up to a point) will be stored in your muscles for *future* fuel. Athletes in ultra-endurance sports such as soccer, basketball, hockey, triathlons, and distance running rely on high-octane muscle fuel for energy. In fact, between the gruelling practice sessions and vigorous competitions, serious endurance athletes are *constantly* depleting and restoring their muscle glycogen stores, so they require much more carbohydrate-rich food than athletes involved in activities that are less aerobic (golf, archery, and martial arts).

Just because you don't compete in an ultra-endurance sport doesn't mean you can fumble in the carb department. Think about all of the laborious *practice* sessions that wrestlers, divers, or short-distance swimmers put in during the week. Bear in mind that it's not just the actual competition that matters, but the intensity of your training as well.

What happens if you don't replenish your muscle-glycogen stores? Simple: If you run out of glycogen, you run out of energy. The amount of muscle fuel you have determines how long you can exercise. Just as a car needs a full tank of gas for a long trip, an endurance athlete requires sufficient "muscle gasoline" to sustain the pace and go the distance. Always tired or run down? Obviously, a vigorous training schedule alone is enough to make you feel that way. You might also want to look into your carbohydrate consumption. Keep a food log and do the math; there could be an easy solution to your problem.

What's Carbo-Loading About?

Carbo-loading is just that—loading your body with large amounts of carbohydrate before an event. Athletes who compete in *extreme* endurance events such as marathons and triathlons can actually manipulate their exercise and eating schedule to help increase the amount of muscle glycogen stored in their body. You see, during intense, prolonged aerobic activity, your muscle-glycogen stores can become severely depleted and cause you to slow down, or worse, drop out. Picture that car running out of gas: *putt, putt, pshh*. By supersaturating the muscles with carbohydrate beforehand, an athlete can ensure that her stores are maximally loaded.

Nutri-Speak

Muscle glycogen is the stored carbohydrate within the muscles. Athletes can use these "energy stores" during prolonged exercise.

Overrated-Undercooked

For you non-athletes who decided to browse through this chapter, remember that not everyone is a candidate for overdosing on carbs. Active people might continuously burn loads of carbohydrate calories, but your muscles can store only a certain amount of carbohydrate. If you're not using what is already there, you'll just end up putting on weight (as fat).

Start this program six days before your event:

Exercise	Schedule	% of Carbs in Daily Diet
Day 1	90 minutes	50
Day 2	40 minutes	50
Day 3	40 minutes	50
Day 4	20 minutes	70
Day 5	20 minutes	70
Day 6	Rest	70
Day 7	Get out there and master your event!	

Personal Protein Requirements

Remember back in the old days when athletes would eat a huge slab of steak with some scrambled eggs for breakfast and then head off to play ball? *Protein power, gotta keep up that strength.* Boy, have things changed.

It's true that athletes do need more protein than sedentary people, but because most people already take in far more protein than the RNI, chances are you're doing fine. (You're okay unless you're one of those "carb-o-holics" who live on the "cereal-bagel-pasta" program, or you're trying so hard to carbo-load that you forget the other key ingredients for optimal performance.)

Athletes do need protein for that competitive edge. You learned the vital roles of protein in Chapter 3, "The Profile on Protein," but let's get sport specific for a minute. Protein is essential for building and maintaining muscle tissue, as well as for repairing the muscle damage you sustain during hard workouts. Remember, dietary protein does *not* automatically build bigger muscles: *You* build bigger muscles through regular exercise and training. Dietary protein simply allows all your hard work to pay off. Go ahead and take the credit; it had nothing to do with all the protein powder you gobbled down each day.

Following are the recommended daily intakes for protein. You'll see that athletes do have greater requirements than the RNIs for the general population (as was also described in Chapter 3). But keep in mind that your total proportion should still be high in carbs, moderate in protein, and low in fat. This is because you're taking in more of everything (especially carbohydrate).

Find your exercise category, and then multiply your weight (in pounds or kilograms) by the number of grams to the right. After you do the math and learn your personal daily requirements, keep a food log for a week and tally up your daily protein totals by checking your foods in the chart located in Chapter 3.

Exercise Category	Recommended Daily Protein (grams per pound)	Recommended Daily Protein (grams per kilogram)
Sedentary people	0.36	0.8
Moderate exercisers	0.36–0.5	0.8–1.1
Endurance athletes	0.5–0.8	1.1–1.8
Strength athletes	0.6–0.8	1.3–1.8
Growing teenage athletes	0.6–0.9	1.3–2.0

Here are some examples:

➤ A 200-pound (91 kg) bodybuilder needs between 120 and 160 grams of protein daily.

➤ A 150-pound (68 kg) triathlete needs 75 to 120 grams of protein daily.

➤ A 14-year-old elite gymnast weighing 92 pounds (42 kg) needs 55 to 83 grams of protein daily.

➤ A casual 120-pound (54 kg) health-club member needs 43 to 60 grams of protein daily.

Notice that even though the growing gymnast might require more protein per pound than the bodybuilder, bodybuilders usually weigh a lot more and therefore tend to have greater protein requirements.

Food Before, During, and After Exercise

This section investigates favourable food choices for your pre-event meal, *and* the recovery foods needed to help your body bounce back after an intense workout. It also lays out the guidelines for fuelling your system throughout prolonged periods of exercise.

Pre-Event Meals

Let me begin by saying that the most outstanding meal before your sporting event won't make up for a week's worth of potato chips, french fries, and cookies! With that in mind, study the following guidelines and help make your pre-event meal a "winning beginning":

➤ Have your large meal (approximately 600–700 calories) at *least* 3–4 hours prior to an event. This will provide adequate time for your food to be digested. (You don't want to feel heavy or nauseated, or have indigestion, while you're running around on the field.)

➤ Stick with carbohydrate-rich foods and moderate amounts of lean protein. The carbs are both loaded with energy and easy to digest. Avoid eating a lot of high-fat foods; they take much longer to leave your stomach, and you don't want food bouncing along on the ride.

➤ Avoid super high-fibre foods that can cause annoying stomach gurgles or send you running to the bathroom right before kickoff.

➤ Also limit gas-producing foods such as beans, Brussels sprouts, grapes, broccoli, and anything else you think might give you stomach pains.

➤ Liquid meals are also fine, especially if you have "pre-game jitters" and can't stomach solid food. Some athletes prefer liquid supplements because they don't leave you feeling as full as a large meal of equal calories does. In fact, they leave your stomach more quickly than solid food.

➤ Also, lay off the salt. As you read in Chapter 5, "Don't As-*salt* Your Body," some people tend to retain a lot of fluid, which can lead to puffiness and discomfort.

➤ Never eat something completely new before an important competition. *Always* try the food during training and see how it settles in your stomach.

➤ Reduce the size of your food intake as you approach the time of your event. For example, 3–4 hours before, you can have a large meal (approximately 600–700 calories); 2–3 hours before, you can have a smaller meal (approximately 400–500 calories); and less than 2 hours before, you can grab some lighter snacks (cereal bars, fruit, flavoured rice cakes, unsweetened fruit juice, yogurt, and so on).

What time is your sporting event? Which meal will be your pre-event send-off: breakfast, lunch, or dinner? Check out the sample menus to get an idea of the foods you should choose. Keep in mind that you should *always* have a well-balanced, carbo-rich meal the night before, especially because on game day, you might get fidgety and lose your appetite.

Q & A

Are there really such things as "winning meals" or "winning foods" that can enhance your performance?

Yes! You see, if a particular food or meal makes you feel *mentally* at your best, then for you, that *is* a winning meal.

Ready-Made Menu

Breakfast

(For a late morning or an early afternoon competition)
Bowl of cereal with low-fat milk
Sliced bananas
Bagel with jam
Glass of orange juice

Lunch

(For a late afternoon or evening competition)
Turkey sandwich on whole-wheat bread
Salad with light dressing
Vanilla-flavoured yogurt with sliced strawberries
Glass of 1% milk or unsweetened orange juice

Dinner

(For an early morning or "any time the next day" competition)
Grilled chicken
Pasta with tomato sauce
Broccoli and carrots
Fruit salad
2 fig bars
Glass of 1% milk

Fuelling Your Body During Prolonged Endurance Activity

Some sports events are so lengthy that you need to eat *during* the event to supply your body with glucose when your glycogen stores are running low. For example, marathon runners (and other endurance athletes such as soccer players) need to take in about 30–60 grams of carbohydrate per hour, which translates into a mere (but important) 120–240 calories. Although it's a minuscule amount, these calories should be spread out over each hour. The simplest method is to drink one of the popular sports drinks during the event. You can "hydrate" and "*carbo*-hydrate" your body at the same time.

Recovery Foods

Now for the last piece of the puzzle—the aftermath nourishment. First, understand that recovery foods are not just for recovering after a competition or game. They're equally important after practice as well. In fact, athletes who regularly train long and hard should replace emptied glycogen stores, fluids, and potassium lost through sweat on a daily basis. What's more, carbohydrate and fluid repletion should begin immediately, within 15–30 minutes of exercising, to promote a quick recovery. Sound unrealistic? Just grab a fruit juice or sports drink while you make your congratulatory high-fives. When you can focus on a real meal, enjoy whatever you fancy; just make sure to include the following essentials:

➤ Plenty of fluids: water, fruit juice, sports drinks, soups, and watery fruits and veggies (watermelon, grapes, oranges, tomatoes, lettuce, and cucumbers).

➤ A lot of carbohydrate-rich foods: pasta, potatoes, rice, breads, fruits, yogurts, and so on.

➤ Moderate amounts of lean protein.

➤ Potassium-rich foods such as potatoes, bananas, oranges, orange juice, dried apricots, and raisins.

➤ Do not attempt to replenish lost sodium by smothering your food in salt or by popping dangerous salt tablets. A typical meal, moderately salted, supplies enough sodium to replace the amount lost through sweat. And if you use sports drinks, they also help replenish lost salt.

As you have read, food can make or break your athletic performance. While training hard is incredibly important, you'll never reach your full potential without paying close attention to making balanced food choices. Remember to focus on the right mix of carbohydrate and protein, and preplan your pre-event and recovery meals. You'll feel great, and you'll have more energy and strength for a winning performance.

The Least You Need to Know

➤ Athletes need carbohydrate-rich foods such as grains, pasta, rice, fruits, and veggies. Carbohydrates supply energy for both gruelling practice sessions and competitions.

➤ Athletes have greater daily protein requirements than sedentary people—roughly 0.5–0.8 grams per pound of body weight (1.1–1.8 g/kg). However, these requirements are easily met because an athlete's greater caloric intake usually provides proportionately more protein.

➤ Your pre-event meal is important, and you need to reduce your food intake as you get close to your event.

➤ During prolonged exercise, your body requires about 30–60 grams of carbohydrate per hour, which translates into 120–240 calories.

➤ Help your body recover after a gruelling workout with plenty of fluids, carbohydrate, and potassium-rich foods.

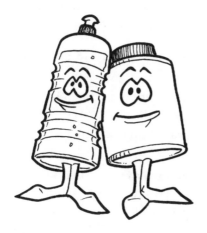

Chapter 17

Going That Extra Mile: Fluids and Supplements

In This Chapter

➤ All about fluids and proper hydration

➤ The nutritional content of popular sports bars

➤ The lowdown on so-called exercise enhancers

Grab your water bottle and guzzle down lots of water. Exercise places such great demands on your body that proper fluid replacement—that is, hydration—before, during, and after intense physical activity is critical. Think about the numerous tasks that depend on fluid: Your *blood* needs fluid to transfer oxygen to working muscles, your *urine* needs fluid to funnel out metabolic waste products, and your *temperature regulating system* needs fluid to dissipate heat through sweat.

You might feel wet, grimy, and sticky on the outside, but sweating helps keep you at a comfortable working temperature. You need to replace the fluids lost through sweat *continuously* so that you can prevent your body from becoming dehydrated and overheated. What's more, athletes who fail to keep up with their water requirements not only jeopardize performance, but also place themselves at risk for injury and serious heat conditions (heat cramps, heat exhaustion, and heat stroke).

Guidelines for Proper Hydration

Unfortunately for athletes, the thirst mechanism is an unreliable indicator for the body's hydration status. First, by the time you feel thirsty, you're already dehydrated; second, the amount of fluid that quenches your thirst might not be enough to quench your body. To ensure adequate hydration, you need to follow a drinking schedule. Here's what's recommended:

Nutri-Speak

Alcohol and caffeinated coffee and tea might cause dehydration because they act as diuretics–substances that cause you to urinate and therefore to lose water.

➤ 2 cups (500 mL) 2 hours prior to exercise

➤ 1–2 cups (250–500 mL) 15–30 minutes *before* exercise

➤ $^2/_3$–1$^1/_3$ cup (150–325 mL) every 15 minutes *during* exercise

➤ 2 cups (500 mL) for every pound (0.5 kg) lost *after* exercise

Here are two quick ways to tell whether you are properly hydrated:

➤ **Weigh in before and after.** Hop on the scale before and after you exercise. For each pound (0.5 kg) of fluid lost (it's just fluid, *not* fat), drink 2 cups (500 mL) of water (or other fluid) to properly *rehydrate* your body (you need to drink 1.1 L of fluid to replace 1 kg of fluid lost). You don't have to gulp it all down at once; just make sure you're fully hydrated by the next day. For example, a soccer player weighs 165 pounds (75 kg) before the game and 162 pounds (73.6 kg) after the game. Therefore, he must drink 6 cups (1.5 litres) of water to replace the 3 pounds (1.4 kg) of lost fluid.

➤ **Check your urine.** The colour of your urine is also a good indicator of hydration. If your urine is voluminous and clear to pale yellow, you're doing just fine. On the other hand, if your urine is dark and concentrated, keep chugging that fluid. The exception to this rule is if you take a multivitamin and mineral—the B-vitamins make your urine a fluorescent yellow (I'm sure you've already noticed!). In this case, judge your hydration status by quantity of urine, not colour.

Sports Drinks Versus Water

Plain old H_2O is cheap, effective, and just fine for most athletes, but in some instances you'll benefit from the added carbohydrate in a sports drink (Gatorade, PowerAde, AllSport, Cytomax, and so on). Go for the loaded stuff when continuous exercise lasts longer than 60 minutes or when you're exercising in extremely hot or humid weather. You see, water can provide straight hydration, but sports drinks can also provide some electrolytes (sodium, potassium, chloride) and carbohydrate—just enough to keep you moving and feeling good during those exceptionally long or hot workouts.

The Bar Exam

Sports bars can be convenient and advantageous for athletes trying to increase their intake of calories, carbohydrates, and protein (depending upon the brand). Here's the nutritional profile on a variety of popular bars on the market. Because most brands come in an assortment of flavours, the information for a specific one might vary slightly from that shown in the list. Also, be sure to sample several brands before you formulate any taste opinion; they vary tremendously!

Cliff Bar
Calories: 250
Fat: 4 g
Sodium: 139 mg
Carbs: 45 g
Protein: 10 g

Sport-Rx
Calories: 337
Fat: 2.8 g
Sodium: 170 mg
Carbs: 48 g
Protein: 30 g

MET Rx
Calories: 340
Fat: 4 g
Sodium: 135 mg
Carbs: 50 g
Protein: 27 g

Bio-X
Calories: 320
Fat: 4.5 g
Sodium: 220 mg
Carbs: 43 g
Protein: 27 g

PromaxBar
Calories: 290
Fat: 6 g
Sodium: 160 mg
Carbs: 39 g
Protein: 20 g

Steel Bar
Calories: 380
Fat: 5 g
Sodium: 35 mg
Carbs: 68 g
Protein: 16 g

Energy Blast
Calories: 225
Fat: 4 g
Sodium: 160 mg
Carbs: 39 g
Protein: 8 g

Balance Bar
Calories: 192
Fat: 6 g
Sodium: 180 mg
Carbs: 23 g
Protein: 14 g

Pure Protein
Calories: 280
Fat: 6 g
Sodium: 80 mg
Carbs: 9 g
Protein: 33 g

Power Bar Harvest
Calories: 222
Fat: 4 g
Sodium: 100 mg
Carbs: 41 g
Protein: 8.3 g

Myoplex Plus
Calories: 344
Fat: 8.4 g
Sodium: 229 mg
Carbs: 44 g
Protein: 24 g

PR Ironman
Calories: 220
Fat: 7 g
Sodium: 200 mg
Carbs: 24 g
Protein: 15 g

Genisoy
Calories: 220
Fat: 3.5 g
Sodium: 150 mg
Carbs: 35 g
Protein: 14 g

SoyOne
Calories: 242
Fat: 6 g
Sodium: 85 mg
Carbs: 29 g
Protein: 18 g

What's the Story on Ergogenic Aids?

Flip through any muscle mag and you'll read plenty of claims regarding substances that can help enhance performance. The word *ergogenic* literally means "work producing," and, unfortunately, there are always far-fetched advertisements selling nutritional pills and potions claiming to beef up performance. To date, there are only a few scientifically proven ergogenic aids, including a proper diet, carbo-loading, a well-trained body, a determined soul, and the right equipment.

Here's what you need to know about ergogenic aids in food and supplement form.

Thumbs Up

To date, the following substances have been shown to improve athletic performance. Of course, this doesn't mean you should start popping pills. In fact, scientists are constantly coming up with new information (good and bad), so stay on top of the current research if you decide to go with one of these supplements. Naturally, *always* check with your dietitian or physician before embarking on anything new:

➤ **Antioxidants** (Vitamins C, E, beta-carotene, and selenium)

Claim: Protects against tissue damage from free-radical formation induced by exercise.

Fact: Antioxidants might protect against tissue damage following prolonged endurance exercise, but they don't improve performance while you are actually exercising. Although the quantities of antioxidants found in food are somewhat small, they do help stop the production and spread of harmful substances in the body. Compared to the other antioxidants, the studies point to vitamin E as an aid in preventing muscle soreness.

➤ **Caffeine**

Claim: Improves endurance.

Fact: Consuming 1.5–3 milligrams of caffeine per pound of body weight (3–6 mg/kg) 1 hour before exercise improves endurance performance without raising urinary caffeine levels above those in the standards set by the International Olympic Committee. Side effects of high caffeine consumption include anxiety, stomach upset, nausea, muscle tremors, palpitations, and headache. Using caffeine in this way is not a good idea if your body is sensitive to it.

➤ **Creatine monohydrate**

Claim: Increases the creatine phosphate content in muscles, improves high-power performance, and increases muscle mass.

Fact: Research has suggested that consuming 20 grams of creatine per day (5 g four times daily) for five days might improve performance in brief, maximal exercise lasting less than 30 seconds (e.g., sprinting, weight lifting). After this loading dose, a maintenance dose of 5 grams per day should suffice. However, not all studies have found that creatine improves strength, sprint performance, or lean muscle mass, so it might not improve all high-power activities. Scientists don't yet know why it's effective in some people and not in others. Nor do we know what taking the stuff over the long term can do to your health. According to current knowledge, taking creatine for a few months appears to be safe. Do not use this supplement if you have kidney problems.

➤ **Sodium bicarbonate**

Claim: Counteracts the buildup of lactic acid in the blood and improves anaerobic ("without oxygen") performance during high-intensity exercise, for example, sprinting and weight lifting, during which your body burns sugar for energy.

Fact: Several studies conducted on sprinters have supported improved anaerobic performance with bicarbonate supplementation. Taking 0.15 grams per pound of body weight (0.3 g/kg) of sodium bicarbonate with water over a 2- to 3-hour period might improve sprinting time by several seconds. However, as many as half of those individuals using sodium bicarbonate experienced urgent diarrhea 30 minutes after loading with this supplement. Obviously, you should be cautious if you use sodium bicarbonate.

➤ **Phosphates**

Claim: Improves endurance.

Fact: Phosphate-loading might increase VO2 max (the maximum amount of oxygen your body can take in and use during exercise, that is, the number of millilitres of oxygen per kilogram of body weight per minute) and decrease the rise of lactic acid during intense exercise. The dose is 1 gram of sodium phosphate four times a day for three days. More research on phosphate-loading is needed.

Thumbs Down

The following so-called exercise enhancers are not backed up by any solid scientific data. Needless to say, they won't improve your athletic performance:

➤ **Amino acids** (arginine, ornithine, and lysine)

Claim: Stimulates the release of human growth hormone, promotes muscle growth, and increases strength.

Fact: These oral amino-acid supplements do not increase growth-hormone levels or muscle mass. Studies have shown that weight lifting and endurance sports alone (without taking in extra amino acids) both significantly increase growth-hormone levels.

➤ **Bee pollen**

Claim: Improves physical performance.

Fact: Bee pollen has no magical quality. It is composed of the same nutrients found naturally in food: starch, sugars, protein, and a small amount of fat. For some people, taking this substance results in an allergic reaction. Anyone with kidney disease or a predisposition to gout should avoid it.

➤ **Brewer's yeast**

Claim: Improves athletic performance (among many other claims).

Fact: Although brewer's yeast is a great source of certain B-vitamins, there's no evidence that it enhances exercise performance.

➤ **Boron**

Claim: Increases serum testosterone levels to enhance muscle growth and strength.

Fact: These claims were based on an American study that showed that boron supplementation increased the levels of testosterone in postmenopausal women. Normal male testosterone is about 10 times that of postmenopausal women, and, in the case of the male population, boron has no effect on testosterone levels, lean body mass, or strength in strength-trained athletes.

➤ **Carnitine**

Claim: Causes an increase in the metabolism of fat, thus promoting a decline in total body fat.

Fact: Carnitine facilitates the transfer of fatty acids into the mitochondria (the location in each cell where metabolism takes place) to be used for energy. There is no evidence that carnitine supplementation promotes increased use of fatty acids during exercise or a decrease in body fat.

➤ **Choline**

Claim: Increases strength and causes a decrease in body fat.

Fact: There is no evidence that choline supplementation increases strength and reduces body fat.

➤ **Chromium picolinate**

Claim: Increases muscle mass, decreases body fat, and promotes weight loss.

Fact: Nutrition Research Centers in Beltsville, Maryland, and Grand Forks, North Dakota, found that a daily supplement of chromium picolinate coupled with weight training for 8–12 weeks did *not* increase strength or muscle mass or decrease body fat. But taking extra chromium might improve endurance performance in athletes who are deficient in this mineral. Chromium works with the hormone insulin to regulate blood glucose (energy) levels. Both heavy training and carbo-loading with refined starches cause chromium loss. Your best bet is to eat more chromium-rich foods such as apples (with the skin), green peas, mushrooms, brewer's yeast, wheat germ, and cheese. If you decide to supplement, 200 micrograms is the recommended daily dose.

➤ **Coenzyme Q10**

Claim: Coenzyme Q10 is used by enzymes that generate energy molecules called ATPs to increase vigour, energy, and stamina.

Fact: There is no dietary requirement for this substance. According to current literature, supplementation with coenzyme Q10 does *not* improve endurance performance, nor does it improve the ability of muscles to use oxygen.

➤ **Ephedra** (Ma huang)

Claim: Promotes weight loss; when combined with caffeine, increases metabolic rate.

Fact: The active ingredients in this herb can increase metabolism but they also stimulate the central nervous system, increase heart rate, and raise blood pressure. The herb is banned in Canada as a single substance but is legal when sold in lower doses as a component in herb combinations. Abuse of this herb is dangerous (potentially life threatening) and can lead to dependency. I strongly recommend you do NOT use products containing ephedra.

➤ **Gamma-oryzanol**

Claim: Increases serum testosterone and growth-hormone levels, enhancing muscle growth.

Fact: Oryzanol is a plant sterol and has a similar structure to cholesterol. Numerous claims have been made that plant sterols (oryzanol is one of them), like cholesterol, can be converted to testosterone. However, oryzanol is *not* muscle building because it cannot be converted to testosterone by the human body and therefore does not promote muscle growth.

➤ **Glandular extracts**

Claim: Enhances the function of the comparable gland in the human body. For example, testes extract enhances testosterone production.

Fact: The glandular extracts are inactive, therefore worthless, when absorbed. They contain no hormones and cannot exert any effect.

➤ **MCT** (medium chain triglycerides)

Claim: Promotes muscle growth and loss of body fat.

Fact: MCT is an inefficient energy source during aerobic exercise. There is nothing in the research to prove that MCT meets its claims in strength-trained athletes. Consuming large amounts can cause gastrointestinal distress and diarrhea.

➤ **Pyruvate**

Claim: Improves endurance performance; promotes fat loss; acts as an antioxidant.

Fact: This by-product of cellular metabolism is used to produce 3-carbon compounds that are used for energy production. Studies giving extra pyruvate to both animals and overweight women have found it to be ineffective in promoting fat loss. Some research suggests that pyruvate may enhance endurance performance but in doses much higher than what's sold as supplements (in such high amounts, pyruvate will cause stomach upset).

➤ **Smilax**

Claim: Increases serum testosterone levels, muscle growth, and strength; also indicated to be a legal alternative to anabolic steroids.

Fact: Smilax does contain saponins—substances that serve as building blocks for the semisynthetic production of certain steroids. But this conversion takes place only in the laboratory, and there is no evidence that Smilax functions as a "legal replacement" for anabolic steroids. What's more, saponins have a strong diuretic action and possible laxative effect, and might also intensify your rate of perspiration.

➤ **Succinate**

Claim: Metabolic enhancer; reduces lactic-acid production and maintains energy production.

Fact: Succinate is a by-product; once it gets formed, it gets converted to other energy-generating compounds. However, supplementation will *not* increase the process of aerobic metabolism or ATP (energy) production; these actions are controlled by enzymes within the pathway.

➤ **Vanadyl sulphate**

Claim: Enhances uptake of amino acids (protein) by the muscles; promotes muscle growth.

Fact: This non-essential trace mineral does have an insulin-like action in the body (it regulates the uptake of blood sugar by cells), but very few studies have tested its effect on sport performance. One 12-week trial found the supplement to have no effect on body composition in weight lifters. Taking this supplement may cause excessive tiredness during and after training.

➤ **Vitamin B-12**

Claim: Enhances DNA synthesis; increases muscle growth.

Fact: Vitamin B-12 is essential in the synthesis of DNA. However, there is no evidence that *extra* B-12 promotes muscle growth or enhances strength.

The appeal of magic pills promising bigger muscles and faster speed is tremendous. However, it's important to know that very few claims about supplements are backed up scientifically—in fact, most of the so-called sport enhancers offer nothing but misleading labels. Without a doubt, the best way to ensure top performance is the old-fashioned mix—a good diet and plenty of hard training.

The Least You Need to Know

➤ Proper hydration is essential for maintaining prolonged activity *and* for optimal performance.

➤ Water is the perfect fluid replacement for exercise lasting under 60 minutes. However, endurance athletes, and anyone exercising in extremely hot or humid weather, will benefit from the added carbohydrate and electrolyte content in the popular sports drinks.

➤ Don't be misled by ads claiming to sell exercise enhancers in the shape of a pill. The way to optimize performance is to eat smart and train hard!

➤ Sports bars can be convenient and advantageous (depending upon the brand) for athletes trying to increase their intake of calories, carbohydrates, and protein. Sample several brands before you form a taste opinion; they vary tremendously.

Part 4

Beyond the Basics: Nutrition for Special Needs

There are so many subspecialties within the world of nutrition. New research comes along all the time and offers us exciting information regarding specialized areas. Among them, I've selected four interesting topics that appear to get a lot of attention; diet and cancer, vegetarian food plans, herbal remedies, and food sensitivities.

Whether you are interested in reducing your risk of cancer, feasting purely on plants, learning some plant-based medicine, or are simply tired of bolting for the bathroom after ingesting dairy products, stayed tuned.

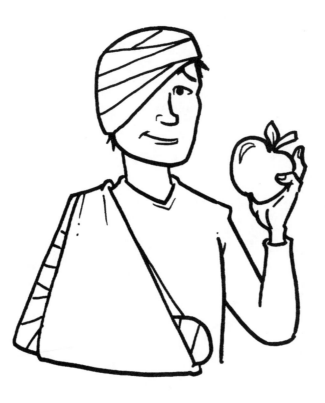

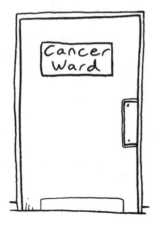

Chapter 18

Diet and Cancer

In This Chapter

➤ Foods that might decrease your risk of contracting certain cancers

➤ Omega-3s, and how they can help

➤ Eating the right fish and getting the most from flaxseed

➤ Your best bets in vegetables and fruit

➤ The many benefits of soy

Over the years, there's been a lot of speculation and controversy about how eating certain foods might prevent cancer. You certainly don't need a preeminent oncologist (or a Toronto nutritionist) to tell you that if you eat in a healthy manner, your body will be stronger, your immune system and organs will be in good shape, and therefore you might be more likely to stay cancer free. But just eating plenty of fruits and veggies and the right kind of nutrients isn't a foolproof way to avoid cancer. Unfortunately, there is no exact science linking food and cancer prevention, although we are constantly researching and studying the subject in the hope of finding some answers.

Nonetheless, while scientists and doctors learn, you can take a proactive approach to feeding your body well, giving it fuel to fight disease, and doing whatever you can to ward off this terrible illness. Even though there is no hardcore proof about which foods offer the best protection against malignancy, research has uncovered how certain foods can hamper the growth of a tumour.

Which Fats Can Help

For years, there has been an incredible amount of hype about fat. Fat clogs your arteries, fat increases your cholesterol, fat causes weight gain—fat is the root of all evil. However, some kinds of fat are not just okay to eat—they are actually good for you. To date, the best type of fat is polyunsaturated and is called omega-3 fatty acids. The omega-3 fats might have the potential to lower the risk of cancer and heart disease, as well as to help ease the pain of rheumatoid arthritis. These fats are found in flaxseed, canola oil, and fish.

The Fatty Fish

Seafood lovers, rejoice! Epidemiological studies have shown a lower rate of cancer in people who eat a lot of fish. The best advice is to have a few servings of tuna, mackerel, sardines, bluefish, striped bass, herring, trout, and salmon—the fish species with a rich concentration of omega-3 fats. Eat such fish at least three times each week (even more if you can).

Flaxseed and Flaxseed Oil

Flaxseed, the light brown seed from the flax plant, has received a lot of attention for its potential for protecting against breast and other hormone-related cancers (in addition to lowering cholesterol and relieving constipation). Rich in omega-3s, antioxidants, lignans-phytoestrogens (which you'll read about later in this chapter), and soluble and insoluble fibre, this impressive seed has been growing in popularity.

You can buy whole flaxseed in most health food stores and grind them with a coffee grinder as needed. Mix them into your cereals, salads, yogurts, cookies, muffins, pancakes, omelets, and even casseroles. Flaxseed oil is ready to pour on salad, but you'll miss out on the lignans and fibre found in whole flaxseed. For more information, visit the Web site of the Flax Council of Canada at www.flaxcouncil.ca.

Fight Back with Antioxidants

Unfortunately, harmful agents called *free radicals* are produced when we breathe and process oxygen. In fact, these destructive molecules can also be produced as a result of pollution, stress, pesticides, asbestos, X-rays, preservatives, exhaust fumes, tobacco smoke, and injury. As discussed in Chapter 7, "Vitamins and Minerals: The Micronutrients," free radicals circulate all through the body and actually destroy the DNA in cells—a cancer-promoting activity. The good news is that we naturally protect ourselves by forming antioxidants, substances that help our body's defence system fight off free radicals and preserve healthy cells. Furthermore, we know that certain foods are rich in nutrients that act as *powerful* antioxidants and might intensify the body's ability to degrade free radicals into harmless waste products that get eliminated before they do any damage.

The following sections list some cancer-fighting ingredients you should include regularly in your diet.

Vitamins C and E, and Beta-Carotene

Vitamins C and E and beta-carotene (a form of vitamin A) are known as dietary antioxidants. You can find them in fruits and vegetables. The best food sources of these antioxidants are the following:

Foods Rich in Vitamin C
Citrus fruits (oranges, grapefruits, and so on)
Melon
Strawberries
Tomatoes
Potatoes
Broccoli
Brussels sprouts
Kiwi
Mango
Papaya
Red peppers

Overrated-Undercooked

Alcohol is not recommended—but if you choose to drink alcohol, limit your consumption to no more than 1 drink per day.

Foods Rich in Vitamin E
Vegetable oils
Margarine
Salad dressings
Whole-grain cereals
Green leafy vegetables
Nuts and seeds
Peanut butter
Wheat germ

Food for Thought

You can buy flaxseed by mail order from the Flax Council of Canada: dial 1-877-BUY-FLAX (1-877-289-3529).

Foods Rich in Beta-Carotene
Cantaloupe
Carrots
Sweet potato
Winter squash
Spinach
Rapini
Broccoli

Green and Black Tea

Both green and black (good old orange pekoe, English Breakfast, or Earl Grey) teas contain potent chemical antioxidants called polyphenols, so drink up. In fact, research has shown that these teas might actually interfere with the ability of cancer-causing agents to bind to our DNA—therefore stopping cancer activity.

Furthermore, you'll want to take it easy with the amount of milk that you pour into your mug because milk proteins might bind with the antioxidants, making them unavailable to your body. For those who prefer lemon and sugar, you're in luck because neither appears to have the same effect as milk on the antioxidants. Unfortunately, herbal teas do not work in the same protective manner as the green teas.

Tomatoes

Tomatoes contain *lycopene*, which is actually the pigment that gives tomatoes their hue. The catch is that tomatoes must be cooked to make the lycopene more available to the body. Grill them, stew them, simmer them in soups, or make a mean pasta sauce—but don't forget to season it with a little garlic. (The allyl sulphides in garlic, chives, and onions might help the body process cancer-causing chemicals more safely.) Also, add a touch of olive oil because a bit of fat will help the lycopene move through your body.

Food for Thought

When taken for many years, folic acid (400 mcg per day) from a multivitamin/mineral pill has been shown to reduce the risk of colon cancer in women.

Can't Get Enough of Those Fruits and Veggies

Everyone knows the nutritional value of fruits and vegetables; that's why at least 5 servings a day are recommended. I've already pointed out that certain plant foods are loaded with vitamins C and E and beta-carotene—helpful vitamins and antioxidants our bodies need to fight disease and stay strong. In addition, plant foods have been shown to play a significant role in the fight against most cancers because they contain phytochemicals and Cox-2 inhibitors—compounds that can stop the growth of new blood cells, which would ultimately impede the growth of a tumour. Let's not forget that vegetables and fruit are naturally low in fat and rich in fibre; that's the icing (fat-free, of course) on the cake, if you will.

Cruciferous veggies such as broccoli, cauliflower, cabbage, bok choy, kale, Brussels sprouts, collards, mustard greens, and turnip greens can also help reduce the risk of cancer by increasing the production of certain enzymes that help carry potential carcinogens out of the body. Make sure you load your stir-fry dishes and salads with the almighty cruciferous vegetables!

Phytochemicals, Phytonutrients, and Phytoestrogens

They sound confusing but they're really quite understandable:

➤ **Phytochemicals**—Phytochemicals (meaning plant chemicals) are another group of compounds in plant foods—legumes, veggies, fruits, and whole grains—that might positively affect your body. They're naturally produced by plants to protect themselves against viruses, bacteria, and fungi. And the bonus is that when we eat these plants, phytochemicals can offer us protection, too. Hundreds of naturally occurring substances, such as carotenoids, flavonoids, indoles, isoflavones, capsaicin, and protease inhibitors, are phytochemicals.

Their exact role in promoting health is still uncertain, but research has suggested that they might help protect against certain cancers, heart disease, and other chronic illnesses. They can act as antioxidants, natural antibiotics, and tumour inhibitors.

Food for Thought

Include plenty of whole grains in your diet. The insoluble fibre in wheat bran can increase the transport of waste products and cancer-causing agents through the gut and lower intestines. The less time waste products spend in your system, the less risk of certain types of cancer, such as colon and rectal cancer.

Food for Thought

Rosemary, turmeric, and red grapes contain Cox-2 inhibitors—compounds that can prevent tumour growth.

Nutri-Speak

Isoflavones are hormone-like substances that are similar to estrogen and are found in plants.

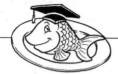

Food for Thought

Make a soy-fruit smoothie: In a blender mix soy-protein powder (made from soy protein isolate) with fruit juice, fresh fruit, and some crushed ice.

➤ **Phytonutrients**—Phytonutrient is a term often used on supplement bottles to indicate that certain botanical supplements extracted from vegetables and other plant foods have been added.

Because there are thousands of phytonutrients, there isn't enough scientific evidence to know whether supplement manufacturers have picked the "right" active substance, or to know if the amount contained in the pill actually offers any benefits.

➤ **Phytoestrogens**—Phytoestrogens are plant hormones similar to, but much weaker than, human estrogens. Phytoestrogens are believed to reduce the risk of breast cancer and prostate cancer; they also might minimize hot flashes and vaginal dryness associated with menopause. Some medical researchers think that phytoestrogens might one day take the place of short-term conventional estrogen replacement therapy (ERT) for some women.

Phytoestrogens, now identified in some 300 plants, are grouped as

Coumestans: bean sprouts, red clover, sunflower seeds

Lignans: rye, wheat, sesame seeds, linseed, flaxseed

Isoflavones: many fruits and vegetables, but most of all, soybeans and soy products

The Story on Soy Products

Replacing steaks, burgers, and franks with tofu, tempeh, miso, and veggie burgers can work to your advantage. (You vegetarians are definitely on to something.) That's because soy foods contain phytoestrogens called *isoflavones*, weak estrogens that might help fight against certain hormone-related cancers, such as breast, uterine, prostate, and possibly ovarian cancer. These weak estrogens bind to the receptors that would otherwise get filled by stronger estrogens—stronger estrogens that have the potential to promote tumour growth. Many experts believe that eating soy foods over a lifetime offers protection from these cancers. So start your kids enjoying soy today!

Although the research is preliminary regarding the amount we should consume, everyone can benefit by shifting from an animal-based to a plant-based diet. The best soy sources include soybeans, tempeh, tofu, dry soy protein isolate, textured soy protein (TVP), dry soy concentrate, and soy milk.

Diet won't eliminate cancer—but we can say that in certain circumstances the foods we eat can certainly help reduce the risk. Try to adopt a cuisine that incorporates some or all of the foods previously discussed, and you will be taking a proactive step toward improving your overall health.

The Least You Need to Know

➤ Your parents knew what they were talking about when they pushed you to eat your veggies; plant foods are especially good for reducing the risk of cancer because they contain antioxidants and phytochemicals—compounds that inhibit the growth of tumours.

➤ Not all fats are taboo; flaxseed, canola, and fish oils are loaded with omega-3 fats, which may actually play a role in the fight against cancer.

➤ Drinking green and black tea, stewing up tomatoes, and eating foods with a high concentration of vitamins C and E and beta-carotene will help fight harmful agents called free radicals and therefore preserve healthy cells and reduce the risk of cancer.

➤ A diet rich in fibre might help decrease your risk of colon and rectal cancer. Insoluble fibre, found in whole grains, wheat bran, and most fruits and veggies, can help the body dispose of waste products and cancer-causing agents from the gut and lower intestines.

➤ Consume more tofu, miso, tempeh, and soy beans; they all contain soy, which may help fight against hormone-related cancers, such as breast, uterine, prostate, and possibly ovarian cancer.

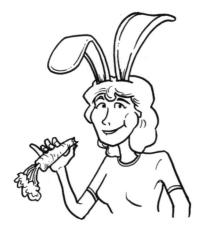

Chapter 19

Going Vegetarian

In This Chapter

➤ The reasons people go vegetarian

➤ The difference between vegans, lacto-vegetarians, and lacto-ovo-vegetarians

➤ Great vegetarian protein and iron sources

➤ What's soy protein all about?

➤ Meatless recipes to tantalize your taste buds

Vegetarian diets are becoming popular, and more and more Canadians are jumping on the "tofu bandwagon." People following vegetarian food plans—or any other prudent diet—must eat well-balanced, varied meals and include fruits, vegetables, nuts, seeds, legumes, low-fat dairy products (depending upon your vegetarian restrictions), and plenty of whole-grain products. Although a typical vegetarian eating plan tends to be very low in saturated fat and cholesterol, it's not automatically low in *total* fat and sugar. Therefore, herbivores, just like carnivores, need to limit their intake of fatty foods, oils, spreads, and sweets.

A Food Guide for Vegetarians

For most vegetarians, following *Canada's Food Guide to Healthy Eating* as outlined in Chapter 1, "Guidelines for Healthy Eating," will address their nutritional needs. Here's what every healthy vegetarian should try to eat each day:

Grain Products: 5–12 servings

Vegetables and Fruits: 5–10 servings

So far, so good, right? These two food groups give you plenty of energizing carbohydrate, fabulous fibre, and essential vitamins and minerals. And such foods are naturally free of animal products. But what happens with the next two food categories?

Meat and Alternatives: 2–3 servings

People who don't eat meat, chicken, or fish can replace these foods with legumes, nuts, seeds, and soy foods found in the meat and alternatives group. These plant foods give you protein, iron, and zinc, so you're not missing out. Easy so far! Let's keep going...

Milk Products: 2–4 servings

Vegetarians who avoid dairy products will be in a calcium bind if they rely on Canada's Food Guide. That's because there are no alternative sources of calcium found in the milk products group. I'm sure many vegetarians are hoping that some day the group will be renamed "Milk and Alternatives." In the meantime, I've listed some calcium equivalents to 1 serving of milk. Keep in mind that 1 serving packs about 300 milligrams of bone-building calcium.

Milk Alternatives	Equivalent Milk Serving
1 cup (250 mL) fortified soy or rice beverage	1 serving
1 cup (250 mL) calcium-fortified orange juice	1 serving
1 cup (250 mL) cooked broccoli, Swiss chard	$1/3$ serving
$3/4$ cup (175 mL) cooked kale, okra	$1/2$ serving
1 cup cooked collard greens	1 serving
$1/2$ cup (125 mL) tofu made with calcium	$1/3$ serving
1 cup (250 mL) cooked tempeh	$1/2$ serving
1 cup (250 mL) cooked legumes (kidney beans, black beans, brown beans)	$1/3$ serving
4 medium figs	$1/3$ serving
$1/4$ cup (50 mL) almonds	$1/3$ serving
1 tbs (15 mL) blackstrap molasses	$1/2$ serving

One downside of high-calcium veggies is that your body absorbs their calcium less efficiently than the calcium in dairy products. To get the most out of them, eat your veggies cooked. Steaming or stir-frying your greens can double the amount of calcium that's available to you!

The Various Types of Vegetarians

A vegetarian diet, when properly followed, can be one of the healthiest diets around. Benefits of the vegetarian diet include the following:

> ➤ **Decreased obesity**—Vegans are rarely obese and, on the average, lacto-ovo-vegetarians are leaner than those who eat meat. However, being vegetarian doesn't guarantee a slim figure. If you eat foods that are high in fat, you may consume as many calories as meat eaters, or even more than they do.

> ➤ **Less risk of coronary heart disease (CHD)**—Vegetarians tend to have lower blood-cholesterol levels and a diet with a lower overall content of saturated fat.

> ➤ **Lower rates of hypertension**—The reason for this is still unknown, but researchers think it might be related to increased intake of potassium, magnesium, polyunsaturated fat, and fibre. All the same, more research is still needed to determine whether the diet itself has anything to do with the lower levels.

Vegetarian eating covers a broad range of people, from those who avoid all animal products to people who simply refrain from eating a few select animal-based foods. Here's a look at the assortment of vegetarian eaters:

> ➤ **Vegans**—This is the strictest type of vegetarian (sort of the granddaddy of all vegetarians). Vegans do not eat or use any animal products; they avoid eating meat, dairy products, and eggs and wearing wool, silk, or leather. If you're a vegan, you'll need to be extra careful about getting adequate protein, iron, calcium, vitamin D, vitamin B-12, and zinc.

> ➤ **Lacto-vegetarians**—This group eliminates meat and eggs but includes all dairy products.

> ➤ **Lacto-ovo-vegetarians**—This group eliminates all meat (red meat, poultry, fish, and seafood) but includes dairy products and eggs.

> ➤ **Semi-vegetarians**—This group does not eat red meat but eats poultry and fish, along with eggs and all dairy products.

> ➤ **Pesco-vegetarians**—This group has chosen to say good-bye to meat and poultry, but eats fish and seafood.

How to Ensure an Adequate Protein Intake

All vegetarians can easily meet their protein needs. Protein doesn't discriminate; it's found in both animal and plant foods. Low-fat dairy products and eggs can provide generous amounts of protein for vegetarians who dare to eat them, and the vegans in the crowd should become closely acquainted with tofu, nuts, seeds, lentils, and tempeh. Flip back to Chapter 3, "The Profile on Protein," to refresh your memory on complementary proteins—that is, making a complete protein (a protein containing all of the essential amino acids) by combining two or more incomplete plant proteins during the day.

Food for Thought

Although tofu and other soy foods contain some fat, it's very low in saturated fat and contains no cholesterol. For recipes, information, and free brochures on soy foods, visit the Web site of the Ontario Soybean Growers' Marketing Board at www.soybean.on.ca or write to

The Ontario Soybean Growers' Marketing Board
P.O. Box 1199
Chatham, Ontario
N7M 5L8

E-mail: cansoy@soybean.on.ca

The Many Faces of Soy Protein

Decades ago, soy foods were one of the world's best kept secrets. Now there are soy products suitable for using in just about any recipe, and soy protein can boost the protein, calcium, and the iron content of almost any dish. Remember that unflavoured soy will take on any flavour you combine it with, particularly if you marinate it. Go ahead and experiment by incorporating some of the following varieties of soy products into your meals:

➤ **Soy beverage**—Start your day with a glass of soy milk, or pour it over your cereal for breakfast. Most brands of soy milk provide about 9 grams of protein per 1-cup (250 mL) serving and are available in low-fat and flavoured varieties.

➤ **Isolated soy protein**—This powdery substance is literally 90 percent pure protein because most of the fat and carbohydrate has been discarded. Isolated soy protein is made from defatted soy flour and can be blended into muffins, pancakes, and cookies to help boost your daily protein intake. A 1-ounce serving (approximately 4 Tbs/50 mL) contains between 14 and 25 grams of protein.

➤ **Soy flour**—Here's another great way to increase the protein content of your baked products. Soy flour can be used for quick breads, muffins, cookies, and brownies, and a $1/2$-cup (125 mL) serving supplies 22 grams of protein. Replace up to one-half of the regular flour called for in your favourite recipes.

➤ **Texturized soy protein (TSP)**—Also called texturized vegetable protein (TVP), this product is made from defatted soy flour and can have a granular, flakey, or chunky texture. TSP comes in both plain and flavoured varieties and can be mixed into chili, tacos, veggie burgers, vegetarian casseroles, and stews. When rehydrated with an equal amount of water, 1 cup (250 mL) prepared TSP solution provides 22 grams of protein.

➤ **Vegetable-type soybeans**—These dry, mature soybeans are loaded with 14 grams of protein per $1/2$-cup (125 mL) serving. What's more, they also contain fibre—a double whammy. Tasting both sweet and buttery, their flavour makes them a nice addition to stir-fry dishes, salads, and soups.

➤ **Tempeh**—This cultured soy food has a tender, chewy consistency that makes it a great candidate for grilled sandwiches, chunky soups, salads, casseroles, and chili.

A 4-ounce (120 g) serving provides 17 grams of protein, about 80 milligrams of calcium, and 10 percent of your daily iron requirement.

➤ **Tofu**—Just about anything goes with this soy protein. "I'll have tofu à la mode!" It's made from soy milk curds and can be blended, scrambled, stir-fried, grilled, and baked; you name it, chances are it can be done with tofu. There are three types of tofu:

> **Firm tofu** is stiff, dense, and perfect for stir-fry dishes, soups, or any dish in which you want the tofu to maintain its shape. A 4-ounce (120 g) serving of firm tofu supplies 13 grams of protein, 120 milligrams of calcium, and about 40 percent of your daily iron requirement.

> **Soft tofu** provides 9 grams of protein, 130 milligrams of calcium, and a little less than 40 percent of your daily iron requirement per 4-ounce (120 g) serving. Soft tofu is good for dishes that require blended tofu, and is commonly used in soups.

> **Silken tofu** is creamy and custard-like and therefore also works well in puréed or blended recipes such as shakes, dips, soups, and pies. Silken tofu doesn't provide as much calcium as the more solid tofu varieties (only 40 mg/4-oz [120 g] serving), but it is the lowest in fat and is packed with $9^{1}/_{2}$ grams of protein per 4-ounce (120 g) serving.

Ironing Out the Plant Foods

Unfortunately for this less carnivorous crowd, the *heme* iron found in animal foods is much more absorbable than the *nonheme* iron supplied from plants. But that's okay; just go out of your way to eat an abundance of iron-rich plant foods and you'll meet your quota. Foods rich in iron include dried beans, spinach, Swiss chard, beet greens, blackstrap molasses, bulgur, prune juice, and dried fruits. You might also find that your favourite breakfast cereals are fortified with this mineral. Another trick of the trade is to boost the amount of iron absorbed at a meal by including a food rich in vitamin C (tomatoes, broccoli, orange juice, and so on). For further information on increasing iron, see Chapter 8, "Mighty Minerals: Calcium and Iron."

Searching for Nondairy Calcium

For the lacto-vegetarians and lacto-ovo-vegetarians, low-fat dairy products are brimming with calcium. For vegans, on the other hand, it takes some planning to get enough calcium, but you too can meet your daily calcium requirements by including collard greens, broccoli, beans, kale, turnip greens, calcium-fortified orange juice, calcium-fortified grains, and, of course, calcium-fortified soy milk products (including tofu, soybeans, and tempeh) in your diet. At the beginning of this chapter, I told you how these foods compare to a serving of a dairy product.

Food for Thought

Vegans who don't eat dairy products and aren't regularly out in the sun should buy foods fortified with vitamin D or speak with their dietitians or doctors about vitamin supplementation.

Have You Had Enough B-12 Today?

Getting enough vitamin B-12 can also be an obstacle for strict vegans, simply because B-12 is derived primarily from animal-based foods. Once again, you lacto-vegetarians and lacto-ovo-vegetarians are off the hook because dairy products and eggs provide enough to satisfy your daily requirements. The vegan eater has to dig a little deeper. Buy food products that are fortified with B-12: cereals, breads, soy and rice beverages, and possibly tempeh. You might also want to take a B-12 supplement or a B complex supplement, just to be safe.

Don't Forget the Kitchen Zinc

Not only do strict vegetarians have to plan their diet to get all the necessary calcium, protein, B-12, and other nutrients, they must also ensure they get adequate zinc. Although this mineral is found in whole-grain products, tofu, nuts, seeds, and wheat germ, our bodies absorb much less "plant zinc" than "animal zinc." This is because *phytic acid* (a substance in the plant fibre) combines with the zinc and prevents it from being fully absorbed. Therefore, vegetarians need to pay particular attention to getting enough of this mineral.

A day in the life of a vegan.

Menu 1

Breakfast

Amaranth flakes with fortified soy milk
Fresh blueberries and raspberries
English muffin topped with peach preserves

Lunch

Peanut butter and banana sandwich (on whole-grain bread, of course!)
Cup of vegetarian chili topped with green onion
Glass of low-fat soy milk

Snack

Mixture of dried fruit and walnuts
Glass of juice or soy milk

Menu 2

Breakfast

Scrambled Tofu (see recipe) with whole-wheat toast
Bowl of oatmeal with chopped dates and almonds
Glass of cranberry-orange juice

Lunch

Bowl of lentil soup with whole-wheat rolls
Carrot sticks with humus dip
Glass of juice or soy milk

Snack

Piece of banana bread
Glass of soy milk

Dinner
Vegetable and tempeh stir-fry (carrots, broccoli,
  cauliflower, and tempeh) with brown rice
Sweet potato
Steamed kale sprinkled with sesame seeds
Glass of soy milk

Dessert
Rice Dream (ice cream substitute)
Sliced bananas

Dinner
Whole-wheat tortilla stuffed with beans, salsa,
  and arugula
Spinach salad drizzled with olive oil and red wine
  vinegar

Dessert
Baked apple with maple syrup and chopped
  walnuts

Tips for the Vegetarian Dining Out

Whether you're dining out to be social or because you just don't feel like cooking, if you're trying to stick to a vegetarian diet, it can be tough to get a satisfying meal, let alone a nourishing one. Here are some tips to get through a night out without starving:

➤ When your dining pals won't have anything to do with a vegetarian restaurant, suggest one that serves Chinese, Vietnamese, Thai, or Italian food. There are always some vegetarian entrées on the menu.

➤ If there aren't any vegetarian entrées, make up a full meal by selecting a few side dishes. For example, have a baked potato or a house salad and ask whether they'll serve a side of beans. Better yet, request a special vegetarian entrée. Most restaurants are pretty accommodating.

➤ Soup can be a great option in any type of restaurant. Remember to ask whether the soup is meat based or vegetable based.

➤ Make substitutions and special requests. For instance, change a bacon, lettuce, and tomato sandwich to a cheese, lettuce, and tomato sandwich, or change an order of chicken fajitas to veggie fajitas.

Q & A

Help, I'm in love with a meat eater! What do I do?

Relax, get with the millennium; mixed marriages are in! If cooking is a major hassle because you and your partner don't eat the same foods, plan some neutral meals that you'll both enjoy. For example, make a large dish of stir-fry vegetables and brown rice. You take a portion and toss in tofu; he or she takes a portion and throws in chicken or beef.

Remarkably Meatless Recipes

Here are some wonderful vegetarian cookbooks available in bookstores (* denotes books by Canadian authors!):

*Becoming Vegetarian: The Complete Guide to Becoming a Vegetarian**
By Vesanto Melina, RD, Brenda Davis, RD, and Victoria Harrison, RD
MacMillan Canada, 1994

*Cooking Vegetarian**
By Vesanto Melina, RD, and Joseph Forest
MacMillan Canada, 1996

*Rose Reisman's Light Vegetarian Cooking**
By Rose Reisman
Robert Rose Inc., 1998

*How It All Vegan! Irresistible Recipes for an Animal Free Diet**
By Tanya Barnard and Sarah Kramer
Arsenal Pulp Press, 1999

*Tofu Mania**
By Brita Housez
Centax Books, 1999

Moosewood Restaurant Low Fat Favorites
Vegetable Kingdom Inc., 1996

Moosewood Restaurant Cooks at Home
Vegetable Kingdom Inc., 1994

Moosewood Cookbook
By Mollie Katzen
Ten Speed Press, 1977

Cajun Red Beans and Rice

Serves four

2 bay leaves

1 can (19 oz/540 mL) kidney beans, drained and rinsed

1 green bell pepper, diced $^{1}/_{4}$ inch (0.5 cm)

$^{1}/_{2}$ onion, peeled and diced $^{1}/_{4}$ inch (0.5 cm)

2 cups (500 mL) water

1 cup (250 mL) canned, crushed tomatoes

1 cup (250 mL) long-grain white rice

2 tsp (10 mL) paprika

1 tsp (5 mL) Worcestershire sauce

$^{1}/_{4}$ (1 mL) tsp garlic powder

Pinch cayenne pepper

$^{1}/_{4}$ cup (50 mL) chopped green onion

Place all ingredients (except for the chopped green onion) in a large saucepan; cover and bring to a boil. Reduce heat and simmer 15–20 minutes until rice is tender and liquid is evaporated. Top each portion with 1 Tbs (15 mL) chopped green onion. Balance out this meal with a dark, leafy green salad tossed with nonfat Italian salad dressing.

<u>Nutrition Analysis for One Serving</u>
Calories: 290
Total fat: 1 gram
Saturated fat: 0 grams
Dietary fibre: 7 grams
Protein: 10 grams
Sodium: 170 mg
Cholesterol: 0 mg

Vegetarian Spinach Lasagna

Serves eight

2 boxes (10–12 oz/284–340 g) frozen spinach, chopped

2 egg whites

1 whole egg

2 lbs (1 kg) low-fat ricotta cheese

4 cups (1 L) grated skim-milk mozzarella cheese

2 tsp (10 mL) oregano

3/4 tsp (3 mL) pepper

Garlic and basil to taste

Nonstick cooking spray

1 jar (32 oz/900 mL) tomato/marinara sauce (low-sodium)

1 package lasagna noodles, uncooked

1 cup (250 mL) water (for cooking only)

Cook and drain spinach well, and then set aside. Mix together the eggs, ricotta cheese, 1/2 of the mozzarella cheese, oregano, pepper, garlic, and basil. Add in spinach and mix again thoroughly. Coat lasagna pan with nonstick spray and preheat oven to 350°F (180°C). Cover the bottom of pan with tomato sauce and then with a layer of the uncooked lasagna noodles. Next, spread 1/2 of the spinach-cheese mixture evenly on top, and repeat the layers (noodles and then the remaining spinach-cheese mixture). Place on top one more layer of noodles (total of 3 noodle layers) and pour on the remaining tomato sauce. Sprinkle on the other 1/2 of the mozzarella cheese. Last, pour the water around the edge of the pan (this will cook the noodles) and cover tightly with tin foil. Bake for 1 hour and 15 minutes, until the cheese is bubbling. Let stand and cool for 15 minutes before slicing.

<u>Nutrition Analysis for One Serving</u>
Calories: 243
Total fat: 7.5 grams
Saturated fat: 3 grams
Dietary fibre: 3 grams
Protein: 19 grams
Sodium: 479 mg
Cholesterol: 43 mg

From the kitchen of Ellen Schloss

Chunky Vegetarian Chili

Serves six

$^1/_2$ cup (125 mL) texturized vegetable protein (TVP)

$^1/_4$ cup (50 mL) boiling water

2 tsp (10 mL) olive oil

1 large onion, diced

3 cloves garlic, minced

2 medium carrots, chopped

2 medium celery stalks, chopped

1 green bell pepper, seeded and chopped

8 oz (250 g) mushrooms, quartered

1 lemon, juiced

$1^1/_2$ tsp (7 mL) chili powder

$1^1/_2$ tsp (7 mL) ground cumin

$^1/_2$ tsp (2 mL) dried basil

$^1/_2$ tsp (2 mL) dried oregano

$^1/_8$ tsp (0.5 mL) red pepper flakes

1 large tomato, chopped

1 can (28 oz/796 mL) crushed tomatoes

1 can (19 oz/540 mL) black beans

1 can (19 oz/540 mL) kidney beans

1 Tbs (15 mL) tomato paste

$^1/_2$ Tbs (7 mL) Marsala wine (optional)

2–4 Tbs (30–50 mL) fresh chives and/or parsley (optional)

Combine the TVP and boiling water in a bowl and set aside. Meanwhile, heat oil in a large stock pot; add onions and sauté until soft (about 3 minutes). Next, add garlic, carrots, celery, pepper, mushrooms, lemon juice, and spices. Cook over medium heat, covered, for 5 minutes.

Stir in TVP, chopped tomato, crushed tomatoes, and beans. Bring to a simmer. Cook uncovered over low heat for 15 minutes, stirring occasionally. Add tomato paste and Marsala wine, and simmer again for an additional 5 minutes. Remove pot from heat and stir in fresh herbs. Ladle the chili into bowls and garnish with a dollop of low-fat sour cream and chopped red onion. Serve with a fresh loaf of whole-grain bread.

Nutrition Analysis for One Serving (Chili Only)
Calories: 330
Total fat: 2.4 grams
Saturated fat: 0 grams
Dietary fibre: 14 grams
Protein: 22 grams
Sodium: 400 mg
Cholesterol: 0 mg

From the kitchen of Meredith Gunsberg, MS, RD

Scrambled Tofu

Serves four

16 oz (500 g) firm tofu

5 Tbs (65 mL) water

2 Tbs (25 mL) mellow barley light miso

$^1/_2$ tsp (2 mL) tumeric

Dash garlic powder

Dash ground cumin

Fresh ground pepper to taste

Mash tofu in a small saucepan. In a separate bowl, whisk together all remaining ingredients. Heat tofu over medium heat, and immediately add the miso mixture. Stir constantly until the scrambled tofu mixture is heated through. Serve hot with toast and ketchup, if desired.

Nutrition Analysis for One Serving (Tofu Only)
Calories: 82
Total fat: 4 grams
Saturated fat: 1 gram
Dietary fibre: 0 grams
Protein: 8 grams
Sodium: 32 mg
Cholesterol: 0 mg

From the kitchen of Meredith Gunsberg, MS, RD

Cucumber Yogurt Dip

Serves four

2 cloves garlic, pressed

1 large cucumber, peeled, seeded, and grated

1 small lemon, juiced

1 cup (250 mL) nonfat plain yogurt

1 Tbs (15 mL) finely chopped fresh dill

1–2 tsp (5–10 mL) finely chopped fresh chives

Combine all ingredients (except chives and dill), and mix thoroughly. Sprinkle dill and chives on top before serving. Serve with pita bread and plenty of raw vegetables. Yields just over 1 cup (250 mL).

Nutrition Analysis for One Serving ($^1/_4$ of Dip)
Calories: 32
Total fat: 0 grams
Saturated fat: 0 grams
Dietary fibre: 0 grams
Protein: 3 grams
Sodium: 270 mg
Cholesterol: 0 mg

From the kitchen of Meredith Gunsberg, MS, RD

If you're thinking of becoming a vegetarian, you now know the basics. If you're already a vegetarian, compare your food with the guidelines presented in this chapter and see how your diet measures up. And if you simply read this chapter because it was between Chapters 18 and 20—try replacing some of your meat meals with plant-based meals. Vegetarian entrées can offer variety, interest, and perhaps a unique experience for your taste buds.

Food for Thought

Pregnant vegetarians need to pay extra attention to their diets. For some further reading, pick up

> *Vegetarian Pregnancy*
> By Sharon Yntema
> McBooks Press, New York
> 1-888-BOOKS11 (1-888-266-5711)

Bringing up infants or kids in a veggie household? For further reading, pick up

> *New Vegetarian Baby*
> By Sharon Yntema and Christine Beard
> McBooks Press, New York
> 1-888-BOOKS11 (1-888-266-5711)

> *Vegetarian Children*
> By Sharon Yntema
> McBooks Press, New York
> 1-888-BOOKS11 (1-888-266-5711)

The Least You Need to Know

➤ Vegans are the strictest vegetarians and avoid all meat, dairy products, and eggs. Lacto-vegetarians eat dairy products but avoid all meat and eggs. Lacto-ovo-vegetarians eat dairy products and eggs but avoid all meat.

➤ Vegetarians (especially vegans) need to be extra responsible about getting enough protein, calcium, vitamin D, vitamin B-12, iron, and zinc.

➤ A lot of non-animal foods provide protein. Nuts, seeds, legumes, and soy-based products are all great sources of protein. The less strict lacto-vegetarians and lacto-ovo vegetarians can also obtain protein from dairy products and eggs. The key for the vegetarian is to eat plenty of complementary proteins to get all that are required.

➤ Soy protein can help boost the protein, calcium, and iron content of almost any meal.

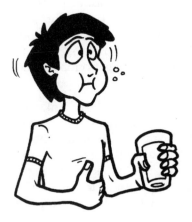

Chapter 20

Food Allergies and Other Ailments

In This Chapter

➤ The lowdown on food allergies

➤ Diagnosing a true food allergy

➤ Different food sensitivities

➤ Living with a lactose intolerance

➤ Learning about celiac disease

Do you break out in hives at the mere mention of a peanut? Do you bolt for the bathroom after ingesting anything made with milk? Does the smell of seafood make your stomach churn? You're not alone! Even my grandmother sneezes repeatedly after eating a bowl of her favourite ice cream.

For millions of Canadians, symptoms such as these turn the pleasurable act of eating into an uncomfortable and sometimes dangerous situation. In fact, an estimated 3.5 million Canadians have some type of food sensitivity, ranging from severe food allergies to less serious (but often still bothersome) food intolerances. This chapter provides an inside look at the variety of food hypersensitivities and sorts through the confusion, controversy, and skepticism in the world of tasty offenders.

Understanding Food Allergies

A true *food allergy* is a hypersensitive reaction that occurs when your immune system responds abnormally to harmless proteins in food. That is, your body misinterprets something good (a protein) as an intruder and produces antibodies to "halt" the

Food for Thought

Statistics report that up to 8 percent of all infants and small children are allergic to certain foods, a much higher incidence than that among Canadian adults (less than 2 percent).

invasion. Remember the episode of *Three's Company* when Jack sneaked in late one night, and Chrissy and Janet mistook him for a burglar and clobbered him over the head? It's the same thing with food allergies, only you're the one who gets clobbered (I guess I'm really dating myself now).

The most common food culprits linked to allergic reactions are wheat, shellfish, nuts, soybeans, corn, cow's milk, and eggs. Furthermore, the organs most commonly affected are the skin (symptoms include skin rashes, hives, itching, and swelling), the respiratory tract (symptoms include difficulty breathing and "hay fever"), and the gastrointestinal tract (symptoms include nausea, bloating, diarrhea, and vomiting). Some allergic reactions are so severe they can even provoke anaphylactic shock, a life-threatening, whole-body response that requires immediate medical attention.

Here's a list of terms to know:

➤ **Food sensitivity** is a general term used to describe any abnormal response to a food or food additive.

➤ **Food allergy** is an overreaction by the body's immune system, usually triggered by protein-containing foods (such as cow's milk, nuts, soybeans, shellfish, eggs, and wheat).

➤ **Anaphylactic shock** is a life-threatening, whole-body allergic reaction to an offending substance. Symptoms include swelling of the mouth and throat, difficulty breathing, a drop in blood pressure, and loss of consciousness. In other words, get help fast!

➤ **Food intolerance** is an adverse reaction that generally does not involve the immune system (lactose intolerance is an example).

➤ **Food poisoning** is an adverse reaction caused by contaminated food (containing micro-organisms, parasites, or other toxins).

➤ **Antibodies** are large protein molecules produced by the body's immune system in response to foreign substances.

Diagnosing a True Food Allergy

Many people view this whole food-sensitivity business as faddism and quackery, and unfortunately, we may have earned this mind-set. Did you know that out of the millions of people who *think* they have a food allergy, a very tiny percentage of the Canadian adult population actually has one? Why does the idea of a food allergy get thrown around so recklessly? One reason may be that people are often quick to blame physical ailments on food. Another aggravating reason for all the misdiagnoses is those so-called allergy quacks that diagnose you with the "allergy of the month" in return for your hard-earned money.

In today's world, a true food allergy can be properly diagnosed with scientifically sound testing. If you think you might suffer from an allergic response to certain foods, get it checked out. The first step is to find a qualified and reputable physician who has been certified by the Canadian Society of Allergy and Clinical Immunology. Ask your family physician for a referral. Next, schedule an appointment. Here's what you can expect:

Nutri-Speak

The word **allergy** comes from the Greek words *allos*, meaning other, and *ergon*, meaning working. In other words, the immune system *is* working other than normally expected.

➤ **Thorough medical history**—You'll give a detailed history of both your and your family's medical background. Special attention will be given to the type and frequency of your symptoms, and to when the symptoms occur in relation to eating food.

➤ **Complete physical examination**—You'll have a routine physical exam, with special focus on the areas of your body where you experience the suspected food-allergy symptoms.

➤ **Food-elimination diet**—The doctor will probably have you keep a food diary while you eliminate all suspicious foods from your diet. The allergist might then tell you to slowly add, one at a time, these foods back into your diet so you can identify which foods specifically might cause an adverse reaction.

➤ **Skin test**—An extract of a particular food is placed on the skin (usually arm or back) and then pricked or scratched into the skin to see if a reaction of itching or swelling occurs. This isn't 100 percent reliable because people who aren't allergic can develop skin rashes. On the other hand, some people don't show skin reactions but do have allergic responses when they eat the food.

➤ **RAST (radioallergosorbent test)**—This test involves mixing small samples of your blood with food extracts in a test tube. If you are truly allergic to a particular food, your blood will produce antibodies to fight off the food extract. One advantage of this test is that it is performed outside your body, so you don't have to deal with the itching and swelling if the test is positive. Note: This test will only indicate an allergy, not the extent of sensitivity to the offending food.

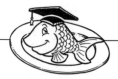

Food for Thought

For further information and educational materials on food allergies, contact the Allergy Asthma Information Association at 416–783–8944. Ask how to contact your regional office.

➤ **Double-blind food-challenge test**—This type of test must be performed under close supervision, preferably in an allergist's office or hospital, and it is considered the "gold standard" in food-allergy testing. Two capsules of dried food are prepared, one with the real food and another with a non-reactive substance. Neither doctor nor patient knows which is which (that's why it's called a double-blind challenge). These challenges can rule out, as well as detect, allergies or intolerances to foods and other food substances such as additives.

Treating a True Food Allergy

What's the treatment once you're diagnosed as having a true food allergy? Avoid the offending food!

Although this list is not a substitute for consulting a registered dietitian, it can provide a pretty good idea of which food ingredients to avoid after you've been diagnosed as having one of the following food allergies:

➤ **Cow's milk**—Check labels carefully and avoid all foods with the following ingredients: milk, yogurt, cheese, cottage cheese, custard, casein, whey, ghee, milk solids, curds, sodium caseinate, lactoglobulin, lactalbumin, milk chocolate, buttermilk, cream, sour cream, and butter.

➤ **Wheat**—Avoid all foods with the following ingredients: wheat, wheat germ, all-purpose flour, Durham flour, cracker meal, couscous, bulgur, whole-wheat berries, cake flour, gluten flour, pastry flour, graham flour, semolina, bran, cereal or malt extract, modified food starch, farina, and graham.

➤ **Corn**—Avoid all foods with the following ingredients: fresh, canned, or frozen corn (regular and creamed), hominy, corn grits, maize, cornmeal, corn flour, corn sugar, baking powder, corn syrup, cornstarch, modified food starch, dextrin, maltodextrin, dextrose, fructose, lactic acid, corn alcohol, vegetable gums, sorbitol, vinegar, and popcorn.

➤ **Soy**—Avoid all foods with the following ingredients: soy, lecithin, tofu, textured vegetable protein (TVP), tempeh, modified food starch, soy miso, soy sauce, teriyaki sauce, and soybean flour.

➤ **Nuts**—People who are allergic to peanuts and other types of nuts not only have to avoid the obvious plain nuts and nut butters, but also need to be on the lookout for "hidden" nuts tossed into baked goods, vegetarian dishes, candies, cereals, salads, and chicken stir-fry meals.

➤ **Eggs**—Avoid all foods whose label lists any of the following ingredients: powdered or dry egg, egg white, dried egg yolk, egg substitute, eggnog, albumin, ovalbumin, ovomucin, ovomucoid, vitellin, ovovitellin, livetin, globulin, and ovoglobulin egg albumin.

➤ **Shellfish**—Avoid all shrimp, lobster, prawns, crab, crawfish, crayfish, clams, oysters, scallops, snails, octopus, squid, mussels, and geoducks.

Some people have such severe food allergies that they can even exhibit symptoms after doing the following:

➤ Kissing the lips of someone who has eaten the offending food

➤ Just smelling and inhaling the offending food while it cooks

➤ Coming into contact with utensils that have touched the offending food

Food for Thought

Some people are diagnosed as having allergies to food additives such as sulphites (food preservatives), tartrazine (food colourings), and MSG (flavour enhancer) and therefore must check ingredient labels with extreme care and ask a lot of questions when dining out.

What's the Difference Between Allergy and Intolerance?

The difference lies in how your body handles the offending food. A food allergy affects the body's immune system; a food intolerance generally affects the body's metabolism. In other words, the body cannot properly digest a food or food substance, resulting in "intestinal chaos"—a.k.a. the gurgles (and sometimes a whole lot more).

Food for Thought

Don't confuse a lactose intolerance with a milk allergy. A lactose intolerance involves difficulty digesting the milk sugar *lactose*; a milk allergy involves an allergic reaction from the protein components in cow's milk. People who suffer from milk allergies cannot tolerate reduced-lactose products because the part of the milk they are allergic to (milk proteins) is still present.

What's Lactose Intolerance All About?

If you can't stomach milk and you experience bloating, nausea, cramping, excessive gas, or a bad case of the runs after eating a dairy food, you are not alone. In fact, it's estimated that 70 percent of the world's population suffers from some degree of lactose intolerance, which is the inability to digest the milk sugar *lactose*. I once had a client tell me he visited so many men's rooms while touring through Europe he was ready to write *The Complete Idiot's Guide to European Bathrooms*.

Why can't some people tolerate dairy foods? People who are lactose intolerant are unable to produce enough of the enzyme *lactase*, which is responsible for the digestion of lactose. Just imagine trying to tear down a skyscraper without a bulldozer; it's not going to happen! Just like the bulldozer, lactase must break down, digest, and absorb lactose in the bloodstream. What's more, this type of intolerance affects people at different levels. Whereas one person might dash for the bathroom after just one sip of milk, others can tolerate small amounts of dairy without any problem.

Who generally tends to have a problem digesting milk?

➤ Individuals of certain ethnic origins, including Native Americans, African Americans, Asians, and South Americans, have more difficulty digesting milk.

➤ In rare cases, some people are born unable to produce the enzyme lactase due to a congenital defect.

➤ People with celiac disease, Crohn's disease, colitis, and irritable bowel syndrome often react to dairy products.

➤ Following gastric surgery, people taking chronic antibiotics or anti-inflammatory drugs might also lose their ability (both short-term and long-term) to digest lactose.

➤ People might develop a temporary lactose intolerance during a bout of the flu or a stomach virus, or when suffering from irritable bowel (spastic colon). During these instances, your doctor will probably tell you to avoid all milk and dairy products because the enzyme lactase is easily destroyed when there is any stomach irritation. In these cases, when you recover, you also recover your ability to produce lactase.

Living with a Lactose Intolerance

Food for Thought

For further information and a free brochure on lactose intolerance, call 1-800-LACTAID (1-800-522-8243).

The following tips are helpful for people who have difficulty digesting lactose. As mentioned earlier, the degree of lactose intolerance can vary from person to person; therefore, not everyone will be able to handle all of these suggestions. Give them each a shot, but be sure that you're in a comfortable place if some seem a bit risky. Keep in mind that lactose-containing foods are generally your best sources of the mineral calcium, so children and women with increased calcium requirements should load up on the nondairy sources of calcium and speak with a registered dietitian about the possibility of calcium supplementation.

➤ Carefully look through the list of food ingredients on the label and check for obvious and disguised lactose: milk, cheese, cream, margarine, sour cream, milk solids, milk chocolate, whey, curds, malted milk, and skim-milk solids. Remember that people with severe lactose problems might not be able to tolerate even the small amounts in pancakes, biscuits, cookies, cakes, instant potatoes, salad dressings, sauces, gravies, lunch meats, soups, powdered coffee creamers, and whipped toppings.

➤ Be aware that a lot of over-the-counter medications have added lactose. Speak with your pharmacist if you're not completely sure.

➤ Although most lactose-intolerant people can't gulp down a straight glass of milk, some can tolerate smaller amounts of dairy products combined with other foods. For instance, try a bowl of cereal with fruit and milk, or a slice of pizza with a lot of veggies (easy on the cheese), or a ham sandwich with one slice of cheese.

➤ Many people with a mild or moderate lactose intolerance can tolerate yogurt because the bacteria in the yogurt actually metabolize the milk sugar lactose for you.

➤ Also try cultured buttermilk and sweet acidophilus milk. Some people find them easier to digest than regular milk.

➤ When real ice cream is a taboo, try a nondairy substitute such as Tofutti or Rice Dream.

➤ Stock up on special lactose-reduced products, including Lactaid milk, Lacteeze yogurt, cottage cheese, and regular yogurts.

➤ Try the special tablets and drops that you can add to regular milk; they will break down the lactose in milk almost completely after about 24 hours in the fridge.

➤ Also look for special lactase enzyme pills in your pharmacy that you can swallow *before* eating or drinking a dairy product. These come in handy when you want to eat dairy products.

➤ In severe cases, even the lactose-reduced products might not be tolerated. But don't cheat your body of calcium just because you can't handle milk products. Buy calcium-fortified juice, calcium-fortified soymilk,

Food for Thought

Despite the widespread notion that chocolate, sugar, dairy products, and other fatty foods are responsible for pimples, most dermatologists today rarely identify an underlying relationship between acne and diet.

Nutri-Speak

Gluten intolerance is an intestinal disorder that involves gluten—a protein component of many grains. Gluten is broken down into two parts; gliadin and glutenin. Gliadin is the portion that can be toxic to the small intestines and may result in malabsorption of vital nutrients.

and any other calcium-fortified food products you can get. Note: Definitely speak with your registered dietitian or physician about calcium supplementation.

Celiac Disease: Life Without Wheat, Rye, Barley, Triticale, and Oats

Another food-related condition (less common than lactose intolerance) is *gluten-sensitive enteropathy*, better known as *celiac disease* or *gluten intolerance*. Celiac disease is a chronic disorder found in genetically susceptible individuals who exhibit severe intestinal distress after eating anything made with *gluten*, a protein found in wheat, rye, barley, triticale, and oats. People with this condition must follow a lifelong diet, avoiding all offending foods, or potentially suffer malnourishment from chronic diarrhea and nutrient malabsorption.

As you can imagine, life on this diet is no picnic: A bowl of pasta, a bagel, cereal, crackers, or even a slice of bread can send a celiac sufferer's intestines on a roller coaster ride. Obviously, with the tremendous number of food restrictions involved, members of the Gluten-Free Club should consult with a knowledgeable nutritionist. What's more, become best friends with your local health food store: It's celiac-friendly and will generally carry the specialty items you need.

Food for Thought

For further info on celiac disease, write to: Canadian Celiac Association National Office 190 Britannia Rd. East, Unit 11, Mississauga, Ontario L4Z 1W6 1-800-363-7296 www.celiac.ca

For further reading on life without gluten or wheat, order these publications, which are available from the Canadian Celiac Association:

Celiac Disease Needs a Diet for Life, 3rd edition, The handbook for celiacs and their families

Growing Up as a Celiac A handbook specifically designed for the celiac child

Pocket Dictionary—Acceptability of Foods and Food Ingredients for the Gluten-Free Diet

Irritable Bowel Syndrome

Although not completely understood, irritable bowel syndrome (IBS) seems to be more common these days than the sniffles. With symptoms ranging from excessive gas, cramping, and bloating to intermittent bouts of constipation and diarrhea, IBS (also called spastic colon) usually has nothing to do with food allergies or intolerances. It's more likely a functional problem with the muscular movement of your intestines, and generally is diagnosed when the serious gastrointestinal ailments are ruled out. Some doctors say that anxious or nervous people can even bring it on themselves.

Dietary treatments that can help alleviate the symptoms of IBS include eating slowly, increasing your fibre intake gradually, drinking more water, reducing your caffeine intake, and avoiding greasy foods. You might also want to keep a food log for a week or two to see whether any particular foods exacerbate the symptoms. (Common culprits include alcohol, tobacco, caffeine, fatty foods, milk, beans, sorbitol, spicy foods, and cruciferous veggies such as cauliflower, cabbage, and broccoli.) See whether there's a correlation between your work schedule and the days you're feeling bad; some people find that the symptoms improve on the weekends when they're relaxing.

You can also try alternative remedies such as taking enteric-coated capsules of peppermint oil three times a day between meals (skip this one if you have heartburn), or explore yoga, meditation, or hypnosis to lessen stress and anxiety, which can sometimes wind up in your gut. Women who notice IBS flare-ups around the time of menstruation should speak to a qualified nutritionist about managing your diet and supplements around your menstrual cycle.

For the Caffeine Sensitive

Some people are extremely sensitive to caffeine; it makes them dizzy, shaky, and sometimes nauseated. Here's a list of some beverages and foods to watch out for:

Food/Beverage	Caffeine (in Milligrams)
Coffee (5 oz/156 mL)	
Drip	110–150
Percolated	40–170
Decaffeinated	2–5
Freeze-dried instant	40–108
Decaffeinated	2–3
Tea (bags or loose, 5 oz/156 mL)	
1-minute brew	9–33
3-minute brew	20–46
5-minute brew	20–50
Iced tea (12 oz/375 mL)	22–36

Food/Beverage	Caffeine (in Milligrams)
Chocolate Items	
Hot cocoa (5 oz/156 mL)	2–15
Dry cocoa (1 oz/30 g)	6
Chocolate milk	8
Milk chocolate (1 oz/30 g)	15
Baker's chocolate (1 oz/30 g)	25
Soft Drinks (12 oz/375 mL)	
Diet and regular	35–60
Caffeine free	0

If you think you may be suffering from a food sensitivity or intolerance, check it out. Keep a detailed food log for a week and include everything you eat and drink—you may even want to include the times of day that you are eating and drinking. Pay close attention to your body's reaction and see if you can find any correlation with a single food (like bell peppers, oranges, beans) or an entire food group (like milk, yogurt, and cheese). Meet with a registered dietitian who can help you determine the foods that are aggravating your system.

The Least You Need to Know

➤ A food allergy occurs when your body misinterprets a harmless food as an intruder and produces antibodies to fight off the foreign substance.

➤ A food allergy affects the immune system, whereas a food intolerance generally affects only the digestive system.

➤ Lactose intolerance is the inability to produce enough of the enzyme *lactase*, which is responsible for digesting the milk sugar *lactose*. Symptoms include bloating, cramping, gas, diarrhea, and nausea.

➤ Celiac disease is a condition that causes severe malabsorption after ingesting the protein gluten, which is found in wheat, rye, oats, triticale, and barley.

➤ Irritable bowel syndrome is a functional problem with the muscular movement of the intestines, resulting in intermittent bouts of constipation, diarrhea, bloating, and gas.

Chapter 21

Herbal Remedies

In This Chapter

➤ What herbal medicine is all about

➤ Alternative therapies for a variety of ailments

➤ The scoop on how much to take—and how often

Herbal remedies were once considered strange, something used only by so-called witch doctors. Now, botanical supplements are moving into the mainstream, and even traditional MDs are learning how to take the alternative route.

Although extensive research on herbal medicine has been done, you should always be wary about taking herbal remedies. Do your homework, know your manufacturers, and read the bottles carefully; some of the herbal remedies out there have not been proven to be safe and effective, and it isn't easy to track problems related to herbal products. If you're looking for an alternative way to relieve a particular ailment, go ahead and learn about herbal supplements. Just tell your physician and pharmacist what you're taking, especially if you're on other medication. Be safe and don't combine several remedies at the same time (which could lead to serious side effects), and never use them when you're pregnant or planning to become pregnant.

This chapter provides the lowdown on popular herbs that have been shown to do some pretty impressive things. Read on to see if one of them might be right for you.

Judging the Quality of Herbal Products

It can be quite overwhelming to choose a particular herb—all those bottles tend to look alike in the health food store, vitamin shop, pharmacy, and grocery store. And although herbs have properties that can affect our bodies' internal functions, there are no regulations on herbal supplements within Canada to date. In fact, this lack of regulation means that different manufacturers use different measures of active ingredient per dose, and some may be unreliable. Here is a list of brand manufacturers (Canadian, American, and European) that you can trust; they probably produce many or all of the herbal supplements discussed in the chapter.

- ➤ Quest Vitamins (Boehringer Ingelheim)
- ➤ Natural Factors
- ➤ Sisu
- ➤ Life Brand (Shopper's Drug Mart)
- ➤ Gaia (primarily tinctures)
- ➤ Nature's Way
- ➤ Pharmaton

If you are seriously interested in the herbal world, find a herb-friendly health professional. You can call the Canadian Herb Society at 604-734-8455 for a list of professional practitioners in your area.

Q & A

Since they are natural, are all herbs safe?

In most circumstances, most herbs can be quite safe if taken as directed. However, because herbs can have medicinal abilities, you should never take them indiscriminately. Read labels closely, follow dosage directions, and discontinue using a herb if you experience any uncomfortable side effects such as throat irritation, upset stomach, diarrhea, and headaches. Also, some people may even experience an allergic reaction to a particular herb.

For Female Health

Over the centuries, many herbal products have been created for the special needs and health concerns of women. This section will cover valerian root, black cohosh, and evening primrose oil.

Valerian Root

Use: Three decades of extensive research have shown that valerian root (*valeriana officinalis*) is like a minor tranquilizer. It is known as a sleeping aid, and it might be useful for treating insomnia and mild anxiety and restlessness, lowering blood pressure, and reducing the negative symptoms of menstruation and menopause. To date, it has not been proven to be habit forming.

Dosage: Tea, *tincture*, or a standardized extract; it can also be added to bath water for external application. Relatively large amounts are required for effectiveness, typically about 50 to 100 drops or 1 teaspoon (5 mL) of dried root for tea. Take one hour before bed. Beware: valerian root has a horrible odour, so you might want to invest in the standardized tablet or capsule version (400–600 mg standardized to contain 0.8 percent valerenic acid). It's not safe for long-term use, and it has no effect with alcohol but might intensify the effect of sedatives.

Standardized extracts are capsules or tablets that contain a concentrated amount of herb. These solid extracts are formulated to contain a set, guaranteed dose of the herb's active ingredient. The advantage of using a standardized extract is that you can be sure you're getting a product with the plant's healing ingredients. The disadvantage is that they are expensive.

Nutri-Speak

A **tincture** is a liquid extract that that contains a combination of ethyl alcohol and water as the solvent. The advantages of using tinctures are that they have an increased shelf life and they do not have to be refrigerated (fresh herbs do!). The disadvantages are that they contain alcohol, which is a problem for people who abstain from it and for children, and they do not taste pleasant. You can buy tinctures that are alcohol free—a great choice for kids!

Black Cohosh

Use: Many women take this herb to relieve symptoms of menopause, and it's especially popular in Europe. Clinical studies have found black cohosh to be as effective as estrogen pills at reducing hot flashes. It suppresses the leutinizing hormone and therefore helps control hormone surges that cause discomforting menopausal symptoms. Relieving physical symptoms can improve emotional symptoms.

Dosage: As a tincture, 10–60 drops; as tea, 1–2 grams; as a standardized extract, 40 milligrams (standardized to contain 2.5 percent triterpene glycosides and 1 milligram of 27-deoxyacteine) twice daily. Black cohosh may cause stomach upset and headache. Note: This herb is safe for women with a history of breast cancer, and can be used for longer than six months.

Evening Primrose Oil

Use: It is a natural source of an unusual fatty acid called gamma-linolenic acid (GLA), which occurs in only a few other plants such as borage and black currant. Evening

Nutri-Speak

Prostaglandins are hormone-like compounds that were first discovered in the prostate gland (*prosto*-glandins). Abnormal secretions of these compounds are thought to contribute to PMS (premenstrual syndrome).

Premenstrual syndrome is a cluster of symptoms, including both physical and emotional pain, that some women experience before and during the onset of menstruation.

primrose oil modifies the synthesis of a group of hormones called *prostaglandins*, which are believed to be involved in a variety of PMS symptoms and are the target of anti-inflammatory drugs such as Advil or Motrin. In simple terms, you can use this oil to help relieve debilitating PMS symptoms, as well as arthritis pains and auto-immune diseases. It's also a great anti-inflammatory, and it promotes healthy growth of hair, skin, and nails.

For Male Health

Like women, men can also benefit from herbs that target their special needs. Although men do not commonly buy and take herbs as often as women, men are doing so more and more. Here are some herbs that are of particular interest to men.

Dosage: The recommended dose is one 500-milligram capsule twice daily; it takes six to eight weeks before you see results.

Saw Palmetto

Use: This herb is used to treat BPH (*benign prostatic hyperplasia*), that is, enlarged prostate. Saw palmetto reduces the size of the prostate and has a diuretic property. It might also stimulate the appetite and enhance the sex drive.

Dosage: The recommended dose is 160 milligrams twice daily of an extract standardized for 85–95 percent fatty acids and sterols. The herb is generally well tolerated and it has not been shown to cause toxicity.

Pygeum Africanum and Stinging Nettle

Use: Like saw palmetto, these two herbs are combined to treat the symptoms of BPH. *Pygeum africanum* is an African evergreen tree whose bark has been used to treat prostate disorders in Europe since the 1980s. It appears to be even more effective when combined with stinging nettle.

Dosage: The recommended dose is 25 milligrams of a standardized extract of pygeum africanum with 300 milligrams of stinging nettle root and 25 milligrams of stinging nettle bark once daily. In Canada, this herbal combination is sold as "Prostatonin."

Yohimbe

Use: This aphrodisiac dilates blood vessels of the skin and mucous membranes (including those of the sexual organs). It is a monoamine oxidase inhibitor, which means that you should strictly avoid nasal decongestants, foods containing tyramine (such as liver, cheese, and red wine), and certain diet aids containing phenylpropanolamine. The drug should not be taken by anyone suffering from hypotension (low blood pressure), hypertension (high blood pressure), diabetes, or heart, liver, or kidney diseases. The effectiveness of this herb/drug has not yet been proven, and in the United States, it has been declared unsafe and is unavailable. If you really want to make it a part of your daily intake, you might need to trek to Germany; it's available in every sex shop!

Dosage: Usually administered in 5.4-milligram doses, yohimbe is available as a prescription drug in many combinations with other so-called sexual stimulants such as strychnine, thyroid, and methyltestosterone.

For Depression, Sleeping, and Aging

Are you feeling restless, tense, or depressed, or having trouble sleeping at night? Or maybe you simply want to defy some of the signs of aging. Read on—this section examines six herbs that may be worth a try: gingko biloba, St. John's wort, kava-kava, Asian ginseng, and chamomile.

Food for Thought

A few drops of lavender oil in the bath can help you to relax. In fact, some say that after massaging your body with the lavender–bath water, you are more apt to have a sound sleep.

Gingko Biloba

Use: Derived from the gingko tree, which originated in China 200 million years ago, gingko biloba has been used for centuries as a digestive aid. Tests have shown that it thins the blood and therefore increases circulation in the brain and extremities, making it good for enhancing the memory and easing symptoms of age-related cognitive decline and early-stage dementia. It may also keep us sharp by acting as an antioxidant and protecting brain cells from free-radical damage. One recent study showed that it slowed the progression of Alzheimer's disease in 27 percent of participants.

Dosage: Large doses are required, which explains why a concentrate is used rather than the herb itself. The typical dose of a standardized extract is 40 milligrams three times daily. If you take blood thinners, let your doctor know you're taking gingko (it can intensify their action and cause serious problems), and look for the standardized leaf extract, containing 24 percent flavone and 6 percent terpenes. (It is available as a tincture, capsules, or tablets.)

St. John's Wort

Use: This herb can be used to treat mild to moderate depression and seasonal affective disorder. Hypericin and hyperforin are the active ingredients, which aid in serotonin re-uptake inhibition in the brain. Although this might be one of the most popular and widely used herbs, its action as an antidepressant is not yet fully understood. Therefore, it is not a miracle drug or something that should be used indiscriminately.

Dosage: The dosage is based on the hypericin and hyperforin concentration in the extract. The recommended dose is 300 milligrams of dried leaf and flower extract standardized to 0.3 percent hypericin and 3 percent hyperforin three times per day; 40–80 drops of tincture three times per day; one or two cups of tea in the morning and evening made with 1–2 heaping teaspoons (5–10 mL) dried herb per cup. It might take several weeks for the effects to kick in. Do not use this herb at the same time as prescription antidepressants. Note: Using St. John's wort might cause photosensitivity in those with particularly fair skin.

Kava-Kava

Use: This herb relieves anxiety, tension, restlessness, stress, and insomnia. The relaxing properties of kava-kava are related to kavalactones, the primary active ingredient. High-quality kava-kava contains 5.5–8.3 percent of these compounds, which create changes in the brain activity that are similar to the effects of anti-anxiety drugs but without their sedative or hypnotic effect.

Dosage: The recommended dose is 100–200 milligrams divided over two or three doses. (Look for standardized extracts of 30 percent kavalactones.) Long-term consumption of very large doses (more than 9 g/day) might turn the skin and nails yellow temporarily. This herb should not be taken with drugs that act on the central nervous system, such as alcohol, benzodiazepines, antidepressants, and barbiturates. Rare side effects include mild gastrointestinal disturbances.

Asian Ginseng (a.k.a. Panax, Korean or Chinese)

Use: Ginseng is used for supporting health; it alleviates fatigue or stress, enhances cognitive function and physical endurance, and aids in resistance to disease. It is widely used by athletes because of its potential to improve aerobic capacity and recovery time following exertion. Ginseng contains panaxosides, which have been shown to exert a hypoglycemic effect and are being studied in the treatment of diabetes.

Dosage: The recommended dose is 100 milligrams once or twice a day, usually used over a two- to three-week period, followed by one to two weeks of "rest" before resuming. In rare cases, ginseng can cause overstimulation, and hence insomnia, and it is not recommended during pregnancy and lactation or for those with high blood pressure. Long-term use might cause menstrual abnormalities and breast tenderness in women.

Chamomile

Use: This herb is known as a "cure-all," like homemade chicken soup. It's a cornerstone of European and North American herbal medicine that has been used to treat irritable bowel syndrome, infant colic, mouth sores, anxiety, insomnia, menstrual cramps, and digestive problems.

Dosage: Because much of the value of the plant lies in its volatile oil, it is unfortunate that even a strong tea, properly prepared in a covered vessel and steeped for a long time, contains only about 10 to 15 percent of the oil originally present in the plant material. Whole extracts of the drug or preparations containing high quantities of the oil are more effective but are generally not marketed in Canada. Boiling water is poured over a heaping tablespoon (15 mL) of dried flowers and strained after 10–15 minutes. You can drink it three to four times daily between meals. It might cause an allergic reaction in those with allergies to similar plants such as ragweed.

Heart Disease

Heart disease remains a leading cause of death in both men and women. The following section provides information on two herbs that may help to fight heart disease; garlic and hawthorn.

Garlic

Use: Garlic contains allyl sulphides, which lower both cholesterol levels and blood pressure. There is evidence that garlic inhibits platelet aggregation (thins the blood) and may therefore help prevent blood clots. It also has an overall positive effect on the cardiovascular system, and, according to many researchers, garlic stimulates the immune system, hence possibly preventing cancer (in particular stomach and colon cancer) by hindering the growth of malignant cells.

Dosage: For therapeutic purposes, chew one-half to one fresh clove daily. (For *breath* purposes, you might want to follow it up with an Altoid, one of those "curiously strong mints!") There are also aged garlic extract supplements, which contain a large amount of protective allyl sulphides; take 300–600 milligrams one to three times daily. Consumption of large quantities of raw or supplemental garlic can result in excessive blood thinning, heartburn, flatulence, and related gastrointestinal problems.

Hawthorn

Use: Hawthorne is taken for cardiovascular ailments, including high blood pressure, hardening of the arteries, and angina, and, potentially, during early stages of congestive heart failure. It is not suitabe for acute attacks because its action is slow. This herb dilates the blood vessels, especially the coronary vessels, reducing peripheral resistance and thus lowering the blood pressure. It has a direct effect on the heart itself, which is especially noticeable in cases of heart damage.

Dosage: The recommended dose is 160 milligrams dried leaves and flowers (higher doses should only be used under strict medical supervision) or 20–40 drops of tincture three times daily.

Liver Disease

The liver is one of the major organs that is affected by alcohol and pharmaceutical drugs. This section reviews milk thistle—an impressive herb that has been shown to protect and regenerate the liver.

Milk Thistle

Use: Milk thistle is taken for chronic inflammatory liver disease, such as cirrhosis and hepatitis, as well as for more acute conditions such as toxic liver damage. Milk thistle protects healthy liver cells or cells that are not yet damaged by the entry of toxic substances.

Dosage: Insoluble in water, milk thistle is ineffective if taken as a tea. (Studies show that less than 10 percent of the active ingredient is available in this form.) Use seed extracts standardized to at least 70 percent silymarin (the antihepatotoxic principle). The suggested daily dose is 200 milligrams of concentrated extract three times daily in the treatment of liver disease, representing 140 milligrams of silymarin per capsule (in total, 420 mg daily). You can use one 200-milligram dose as part of a cleansing/detoxification program. It might have mild laxative effects in some people.

Respiratory Ailments

One of the top-selling herbs in Canada, echinacea has become an everyday household name. This section will run through everything you'll need to know, from fighting colds and flu to treating ear infections.

Echinacea

Use: Echinacea is popular for the prevention and treatment of the common cold and flu and adjunctive treatment in recent infections (such as those of the middle ear, respiratory tract, urinary tract, and vaginal candidiasis). It is also an immunity booster. The myth that it's more effective with goldenseal is not true.

Dosage: The recommended dose is 15–30 drops of tincture up to five times a day at the onset of cold symptoms and continued for least 10–14 days after. Or, buy capsules standardized to 4 percent echinsacosides and take 250–500 milligrams up to five times a day. The dosage varies, however, with the potency of the product—so read the product label. Teas are not recommended because some of the active ingredients are not soluble in water. If you use echinacea to prevent a cold, take it three times daily for six to eight weeks. A "rest" period is recommended after eight weeks because the effects of this herb might diminish if it is used for longer periods. Caution: Do not take echinacea if you have an auto-immune disease (MS, HIV, lupus) or if you are allergic to plants in the daisy family (such as ragweed).

Arthritis

Arthritis involves the painful inflammation of joints, and can be caused by various conditions. If you are suffering from a form of arthritis, you may want to try one of these two supplements: boswella and glucosamine sulphate with chondroiten. Of course, before you pop any pill, check with your physician, especially if you are already taking other medication.

Boswella

Use: Boswella is intended for the treatment of rheumatoid arthritis and osteoarthritis. It is a nonsteroidal, anti-inflammatory agent that improves mobility and decreases joint pain and stiffness. At this point, it is still unclear whether long-term effects will reduce joint destruction.

Dosage: The recommended dose is 150 milligrams three times per day, for 8–12 weeks.

Glucosamine Sulphate with Chondroiten

Although this supplement is *not* herbal, it's still considered to be an alternative remedy and is definitely worth mentioning in this chapter.

Use: The combination of glucosamine sulphate with chondroiten is shown to slow and eventually eliminate the pain of osteoarthritis in many patients. In fact, it's estimated that up to 40 percent of osteoarthritis sufferers might see marked improvement after taking this supplement for approximately six weeks.

Glucosamine stimulates the production of collagen, which is the protein portion of a fibrous substance that holds the joints together, as well as being the main shock-absorbing substance that acts as a cushion between our joints. Hence, glucosamine helps the body repair damaged cartilage and eases the pain of osteoarthritis. It also has an anti-inflammatory effect that eases joint pain.

Chondroiten sulphates act as "liquid magnets," helping to attract fluid to the cartilage, which acts as a buffer. Chondroiten might also protect existing cartilage from premature breakdown by inhibiting certain enzymes that can destroy the cartilage.

Dosage: 1,500 milligrams per day of glucosamine and 1,200 milligrams per day of chondroiten. These amounts are divided into three doses. Note: The initial dosage should be adjusted according to your weight, and you should speak with your rheumatologist about adjusting the dosage when you are ready for a maintenance level.

Migraines

Migraines are characterized by severe head pain, plus one or more of a range of symptoms including nausea, vomiting, and sensitivity to light. A migraine attack can last up to 72 hours and leave a person completely immobile. This sections provides information about feverfew, a herb that may help alleviate these debilitating headaches.

Feverfew

Use: This herb inhibits platelet aggregation and also helps prevent the blood vessels from constricting. The result is a reduction in severity, duration, and frequency of migraines and an improvement in blood-vessel tone.

Dosage: The recommended dose is 125 milligrams of dried authentic feverfew leaf, containing a minimum of 0.2 percent of panthenolide, taken over a period of four to six weeks. The most common side effect is mouth ulceration, predominantly found in those who chew the leaves. (This herb should not be used by children.)

Cancer

The incidence of cancer is quite low in Asian countries. Therefore, scientists constantly conduct research to investigate which cultural practices in these countries may help ward off this terrible illness. This section will provide you with some exciting news about green tea, which was also discussed in Chapter 18, "Diet and Cancer."

Chinese Green Tea

Use: Green tea has cancer-fighting properties that inhibit the interaction of tumour promoters, hormones, and growth factors with their receptors, in effect sealing off the tumour and preventing it from growing.

Dosage: The more tea you drink, the better. It's nontoxic, but watch out for the caffeine (a cup has 25 mg—a fraction of that found in coffee).

More Herbal Remedies Worth Mentioning

Yes, there are even more herbs to talk about. Find out how ginger can settle your stomach, bilberry can help your eyes, rosemary can get your blood pumping, peppermint can aid in indigestion, and aloe can heal your wounds.

Ginger

Use: Ginger might relieve motion sickness, nausea from morning sickness, and indigestion or an upset stomach. It has an overall calming effect on the digestive system because it increases the secretion of digestive juices, including saliva, neutralizing stomach acids, and toxins.

Dosage: Take capsules containing 500 milligrams of the powdered herb; the total daily dose should not exceed 1,000 milligrams. Ginger can also be consumed in the form of a tea or as candied ginger. Take 1,000 milligrams 30 minutes before travelling for motion sickness; two cups of tea using 1 teaspoon (5 mL) of fresh root or $1^1/_2$ teaspoons (7 mL) of powdered root per cup; or two 1-inch (0.5 cm) squares of candied ginger.

Bilberry

Use: Bilberry is useful for treating retinopathy and preventing age-related cataracts and macular degeneration, as well as for treating peripheral vascular disease, varicose veins, and hemorrhoids. Bilberry promotes the formation of normal connective tissue and protects from damage secondary to inflammation.

Dosage: Extract standardized to 25 percent anthocyanoside content is recommended at a daily dose of 480–600 milligrams in two to three doses, which may be reduced to a maintenance dose of 240 milligrams per day. The lower dose can be used by those interested in the prevention of eye or circulation disorders.

Rosemary

Use: Rosemary is not just for putting on roast chicken—this herb will spice up your entire circulatory system! Recommended for its tonic, astringent, and diaphoretic effects (it increases perspiration), rosemary is said to aid in digestion and can be made into a hair tonic that will prevent baldness. It is also great for those with low blood pressure and can be used to stimulate menstruation.

Dosage: Infuse rosemary in tea, wine, a spirit, or a bath. Large quantities of the oil are needed for therapeutic purposes, and it's not safe when taken internally. (It can irritate the stomach, intestines, and kidneys.)

Peppermint

Use: Peppermint has served as a treatment for indigestion, flatulence, colic, and even menstrual cramping. Menthol, the active ingredient, can aid in digestion because it reduces tonus of the lower esophageal sphincter and facilitates belching, which brings relief.

Dosage: Drink several cups of tea prepared from the leaves. To relieve spasms of irritable bowel syndrome, take one enteric-coated peppermint oil capsule before meals.

Aloe

Aloe is used to make two products that are completely different in terms of usage and chemical composition.

Aloe vera gel or mucilage is a thin, clear jelly—like substance that is used externally to treat wounds and sunburn. Although there is controversy about whether aloe gel retains its properties in preparation, fluid from a fresh leaf has been shown to promote attachment and growth of normal human cells. This type of aloe is recommended for healing external wounds.

Aloe latex or juice is quite different. In fact, it acts as a laxative and is clearly not recommended.

...And Stay Away from These!

The following herbs might appear in over-the-counter products. Read labels and stay away from these products; they have been shown to be dangerous!

Ephedra/Ma Huang

Use: This herb has been taken to relieve constriction and congestion associated with bronchial asthma. It is also used as a nasal decongestant, to treat certain allergies, and to promote weight loss.

The real story is that ephedra increases both systolic and diastolic blood pressure as well as the heart rate, which causes palpitations, nervousness, headaches, insomnia, and dizziness. Using ephedra can be harmful and life threatening—especially for those who suffer from heart conditions, hypertension, diabetes, and thyroid disease.

Dong Quai

Use: Some women have taken this herb to treat gynecological complaints, such as irregular periods and menopausal symptoms.

The real story is that dong quai can negatively affect blood pressure, heart rhythm, and respiration.

Using herbs can be a convenient way to alleviate everything from headaches to upset stomachs. Use this chapter as a reference guide, and look things up when you are searching for a remedy to a particular ache or ailment. Once again, I cannot stress the importance of checking things out with your health care practitioner, especially if you are taking medication or have a serious illness.

The Least You Need to Know

➤ In the last decade, herbal remedies have become popular treatments for a variety of ailments. If you want to get into herbal culture, do it slowly, get expert advice, and monitor your body as you go along.

➤ Never indulge in herbal remedies when you're pregnant, planning to become pregnant, or lactating.

➤ Always consult with a physician or pharmacist before using herbs, especially if you're already taking other prescription drugs.

➤ Do some research: Know your manufacturers, be aware of what you're taking, read the bottle labels, and follow the instructions carefully. Adverse reactions are not uncommon.

➤ Avoid using products with ephedra (ma huang); it can negatively affect blood pressure and heart rate.

Part 5

Pregnancy and Parenting

Let the cravings begin! Being pregnant is both exciting and overwhelming, and the importance of good nutrition for mothers-to-be has been stressed over and over again. What's more, today most health experts also encourage exercise, which can help keep moms feeling more fit and mobile during their nine months of growing girth. Read on; in this section, I provide a lot of essential information that will help to manage your and your child's health.

Part 5 is also dedicated to the younger folks. I certainly understand that sometimes it can be quite a challenge to get your kids to eat healthy. If we could only mould carrots and bananas into log shapes and pop a "Snickers" wrapper on top, life would be so much simpler. In this section, I'll offer creative suggestions for sneaking veggies into meals and making lower fat after-school snacks, and provide tips to help you encourage your kids to be more physically active.

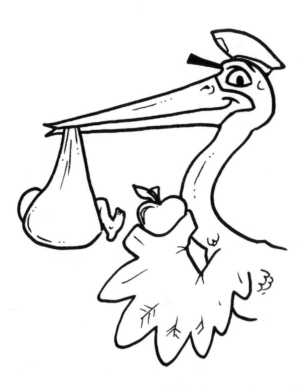

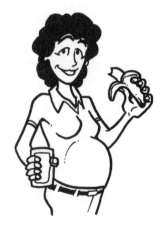

Chapter 22

Eating Your Way Through Pregnancy

In This Chapter

➤ Eating for a healthy pregnancy

➤ How much weight should you gain?

➤ Boosting your intake of protein, dairy products, iron, and fluids

➤ Strategies to reduce constipation, nausea, heartburn, and water retention

➤ A comprehensive five-day meal plan—with recipes and nutritional information

---

Yippee, you're pregnant—congratulations on your exciting news! This chapter provides all the info you'll need to nourish yourself and your growing baby properly.

Are You Really Eating for Two?

Has anyone ever said, "Go ahead and pack it in; you're eating for two"? Well, that's both true and false. *True* because your food selections will directly affect your growing baby. In other words, eat plenty of quality foods loaded with nutrients, and you'll shower that growing bambino with all the right ingredients. If you miss out on nutrients, your baby misses out too!

On the other hand, this statement is also *false* because you're clearly *not* eating for two adults. In fact, your growing baby is only a fraction of your size, so it's not the time to win a gold medal in the food Olympics.

Increased Calories and Protein

It's true that you do require more calories. In fact, over the course of your pregnancy, you'll need to consume about an extra 63,000 calories. Obviously, this caloric increase

Food for Thought

You don't need to gain that much weight during the first trimester of your pregnancy. In fact, aim for a total weight gain of 3–5 pounds (1.4–2.3 kg).

is spread out over nine months: It amounts to approximately 100 extra calories a day during the first trimester (the first three months) and around 300 extra calories a day during the second and third trimesters (the last six months).

For the first, second and third trimester, you'll also need an additional 5, 20, and 24 grams of protein respectively within those extra calories. Your daily requirement goes from 44 to 68 grams when you're pregnant, for the development of your precious fetus. Getting this increased protein is typically not a problem. Most women already overshoot their needs, and consuming extra dairy products and larger servings of lean meat, fish, poultry, eggs, and legumes will ensure that you get enough. For a more detailed description of how much protein you'll need, see the section "Adjusting Your Eating Plan" later in this chapter.

A Weighty Issue: How Much Weight Should You Gain?

It seems like the first thing people ask when you return from your doctor's office is "How much weight did you gain?" None of their business! Understand that all women are different, and the rate and speed of weight gain will vary from person to person. Some women gain a lot in the second trimester, and then weight gain slows down drastically in the third, whereas others gain weight evenly throughout their pregnancy. Here's what's recommended for most healthy women:

Pre-Pregnancy Weight	Suggested Gain	Weekly Gain in Second and Third Trimester
Underweight	28–40 pounds (12.7–18.0 kg)	> 1 pound (> 0.5 kg)
Normal, healthy weight	25–35 pounds (11.4–16.0 kg)	0.8–1.0 pound (0.4–0.5 kg)
Overweight	15–25 pounds (6.8–11.4 kg)	0.7 pound (0.3 kg)
Obese	15–20 pounds (6.8–9.0 kg)	0.5 pound (0.2 kg)

Understand that there are special circumstances in which some women will need to gain more, some less. For instance, women carrying twins will need to gain about 35–45 pounds (16–20 kg), and although women with triplets almost never carry full term, (they typically deliver around 33 weeks) if they did, they would need to gain about 50–70 pounds (23–32 kg) and hire three full-time nannies and a massage therapist. Speak with your doctor and listen to his or her advice on this weighty issue.

Q & A

Where does the extra weight go?

Baby: 7–8 pounds (3.5 kg)

Placenta: 1–2 pounds (0.5–0.9 kg)

Amniotic fluid: 1 1/2–2 pounds (0.7–0.9 kg)

Uterine tissue: 2 pounds (0.9 kg)

Breast tissue: 1–2 pounds (0.5–0.9 kg)

Fluid volume: 6–10 pounds (2.7–4.5 kg)

Fat: 6+ pounds (2.7+ kg)

Total: 25–35 pounds (11.4–16.0 kg)

Adjusting Your Eating Plan

Let's ensure that you're gaining weight by eating the proper foods. Remember those four friendly food groups that have haunted you since page 1? *They're baa-ack.* Although women's individual requirements vary depending on caloric needs, the following chart gives some guidance in determining the basics of your diet:

Food Group	Daily Servings	Sample Servings
Grain Products	6+	1 slice bread, or
		1/2 small bagel, or
		1 serving cereal, or
		1/2 cup (125 mL) cooked rice or pasta
Fruits	3+	1 medium fruit, or
		1 cup (250 mL) berries or melon, or
		1/2 cup (125 mL) fruit juice

Food Group	Daily Servings	Sample Servings
Vegetables	3+	1 cup (250 mL) raw leafy veggies, or $^1/_2$ cup (125 mL) cooked veggies
Milk Products	3–4	1 cup (250 mL) milk, or 1 cup (250 mL) yogurt, or $^3/_4$ cup (175 mL) cottage cheese, or $1^1/_2$ ounces (45 g) hard cheese
Meat/poultry/ fish/beans/eggs/ nuts	2–3	2–3 ounces (60–90 g) lean meat, or 2 eggs , or $^2/_3$ cup (165 mL) tofu, or 2–3 ounces (60–90 g) fish or poultry
Fluids	8+	8 ounces (250 mL) water, seltzer water, and other beverages
Other foods (fats, sweets)	Moderation	Try your best to keep these foods to a minimum.

Overrated-Undercooked

Don't think, "Great, I'm pregnant; I can eat *whatever* and *whenever* I want!" With pregnancy come increased caloric and nutrient requirements, but you can meet these needs without putting on 20 pounds of flab. Don't deprive yourself of satisfying your cravings; that's one of the fun things about pregnancy. Just don't go overboard. Extra weight gained during your pregnancy is extra weight you'll be wearing *after* the baby is born.

Why All the Hype About Calcium?

Although calcium is needed throughout life, it is particularly important during pregnancy. (At last, you finally learn why everyone pesters you to drink your milk.) Your daily requirement remains at 1,000 milligrams, but some experts recommend up to 1,500 milligrams. That's approximately 3–4 servings of dairy products, for example, 1 cup (250 mL) milk + 1 cup (250 mL) pudding + 1 cup (250 mL) fruit yogurt + $1^1/_2$ ounces (45 g) hard cheese.

As you learned in Chapter 8, "Mighty Minerals: Calcium and Iron," calcium is responsible for strong bones and teeth and for the proper functioning of blood vessels, nerves, and muscles, as well as for maintaining healthy connective tissue. During pregnancy, calcium is especially critical because you have to worry about your own bones *and* your growing baby's bones, tissues, and teeth. In fact, your baby counts on *your* calcium for normal development; therefore, when you skimp on the calcium-rich foods (and don't take supplements), the calcium in your bones will be used to meet the increaseing demands of the growing fetus. In other words, you'll be placing yourself at a much greater risk for osteoporosis. See Chapter 8 for the calcium content of various foods, both dairy and nondairy.

Hiking Up the Iron

Ever wonder why the prenatal vitamins are loaded with iron? It's because during pregnancy, your body requires about double the usual amount of this mineral. In fact, when you're expecting you go from needing 13 milligrams to requiring a daily dose of 23 milligrams.

Why do pregnant women require more iron? Remember, iron is found in your blood and is responsible for carrying and delivering oxygen to every cell in your body. Pregnant women have an *expanded* blood volume, so it makes sense that more blood requires more iron. Also, you have to supply oxygen to both your cells *and* the cells of your growing baby. Once again, this greater demand for oxygen requires greater amounts of iron.

Because nursing your baby *also* requires an increase in a variety of nutrients, nursing women will also benefit from following the same general eating guidelines discussed in this chapter. Take a look:

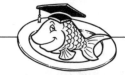

Food for Thought

Pregnant women with lactose intolerance should eat plenty of *nondairy* calcium-fortified foods, along with special lactose-reduced products. Also, speak with your dietitian about calcium supplementation. (For further information on lactose intolerance, see Chapter 20, "Food Allergies and Other Ailments.")

Q & A

Won't the prenatal vitamins cover all the calcium my baby will need?

Definitely not! Prenatal supplements supply about 200–250 milligrams per pill; that doesn't even equal 1 serving from the milk group.

	Before	Pregnant	Lactating
Calories		+300	+500
Protein (g)	44	68	68
Calcium (mg)	1,000	1,000	1,000
Folic acid (mg)	400	600	500
Iron (mg)	13	23	13

These requirements are for healthy women age 19–50 years of age.

Just because the prenatal vitamins are brimming with the stuff, don't think you can slack off in the food department. Understand that prenatal supplements (providing around 30–60 milligrams) are merely "just in case"—you still need to eat a lot of iron-rich foods. On the eating plan, you require 2–3 servings of protein foods each day. This will help satisfy your body's extra demand for *both* protein and iron because the best absorbable iron is found in the foods within this group. For further tips on boosting your iron, flip back to Chapter 8.

➤ **Best sources of heme iron**—Animal foods such as liver, beef, pork, lamb, veal, chicken, turkey, and eggs

➤ **Good sources of nonheme iron**—Non-animal foods such as enriched breads and cereals, beans, dried fruits, seeds, nuts, broccoli, spinach, collard greens, broccoli, barley, chickpeas, and blackstrap molasses

Blast Your Baby with Vitamins!

During pregnancy you want to provide your growing baby with plenty of nutrients, including the antioxidants vitamin C and beta-carotene. Read on and learn which fruits and vegetables supply the biggest bang for your buck.

➤ **Fruits rich in vitamin C**—Oranges, grapefruit, mango, strawberries, papaya, raspberries, tangerines, kiwi, cantaloupe, guava, lemons, orange juice, grapefruit juice, and other vitamin-C-fortified juices

➤ **Vegetables rich in vitamin C**—Broccoli, tomatoes, sweet potato, pepper, kale, cabbage, Brussels sprouts, rutabaga, cauliflower, and spinach

➤ **Fruits rich in beta-carotene**—Apricots, cantaloupe, papaya, mango, prunes, peaches, nectarines, tangerines, watermelon, and guava

➤ **Vegetables rich in beta-carotene**—Broccoli, Brussels sprouts, carrots, collard greens, escarole, dark green lettuce, spinach, sweet potato, kale, butternut squash, chicory, red pepper, and tomato juice

Keep on Guzzlin' Those Fluids!

Proper hydration is another vital necessity for a healthy pregnancy. Did you know that the average female is about 55–65 percent water, and the average newborn is about 85 percent water? During this nine-month period of bodily change, shift, and growth (to put it mildly), your fluid demands skyrocket for the following reasons:

➤ You need to maintain your *expanded* blood supply and fluid volume. You see, through the blood and lymphatic system, water helps deliver oxygen and other nutrients all over your body.

➤ As always, fluids are needed to help wash down your food and assist in nutrient absorption.

➤ Extra fluids, along with fibre, can help alleviate some of the bothersome plumbing problems (alias "mom-to-be" constipation).

➤ Fluid provides a cushion for the developing fetus and also helps lubricate your joints.

➤ Lastly, fluid is needed for the normal functioning of *every* cell in your body.

"Favourable fluids" you should be gulping down include water, club soda, bottled water, vegetable juice, seltzer water, unsweetened fruit juice, and low-fat milk.

Liquids you should steer clear of are alcohol, coffee, tea, soft drinks, diet cola (and other artificially sweetened drinks), and questionable herbal teas.

Also realize that in some instances, you might need even *more* than the already increased amount: for example, when you're perspiring in hot weather, or when you're exercising, or if you have any type of fever, vomiting, or diarrhea. (Obviously, in the last case, contact your doctor immediately.)

Foods to Forget!

The following is a suggested list of foods to *avoid* until after the baby is born:

➤ **Raw foods**—Because these foods can increase your risk for bacterial infection, avoid anything raw, including sushi and other seafood, beef tartare, undercooked poultry, raw or unpasteurized milk, soft-cooked and poached eggs, or raw egg that may be found in eggnog, cookie dough, Caesar salads, and milkshakes.

➤ **Nitrates, nitrites, and nitrosamines**—These are possible cancer-causing chemicals and are found in hot dogs, bacon, bologna, and other processed cold cuts.

➤ **Alcohol**—Because alcohol can damage the developing fetus (fetal alcohol syndrome), avoid all beer, wine, and liquor.

➤ **Caffeine**—Although there is insufficient evidence to conclude that caffeine adversely affects reproduction in humans, it does pass through the placenta and

Q & A

What is gestational diabetes?

Gestational diabetes is the onset of high blood sugar (or carbohydrate intolerance) that is generally detected around the 28th week of pregnancy. Because this condition is caused by the placenta putting out large doses of anti-insulin hormones, as soon as the placenta is removed (during the baby's delivery), the condition disappears in almost all cases. Women diagnosed as suffering from gestational diabetes have very specific dietary concerns and should work with a qualified nutritionist (registered dietitian) on appropriate meal planning.

Food for Thought

Getting enough of the vitamin folate (folic acid) can *drastically* reduce the risk of a baby being born with neural-tube defects such as spina bifida. So fill up on the green leafy veggies and get precautionary backup from a prenatal vitamin that supplies folic acid.

into the baby's body. Therefore, it is smart to avoid coffee, tea, and other highly caffeinated beverages. Speak with your personal nutritionist about caffeine.

➤ **Herbal teas**—Some herbal teas can have medicinal properties. Check out herbal teas with your nutritionist or physician before assuming that they're okay to drink.

➤ **MSG**—Monosodium glutamate can cause uncomfortable side effects in pregnant women, including headaches, dizziness, and nausea.

➤ **Artificial sweeteners**—This is a tough call. Although some health professionals claim artificial sweeteners are perfectly safe during pregnancy, others say you should completely avoid them. In my opinion, why play around with your baby's health? You can live without them for nine months.

The Many Trials and Tribulations of Having a Baby

When embarking on the road to motherly bliss, some women glow and others, shall I say, turn green. Although agonizing and uncomfortable (to put it *mildly*), these lousy side effects, including constipation, nausea, water retention, and heartburn, are merely normal occurrences of pregnancy and most certainly worth the beautiful result—your baby.

The "Uh-Oh, Better Get Drano" Feeling

Most pregnant women experience the constipation blues at one time or another during the nine-month haul. Why does food tend to stop dead in its tracks before reaching its final destination, anyway? Unfortunately, there are a bunch of explanations:

➤ Hormonal changes

➤ The increased pressure on your intestinal tract as your baby grows

➤ All of the extra iron in your prenatal supplements

➤ Not enough fibre in your diet

➤ Not drinking enough fluids

➤ Plain old lack of exercise

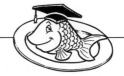

Food for Thought

Sometimes, the increased iron can cause constipation, diarrhea, dark coloured stools, and abdominal discomfort. Don't be alarmed; these are just par for the course. Be sure to increase your intake of fibre and fluids and move around as much as possible.

Yes, it's true that the first three circumstances are completely uncontrollable, but let's focus on the last three, fibre, fluid, and exercise, which are quite controllable and can *dramatically* decrease your plumbing problems.

First, increase your dietary fibre by eating more fresh fruit, veggies, and whole-grain foods. Better yet, flip back to Chapter 6, "The Facts on Fibre," and read the tips for boosting your daily intake. Next, drink a ton of fluids. Stay tuned for Chapter 23, "Exercising Your Way Through Pregnancy," which provides exercise guidelines during pregnancy.

Ugh! That Nagging Nausea

Commonly known as "morning sickness," nausea and vomiting can occur at any time of the day, so don't be misled. One bit of reassuring news: Although horridly unpleasant, nausea and vomiting are *normal* and thought to be simply a side effect of the hormonal changes that take place during pregnancy. If you're on a first-name basis with your toilet, hang in there; the nausea usually disappears by week 14.

Here are some tips to help reduce nausea:

➤ Nibble on carbohydrate-rich foods throughout the day. They are easy to digest and will provide your body with some energy (calories). For example, bagels, pretzels, crackers, cereal, and rice cakes are all great snacks that keep the nausea at bay.

➤ If you tend to be nauseated in the early morning, keep some of the carbs just mentioned by your bed. Pop something into your mouth *before* getting up; this will start the digestive process and get rid of excess stomach acid.

➤ Most women find cold foods easier to tolerate than hot foods; however, everyone is unique. What makes one woman sick might be soothing to another. In other words, listen to your body and go ahead with whatever works best for you.

➤ Avoid any strong cooking odours, and open the windows for some fresh air.

➤ When you just can't take solid foods, suck on a Popsicle or frozen fruit bar or sip lemonade and fruit juice.

➤ Avoid high-fat foods because they stay in your stomach longer and can exacerbate the nausea.

➤ Sometimes iron supplements can intensify nausea. If you are taking iron pills, take them with a snack or two hours after a meal with some ginger ale. If the nausea persists, you might also want to speak with your doctor about possibly holding off on the iron until you feel better.

➤ Do *not* take prenatal vitamins on an empty stomach; take them with a meal or snack.

Contact your doctor immediately if you have persistent vomiting, are losing weight, or are too nauseated to take in fluids.

What's All the Swelling About?

Edema is the uncomfortable swelling, or retention of water, that occurs primarily in your feet, ankles, and hands during pregnancy. As long as there's no increase in blood pressure or protein in the urine, edema is normal and, unfortunately, tends to get worse in the last trimester. However, there is no need to panic; most of this bothersome fluid will be lost during and shortly after your baby's delivery.

Make yourself more comfortable; the following can alleviate the effects of edema:

➤ Lie down with your feet elevated on a pillow.

➤ Remove all of your tight rings.

➤ Wear loose, comfortable shoes.

➤ Ease up on the salty stuff such as sauerkraut, pickles, soy sauce, salty pretzels, and chips.

➤ Never restrict your fluid intake; always continue to drink plenty of fluids.

Oh, My Aching Heart

Contrary to its name, heartburn is actually a burning sensation in your lower esophagus that is usually accompanied by a sour taste. Although this dreadful feeling can happen at any time during your pregnancy, it's most common during the last few months, when your baby is growing rapidly and exerting pressure on your stomach and uterus. What's more, during pregnancy, the valve between your stomach and esophagus can become relaxed, making it easy for the food to occasionally reverse directions.

Here are some simple remedies to ease heartburn:

➤ Relax and eat your food slowly.

➤ Instead of eating a lot at one sitting, eat several smaller meals throughout the day.

➤ Limit fluids with meals, but increase fluids between meals.

➤ Chew gum or suck candy. Of course, your dentist will berate me, but it can help to neutralize the acid.

➤ Never lie flat after you have eaten. When you sleep, keep your head elevated with the help of extra pillows and by placing a couple of books underneath the mattress to help tilt it slightly upward.

➤ Avoid wearing tight clothing. Stick with items that are loose and comfortable.

➤ Stand up and walk around. This can help encourage your gastric juices to flow in the right direction.

➤ Keep a log and track foods that might be triggering your heartburn. Some common culprits include regular and decaf coffee, colas, spicy foods, greasy fried foods, chocolate, citrus fruits and juices, and tomato-based products.

➤ Do not take any antacids without your doctor's approval.

Five-Day Pregnancy Meal Plan

Here's a five-day meal plan to get you started on your healthy eating track. You'll notice the adjustments for the first trimester at the bottom of each menu; this is because your body requires fewer calories during the first three months and more during the last six months.

Menu 1

<u>Breakfast</u>

1 cup (250 mL) whole-grain cereal topped with
1 cup (250 mL) 1% low-fat milk and 1 Tbs (15 mL) chopped nuts
$^1/_2$ cantaloupe (or 1 cup/250 mL berries)
8 ounces (250 mL) grapefruit juice

<u>Lunch</u>

Turkey/cheese sandwich (2 oz/60 g turkey, $1^1/_2$ oz/45 g cheese, with roasted peppers on 2 slices whole-wheat bread)
1 cup (250 mL) vegetable soup
Glass of seltzer water with 4 ounces (125 mL) cranberry juice

<u>Snack</u>

Yogurt/fruit shake (blend 1 cup/250 mL low-fat frozen yogurt, 1 banana, and $^1/_2$–1 cup/125–250 mL strawberries or blueberries)

<u>Dinner</u>

Tossed salad with 2 Tbs (25 mL) dressing
5 ounces (150 g) grilled chicken breast, cut into chunks and stir-fried with
1 cup (250 mL) assorted veggies (with 1 Tbs/15 mL olive oil and 1 tsp/5 mL low-sodium soy sauce)
1 cup (250 mL) brown rice
Seltzer water or water with fresh lemon

<u>Snack</u>

1 cup (250 mL) 1% low-fat milk
4 graham crackers topped with 1 Tbs (15 mL) peanut butter

<u>Nutrition Information:</u>

Calories: 2,544

Fat: 26% (74 grams)

Carbohydrate: 53%

Fibre: 38 grams

Protein: 21%

Iron: 25 mg

Calcium: 1,645 mg

Folic acid: 465 mcg

B-6: 4.7 mg

Zinc: 18 mg

For the first trimester, skip the midnight snack of milk, graham crackers, and peanut butter, and you'll have the following nutrition information:

Calories: 2,288

Fat: 24% (62 grams)

Carbohydrate: 54%

Fibre: 37 grams

Protein: 22%

Iron: 24 mg

Calcium: 1,335 mg

Folic acid: 438 mcg

B-6: 4.5 mg

Zinc: 16 mg

Menu 2

Breakfast

1 cup (250 mL) oatmeal with $^1/_4$ cup (50 mL) raisins
Whole-wheat pita bread
2 tsp (10 mL) reduced-fat margarine and 1 Tbs (15 mL) jam
1 cup (250 mL) 1% low-fat milk

Lunch

Tuna Salad Melt (see recipe in Chapter 11, "Now You're Cooking")
Carrot sticks with 2 Tbs (25 mL) low-fat dressing
8 ounces (250 mL) unsweetened orange juice
Apple

Snack

1 cup (250 mL) low-fat fruit yogurt
2 oatmeal raisin cookies
Seltzer water with lemon

Dinner

4 ounces (120 g) broiled beef sirloin
$1^1/_2$ cups (375 mL) linguine with $^1/_2$ cup (125 mL) tomato sauce
1 cup (250 mL) steamed spinach with garlic and 1 tsp (5 mL) olive oil
1 cup (250 mL) fruit salad with 1 Tbs (15 mL) chopped walnuts
Seltzer water or water

Snack

Frozen yogurt bar
6 flavoured mini rice cakes

Nutrition Information:

Calories: 2,517	Iron: 20 mg
Fat: 24% (67 grams)	Calcium: 1,772 mg
Carbohydrate: 55%	Folic acid: 406 mcg
Fibre: 34 grams	B-6: 2.5 mg
Protein: 21%	Zinc: 19 mg

For the first trimester, skip the nighttime snack of frozen yogurt and rice cakes, and you'll have the following nutrition information:

Calories: 2,342	Iron: 20 mg
Fat: 24% (63 grams)	Calcium: 1,667 mg
Carbohydrate: 54%	Folic acid: 402 mcg
Fibre: 34 grams	B-6: 2.4 mg
Protein: 22%	Zinc: 19 mg

Menu 3

Breakfast

2 whole-grain waffles
1 Tbs (15 mL) margarine
1 cup (250 mL) strawberries (or small banana)
1 cup (250 mL) low-fat fruit yogurt
1 cup (250 mL) 1% low-fat milk

Lunch

Mexican Style Egg-White Omelet (see recipe in Chapter 11, "Now You're Cooking")
Toasted bagel with 2 Tbs (25 mL) cream cheese and 1 Tbs (15 mL) jam
1 serving canned peaches in light syrup
Seltzer water or club soda

Snack

Granola bar
1 cup (250 mL) frozen seedless grapes
8 ounces (250 mL) orange juice

Dinner

Tossed salad with 2 Tbs (25 mL) dressing
4–5 ounces (120–150 g) grilled fish
1$\frac{1}{2}$ cup (375 mL) couscous
Steamed carrots
Frozen fruit bar
Seltzer water or water with lemon

Snack

1 slice of whole-grain toast
1$\frac{1}{2}$ ounces (45 g) low-fat cheese

Nutrition Information:
Calories: 2,554
Fat: 25% (70 grams)
Carbohydrate: 55%
Fibre: 30 grams
Protein: 20%

Iron: 15 mg
Calcium: 1,827 mg
Folic acid: 457 mcg
B-6: 2.1 mg
Zinc: 10 mg

For the first trimester, skip the nighttime snack of whole-grain toast and cheese, and you'll have the following nutrition information:

Calories: 2,322
Fat: 24% (63 grams)
Carbohydrate: 57%
Fibre: 27 grams
Protein: 19%

Iron: 13 mg
Calcium: 1,363 mg
Folic acid: 435 mcg
B-6: 2.0 mg
Zinc: 8 mg

Menu 4

Breakfast

Vanilla French Toast with Fresh Fruit (see recipe in Chapter 11, "Now You're Cooking")
8 ounces (250 mL) grapefruit juice

Lunch

Chef salad with lettuce, tomato, carrots, and 1 ounce (30 g) roast beef
2 ounces (60 g) turkey breast
$1^1/_2$ ounce (45 g) Swiss cheese
2 Tbs (25 mL) vinaigrette dressing
Whole-grain roll
$^1/_2$ cup (125 mL) dried apricots mixed with 2 Tbs (25 mL) almonds
Club soda

Snack

1 cup (250 mL) frozen yogurt topped with granola
Nectarine

Dinner

$1^1/_2$ cups (375 mL) cooked pasta with 3 ounces (90 g) shrimp, 1 cup (250 mL) cooked broccoli
 (or peapods and carrots), $^1/_2$ cup (125 mL) tomato sauce
1 cup (250 mL) fresh strawberries with 3 Tbs (45 mL) whipped cream
Club soda with lemon

Snack

Slice of angel-food cake
1 cup (250 mL) low-fat milk

Nutrition Information:

Calories: 2,550	Iron: 23 mg
Fat: 25% (71 grams)	Calcium: 1,764 mg
Carbohydrate: 55%	Folic acid: 446 mcg
Fibre: 32 grams	B-6: 2.3 mg
Protein: 20%	Zinc: 14 mg

For the first trimester, skip the granola on the frozen yogurt at midday and the nighttime snack of angel-food cake and milk, and you'll have the following nutrition information:

Calories: 2,232	Iron: 21 mg
Fat: 25% (61 grams)	Calcium: 1,400 mg
Carbohydrate: 55%	Folic acid: 406 mcg
Fibre: 29 grams	B-6: 2.0 mg
Protein: 20%	Zinc: 12 mg

Menu 5

Breakfast

1 cup (250 mL) whole-grain cereal
1 cup (250 mL) 1% low-fat milk
1 cup (250 mL) raspberries
1 slice of raisin bread with 1 Tbs (15 mL) peanut butter
8 ounces (250 mL) orange juice (calcium-fortified)

Lunch

1^1/$_2$ cup (375 mL) rice and 1 cup (250 mL) black beans
1 cup (250 mL) fresh fruit salad topped with 2 Tbs (25 mL) granola and 1 Tbs (15 mL) chopped walnuts
Club soda

Snack

Yogurt/fruit shake
1 chocolate chip cookie

Dinner

Seasoned swordfish steaks (5 oz/150 g)
1 cup (250 mL) steamed kale with 1 tsp (5 mL) olive oil and garlic
Baked sweet potato with 2 tsp (10 mL) margarine
Baked apple with cinnamon
Water

Snack

1 cup (250 mL) frozen seedless grapes or a frozen fruit bar
1 cup (250 mL) 1% low-fat milk

Nutrition Information:
Calories: 2,485
Fat: 25% (69 grams)
Carbohydrate: 58%
Fibre: 53 grams
Protein: 17%

Iron: 26 mg
Calcium: 1,443 mg
Folic acid: 642 mcg
B–6: 3.4 mg
Zinc: 16 mg

For the first trimester, skip the chocolate chip cookie at midday and the nighttime snack of milk and grapes and you'll have the following nutrition information:

Calories: 2,246
Fat: 25% (62 grams)
Carbohydrate: 58%
Fibre: 51 grams
Protein: 17%

Iron: 26 mg
Calcium: 1,100 mg
Folic acid: 625 mcg
B–6: 3.2 mg
Zinc: 15 mg

Eating a balanced and varied diet will provide you and your baby with the 40 or so nutrients important for good health. Pay extra attention to folate, iron, calcium, and protein, and take good care of yourself by monitoring your weight gain and being physically active. Pregnancy is one of the most exciting times in a woman's life-enjoy it!

The Least You Need to Know

➤ You'll need about an extra 63,000 calories during the entire nine-month haul! That's about 100 extra calories each day during the first trimester and around 300 extra calories each day during the second and third trimesters.

➤ Adequate protein, calcium, iron, folate (folic acid), and a variety of other nutrients are required throughout your pregnancy to cover the increased demands of the growing fetus.

➤ Healthy, normal weight women should aim for a weight gain of 25–35 pounds (11.4–16.0 kg).

➤ Although nausea, constipation, water retention, and heartburn can be quite unpleasant, rest assured they are generally normal side effects of pregnancy.

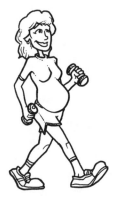

Chapter 23

Exercising Your Way Through Pregnancy

In This Chapter

➤ The pros of exercising through pregnancy

➤ How much and how hard to exercise

➤ Important tips for safety

➤ Appropriate exercise programs

Way back in the olden days (you know, when our parents had us), pregnancy was a time for rest—not exercise. *You're pregnant? Relax, put your feet up, and have a few bonbons.* Today, we know better. Research shows that pregnant women who regularly exercise have fewer aches and pains, better self-esteem, more stamina, strength, and energy, and perhaps less fear of the delivery.

Naturally, pregnancy is not the time to beat the world record in the high jump or place in the Boston marathon, but you can certainly continue with a modified version of your regular exercise regimen. You can even begin a prenatal exercise program if you're a newcomer to the world of fitness. Compare delivering a baby to participating in an Olympic event: The nine-month pregnancy is your chance to train for the big day.

Most Doctors Give the Green Light to Exercise

Most obstetricians today are keen on the idea of pregnant women exercising their way to the delivery room—within the limits of common sense, of course. However, because certain medical instances rule out exercise, and nobody knows you better medically than your obstetrician, never begin exercising without first discussing it with that person.

Q & A

Can you start exercising for the first time when you're pregnant, even if you're totally out of shape?

Yes! In fact, studies report that beginners can safely reap the benefits of exercise as long as they take it easy, warm up and cool down appropriately, keep their heart rate within a safe range, and have appropriate supervision for at least the first few sessions. Naturally, fitness novices must get the okay from their doctors before jumping in. Consult a certified personal trainer who specializes in prenatal fitness.

Food for Thought

Pick up *Fit Pregnancy* magazine and get the latest scoop on keeping fit while you're expecting. It hits the newsstands three to four times a year.

What Do the Experts Say?

This is a summary of the appropriate guidelines and recommendations from the Society of Obstetricians and Gynaecologists of Canada (SOGC) on exercise during pregnancy and postpartum.

For healthy pregnant women who have no additional risk factors, SOGC recommends the following:

1. During pregnancy, women can continue to exercise and derive health benefits even from mild to moderate exercise routines. Regular exercise—at least three times per week—is preferable to intermittent activity.

2. Avoid exercise in the supine position (lying on your back) after the first trimester. This position can decrease the cardiac output (blood flow) to the uterus. Also, avoid prolonged periods of motionless standing.

3. Pregnant women have less oxygen available for aerobic activity and therefore should not expect to be able to do what they did pre-pregnancy. Pay close attention to your body, and modify the intensity of your exercise according to how you feel. Always stop exercising when you feel fatigued and *never* push your body to exhaustion.

Although some women might be able to continue with their regular weight-bearing exercises at the same intensity as they did pre-pregnancy, non-weight-bearing exercises such as swimming and biking might be easier to do and present less risk of injury.

4. Your changing size, shape, and weight can make certain exercises difficult. Avoid activities that can throw off your balance and possibly cause you to fall. Furthermore, avoid any exercise with the potential for even mild abdominal trauma.

5. Pregnancy requires an additional 300 calories a day. Thus, women who exercise during pregnancy should be particularly careful to eat an adequate diet.

6. Pregnant women who exercise in the first trimester should stay cool by drinking plenty of water, wearing appropriate clothing, and avoiding very humid or hot environments.

7. Resume your pre-pregnancy exercise routines gradually after giving birth. Many of the physical changes that take place during pregnancy persist for four to six weeks after delivery.

You should not exercise during pregnancy if you have any of the following conditions:

➤ Pregnancy-induced hypertension (high blood pressure)

➤ Preterm rupture of membranes

➤ Preterm labour during prior or the current pregnancy

➤ Incompetent cervix or cerclage (a surgical procedure to close the cervix to keep the fetus intact in utero)

➤ Persistent second- or third-trimester bleeding

➤ Intrauterine growth retardation

In addition, women with certain other medical or obstetric conditions, including chronic hypertension or active thyroid, cardiac, vascular, or pulmonary disease, should be evaluated carefully to determine whether an exercise program is appropriate for them.

Q & A

Do fit women have easier deliveries than unfit women?

I hate to say it, but probably not. An easy delivery has more to do with genetics, the positioning of the baby, and a lot of luck. I've heard of "super fit" women who had labours from hell, and I've heard of sedentary women who popped out babies with just four pushes. Go figure.

However, one thing is for sure: Fit moms can better handle prolonged, agonizing labour and bounce back more quickly during the recuperation period than unfit moms.

Warming Up, Cooling Down, and All the Stuff in the Middle

Food for Thought

The mysterious art of yoga involves breathing, relaxation, stretching, and body awareness. Therefore, yoga can play a magical role in making you feel terrific during and after your pregnancy.

Pregnant or not, the ABCs of exercise remain the same. Be sure to begin each session with an appropriate warm-up—some light aerobic activity that will rev up your system and prepare your body for the exercise to follow. Next, continue with low- to moderate-intensity aerobic exercise and pay close attention to the cues your body gives you. During pregnancy, work at a comfortable pace, stop when you feel fatigued, and never push yourself to exhaustion. Lastly, always end your aerobic session with a proper cool-down period; gradually slow down the pace to bring your heart rate back to a resting level. See Chapter 14, "Getting Physical," for further details on exercise programs.

Stretch Your Body...Carefully

Regular, consistent stretching can help to maintain your flexibility and prevent some of the muscle tightness that typically sneaks up on you during the last trimester. As always, stretching must be preceded by some type of warm-up activity to increase your circulation and internal body temperature. Also, be sure to ease into each stretch gradually and hold for 10–30 seconds; never bounce! During pregnancy, the objective is for nice and easy stretching. Don't ever push a stretch past the point of your pain-free range of motion.

Keep a Check on the Intensity

As of 1994, the American College of Obstetricians and Gynecologists (ACOG) lifted the rule that limited pregnant exercisers to a heart rate of 140 beats per minute or less. Canadian personal trainers and fitness consultants have adopted the college's guideline and today, there are no limitations on heart rate: You can monitor the intensity of your exercise as long as you use common sense. Keep in mind that you should *always* be able to carry on a conversation comfortably while you exercise; if you can, you are working in a safe aerobic range. Never push through fatigue, cramping, or any other discomfort. (Review the section on checking your heart rate in Chapter 14, "Getting Physical.")

Understand that being pregnant means that typically you will fatigue more easily. Therefore, be cautious in the gym and modify your pre-pregnancy routine by decreasing both the intensity and length of your workout. Also, don't expect to keep up with those nonpregnant jocks; work out with some less competitive people.

Q & A

What should I expect during the first, second, and third trimesters?

During the first trimester, size is not the issue; your raging hormones are! Because some women feel incredibly tired and queasy, listen to your body and do whatever activity you can manage until you feel better.

During the second trimester, most women bounce back and feel like themselves again. If you feel up to it, this is a terrific time to incorporate regular exercise into your weekly schedule.

During the last trimester, your increasing waistline and weight might affect your stamina, agility, and balance. Think about switching to gentler activities that won't strain your joints and muscles (for instance, swimming and walking).

"Energize" Without the Slamming and Jamming!

When it comes to selecting the type of exercise, every woman is different. One woman might be perfectly okay with modifying her usual sport (for instance, a runner might continue to jog at a slower pace), but other women are uncomfortable with the jarring and jolting on the joints, especially in the last trimester, when weight begins to climb. Think about switching to gentler activities, such as walking instead of running, swimming instead of high-impact aerobics, or riding a stationary bike.

Food for Thought

Don't wait to get thirsty: Keep a water bottle close by and drink before, during, and after your workouts to ensure that you and your baby are adequately hydrated.

Take a Walk with Your Baby

Walking is great: there's no crashing impact, you can select your own pace and distance, you get quality "think time" (a precious commodity after the baby arrives), and you can do it just about anywhere. For some fresh air, go for a trek around the neighbourhood or hit a scenic trail. If the weather doesn't suit, try a treadmill, or wander about your local shopping mall. Anything goes; just remember these key points:

➤ You need to keep a strong, upright posture; lead with your chest.

➤ Rhythmically move your arms forward and back from the shoulders. Do not swing them higher than your chest or across your midline.

➤ Do not walk outdoors when the ground is icy. Remember, your balance is not as keen as it used to be.

➤ Don't try to conquer steep hills that can send your heart rate soaring or place a lot of stress on your back.

➤ Do not walk in steamy, hot, or humid weather.

➤ Keep your body and baby well hydrated. Drink before, during, and after your walk.

➤ Eat a snack before you start your walk to prevent a drop in your blood sugar level.

➤ Wear comfortable shoes with good support. Some women's feet swell during pregnancy, so you might need shoes or sneaks at least a half size bigger.

➤ Wear appropriate clothing. On cold days, wear layers that can be shed and tied around your waist as you heat up.

Overrated-Undercooked

Reduce your risk of injury by avoiding activities that require a lot of balance and coordination because, as your body shifts, so does your centre of gravity due to your enlarged belly, breasts, and uterus. Back off from things that might land you on the ground: skiing, horseback riding, biking, and skating. Avoid sports that involve sharp, jerky movements such as tennis, volleyball, bowling, and so on.

Sign Up for a Prenatal Exercise Class

Prenatal exercise classes are specially designed for expectant women and take into consideration your shifting centre of gravity, reduced stamina, and ever-changing figure. Generally, these specialty classes focus on thorough warm-ups, cool-downs, aerobic workouts, and stretching. In some instances, they might also include strength training and yoga. All exercises are carefully choreographed to keep you energized, but in a comfortable and appropriate fashion. Furthermore, you won't feel self-conscious because everyone in the class is in the same boat—give or take a few inches (or yards) around the waist. In other words, it's highly unlikely that the woman standing next to you will be wearing a thong leotard (and if she is, more power to her). It's also a nice place to bond, swap pregnancy war stories, and meet other women who, like you, are soon to have a baby.

You can find out about prenatal exercise classes in your area by checking with the local community centres, health clubs, hospitals, birthing centres, or even your obstetrician's office.

Q & A

What the heck are Kegals?

Kegals are exercises to strengthen the muscles within the pelvic floor (deep inside, between your vagina and belly button). To figure out where these muscles are, stop and start your urine flow when you're sitting on the toilet. Once you find them, regularly strengthen your pelvic-floor muscles with tightening and relaxing exercises. Pull upward and inward toward the body's midline, hold for about 5–10 seconds, and then relax. Repeat these exercises for as many times as you can, as often as you are willing. Kegal exercises can be done sitting, standing, or lying down and can drastically help to increase genital circulation, strengthen and maintain the pelvic-floor muscles, and prevent incontinence after the baby is born.

Yes, Moms-to-Be Can Lift Weights

Being pregnant doesn't necessarily mean passing up the weight room. In fact, some light weight training might cut back on some of the back and shoulder pain associated with enlarged breasts, extra weight, and a growing uterus. It might also reduce the leg cramps and neck strain that some women experience toward the last trimester. One great benefit of prenatal weight lifting is that your muscles will be primed for the "baby *aftermath*." That is, you'll be ready to lug around your purse, diaper bag, and stroller on one arm while carrying your baby on the other. You'll amaze your friends with the amount of equipment you can juggle with just two arms!

If you're experienced with weights, you can continue with a modified version of your regular routine. (Adjust the amount of weight and number of reps according to how you feel.) However, if you are a novice with the dumbbells and machines, this is definitely not the time for unsupervised weight lifting. You can ask a qualified trainer who is experienced with pregnant women to show you the ropes.

Some things to consider:

➤ Regroup your weight-training goals. Instead of focusing on intense workouts that will increase strength and define your muscles, relax, take it easy, and simply concentrate on strength maintenance.

➤ Because you might become less agile and coordinated due to the extra weight you are carrying, consider sticking with machines. They offer much more support and require less balance than free weights.

➤ Be aware that some machines require inappropriate positioning, and, as your belly expands in front, you might not be able to fit on some of the machines comfortably. (Ah, isn't pregnancy fun?) But don't let that halt the workout: Ask a trainer to show you some safe (perhaps nonmachine) exercises. Or simply forget about that exercise until you're back to your postpregnancy routine.

➤ The amount of weight you should lift depends on your strength pre-pregnancy and how you feel during your pregnancy. Lift what feels slightly challenging during the last few reps, not an amount that really pushes your limit.

➤ Pay close attention to your form and concentrate on smooth and steady breathing.

➤ Don't be discouraged if you have to cut back on the weights as you get further into your pregnancy. In fact, expect to cut back. Remember, you're pregnant, not Wonder Woman. Women typically get more tired and have less agility and balance toward the end of the nine-month term.

➤ If at any point you feel nauseated, dizzy, overly fatigued, or any other uncomfortable sensation (cramping, knotting, tingling), stop exercising immediately and consult your doctor before continuing.

Q & A

Can I lie on my back and do sit-ups?

Yes, but only during the first trimester. After the fourth month, you risk pinching off the inferior vena cava, an important large vein that carries blood back to the heart. During pregnancy, the weight of your growing uterus might compress this vein and cause you to feel faint. Ask a trainer to show you how to work your abdominals while you're on your side or standing up, instead of on your back.

Bouncing Back After the Baby Arrives

Generally, five to six weeks after delivering your bundle of joy, your doctor will give you the okay to resume all exercise—which is easier said than done. Between the sleep deprivation and feeling like your body's been through a war, merely scheduling the time and getting the motivation is a feat in itself. Take a deep breath and round up some energy because exercise can do wonders for both your mind and body. Start slowly, go at your own pace, and gradually ease back into your pre-pregnancy routine.

The Least You Need to Know

➤ Women who exercise regularly during pregnancy tend to have fewer aches and pains, better self-esteem, and more stamina, strength, and energy.

➤ Because some medical instances rule out exercise, always get the okay from your doctor before beginning an exercise program.

➤ Because pregnancy generally reduces your stamina, speed, and agility, expect to modify your pre-pregnancy routines by decreasing the intensity and length of your workouts. Always keep your heart rate within a comfortable working range and never push your body to exhaustion.

➤ Most pregnant women prefer gentler activities that do not strain the joints, such as swimming, walking, and riding a stationary bike, especially during the last trimester when their girth and weight start to increase.

➤ Drink plenty of water before, during, and after exercise to ensure that you and your baby are well hydrated.

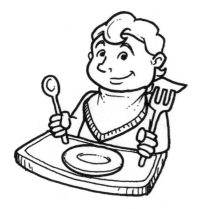

Chapter 24

Feeding the Younger Folks

In This Chapter

➤ Foods for the first year of life

➤ Nutrition guidelines for growing kids

➤ Involving your kids in the kitchen

➤ Healthy snack attacks

➤ Getting your couch potato to exercise

Being a kid these days is a pretty demanding job. It's especially important that the younger folks learn to keep their bodies fit and healthy so that they're better equipped to take on the world—and homework, after-school activities, sports, being popular, and keeping up with fashion.

Nobody knows your children better than you do. Therefore, this chapter does not tell you what you should and shouldn't feed your kids but merely offers suggestions and guidelines to help you in this endeavour. Read on to learn how to encourage your kids to eat nutritious foods and get plenty of physical activity. Bear in mind that healthy kids grow up to be healthy adults.

Your Very First Food Decision: Breast Milk or Formula?

Most pediatricians and nutritionists agree that breast milk is the food of choice for growing babies. First, nursing is a beautiful mother-baby bonding experience, and it's economically savvy. In other words, it's cheap! But most importantly, breast milk can protect your baby from several infections because, or so it is believed, it carries antibodies (protective substances) from mother to infant. *Colostrum*, the yellowish pre-milk substance secreted in the first few days after delivery, might carry even more antibodies, and it's loaded with protein and zinc.

All you women who choose not to nurse, or aren't able to nurse, don't lose any sleep. Companies today make sophisticated baby formulas that closely mimic the components in human milk. What's more, babies that are formula-fed can receive just as much "snuggling time" and form as close bonds with mom as babies that are breast-fed. Whatever feeding method you decide on (the bottle or the breast), rest assured that all kids have a shot at a Nobel prize and a spot on an Olympic soccer team!

When and How to Start Solid Foods

Although you might choose to nurse past six months, at this point your growing baby will need more calories and iron than breast milk or formula alone can supply. Generally, pediatricians recommend beginning solid foods when your baby is between four and six months old. Here are some strategies for getting started:

➤ A general rule is to introduce only one new food at a time (over three to five days) to rule out food allergies and intolerances. If your baby tolerates a food, and you don't notice any adverse reactions (skin rashes, wheezing, diarrhea, stomach aches), you can try the next food item.

As your baby gets older and tries more varieties of food, keep a watchful eye on highly allergenic items such as wheat, egg white, nut butters, and cow's milk. Avoid giving your baby egg whites, regular dairy products, and peanut butter until after the first year.

➤ Rice cereal is usually recommended as the first food to introduce because it is the least allergenic. Follow the directions on the box (usually 3–5 Tbs/45–75 mL dry cereal is mixed with breast milk, formula, or water). Although it might seem bland to you, don't add anything else (such as sugar, salt, or honey) to the cereal. Your baby will find it perfectly fine, and it's really the texture that you want him or her to get used to.

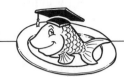

➤ After cereal has passed the test, try some puréed fruit and puréed veggies. (I recommend that you start with the veggies.) Watch how your baby starts to master the art of pushing the food back into the mouth with the tongue; what a genius! You can also give your baby unsweetened 100 percent fruit juice at this point, but be sure to dilute it to half-strength with water.

Food for Thought

It's a good idea to start with vegetables *before* fruit. After tasting the sweetness of fruit, some infants are not so willing to eat vegetables.

➤ By age 6 to 10 months, your baby's digestive system is maturing and it's time to introduce all sorts of mashed concoctions. Try strained meats, chicken, turkey, egg yolks (continue to avoid egg whites), and mashed lentils and beans.

➤ By 12 months, you can go ahead and substitute regular cow's milk for formula, with your pediatrician's okay. Encourage your baby to drink at least 3 full cups (750 mL) of milk per day, but not so much that he or she will be too full for the solid foods that supply the necessary calories and iron. You can also go ahead and add cheese and plain yogurts.

➤ Go at your own pace, and listen to what your pediatrician has to say about the growth and development of your little one, which is clearly the best indication of your baby's nutritional status.

These are popular first-year foods:

➤ Rice cereals	➤ Barley cereals	➤ Oat cereals
➤ Squash	➤ Sweet potato	➤ Carrots
➤ Green beans	➤ Peas	➤ Avocado
➤ Yogurt, plain	➤ Applesauce	➤ Bananas
➤ Peaches	➤ Plums	➤ Pears
➤ Chicken	➤ Beef	➤ Lamb
➤ Turkey		

The Wrong Stuff

Watch out for certain foods. During the first year, avoid foods that are difficult to chew and could cause choking, such as nuts, popcorn, hard candy, and raw carrots. Also avoid foods that have tough outer skins, such as grapes and hot dogs, and foods that are thick and sticky, such as peanut butter.

Honey should definitely not be given to children under age 1 because it can cause botulism. Honey is sometimes contaminated with spores of clostridium botulinum, and in an infant's intestine, these spores can grow and produce a toxin that can make a baby sick and—in extreme cases—can cause death. Adults need not worry because "friendly" bacteria present in their intestines prevent these spores from growing.

Be extra cautious when introducing foods that tend to be highly allergenic, such as egg whites, wheat, corn, nuts, seafood, citrus fruits, cow's milk, chocolate, cocoa, seafood, pork, berries, soy, and tomatoes. If you're allergic to one of these foods, there's a greater chance your child will also react to them. Hold off introducing the food until your little one is 18 months or older.

The Right Stuff for Growing Kids

These are the basic guidelines for children age 3 and older. Keep in mind that this chart represents the minimum requirements. Obviously, active kids who participate in after-school sports (or kids who just plain run around a lot) will need more food than the average couch potato. Also, expect the portion sizes to vary; younger children generally eat much smaller portions than older kids.

Food Group	Suggested Servings/Day	Key Nutrients
Grain products	6+	Carbohydrates, B-vitamins, iron
Vegetables and fruit	5+	Vitamins C and A, folate, magnesium, potassium, fibre
Milk products	3+	Calcium, riboflavin, protein
Meat and alternatives	2	Protein, B-vitamins, iron, zinc

Q & A

Should I worry if my kids aren't getting enough food?

Probably not. Children generally eat when they are hungry and stop when they are full. You might, however, want to pay attention to daily food choices among various food groups. If certain foods are consistently left out, try to find creative ways to work them into the day.

Be a Healthy Role Model

Monkey see, monkey do! As your children grow, they observe and copy everything you do—eating habits included. Remember, actions speak much louder than words, so start munching on those fruits and vegetables.

Cook with Your Kids, Not for Them!

Introduce your kids to healthy eating and the kitchen! I've found that children are more interested and willing to eat unfamiliar foods when they participate in the preparation. Try some of the following suggestions:

➤ Select a few nights each week and involve your kids with dinner planning and preparation. Designate different jobs for each child.

➤ You might prefer to cook with one child at a time. For instance, Tuesday night might be the night you and your son whip up a creative dinner concoction for the family. Thursday night might be a special night for just you and your daughter to plan the evening spread.

➤ How about an entire "theme night"? For example, one night might be Japanese. Make chicken teriyaki over rice; you can set up a table on the floor, sit on pillows, and use chopsticks instead of forks. Or make it Greek night: wear a toga and serve Greek salads.

Healthy after-school snacks include the following:

➤ Fresh fruit
➤ Veggies and low-fat dip
➤ Yogurt and granola
➤ Fig bars and low-fat milk
➤ Fruit cocktail in light syrup
➤ Bananas and apple slices with peanut butter
➤ Carrots and celery with salsa
➤ Whole-wheat toast with apple butter

Food for Thought

Until they reach age 24, kids and young adults are laying down the foundation for a lifetime of strong, healthy bones, so discourage sugary beverages and encourage them to drink milk and calcium-fortified juice.

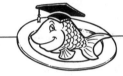

Food for Thought

Make mealtime fun for your younger kids: Set a place at the dinner table for a special doll or stuffed animal.

➤ Trail mix (nuts and raisins)

➤ Dried fruit

➤ Cereal with fruit and low-fat milk

➤ English muffin pizzas

➤ Frozen fruit bars

➤ Frozen yogurt pops

➤ Banana-Berry Frosty (see recipe in this chapter)

➤ Peanut Butter Yogurt Milkshake (see recipe in this chapter)

➤ Animal crackers and graham crackers

➤ Pretzels and fruit juice

➤ Vegetable soup and pita

➤ Flavoured rice cakes

➤ Jazzed-Up Popcorn (see recipe in this chapter)

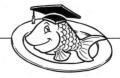

Food for Thought

Typically, the more colour on your plate, the more vitamin content. For example, a plate of noodles with broccoli, tomato sauce, and parmesan cheese will have a lot more colour and vitamin content than a plate of plain noodles with butter.

Fun and Easy Recipes

Here are a few recipes that will help your kids enjoy cooking.

Breakfast Berry Crêpes

Serves four

2 cups (500 mL) whole-grain flour

1 egg, beaten

2^1/$_2$ cups (625 mL) low-fat milk

Nonstick vegetable spray

^{1}/$_2$ cup (125 mL) blueberries

^{1}/$_2$ cup (125 mL)raspberries

^{1}/$_2$ cup (125 mL) sliced strawberries

Place flour in a bowl and add egg plus 2 cups (500 mL) of the milk (save ^{1}/$_2$ cup [125 mL]). Beat with a wire whisk until all lumps are gone and the mixture is completely smooth. Gradually add the remaining ^{1}/$_2$ cup (125 mL) of milk to make a thin batter. Use nonstick cooking spray on hot skillet (medium-high temperature), and pour enough batter in the pan to make a large circle. Sprinkle the desired amount of fruit on top and press down into the crêpe. Cook for approximately 2–3 more minutes and then flip the crêpe and cook the other side. Carefully lift onto a plate and roll the crêpe all the way up.

From the kitchen of Andrea Mendonca

Jazzed-Up Popcorn

Make air-popped popcorn, spray on some nonstick cooking spray, and then jazz it up with one of the following ingredients:

Parmesan cheese

Chili powder and garlic

Ground cinnamon

Low-sodium soy sauce

Tuna Salad Cones

Serves four

Open a can of water-packed tuna and drain off liquid. Mash up tuna and mix in grated carrots, chopped tomatoes, and some shredded low-fat cheddar cheese (optional). Mix with a little light mayonnaise or Italian salad dressing, and scoop into flat-bottomed ice cream cones (not the sugar kind). Serve for lunch or at a party; your kids will love them!

From the kitchen of Lisa, Jason, and Harley Bauer

Banana-Berry Frosty

Serves two

3–4 ice cubes

$^{1}/_{2}$ banana

1 cup (250 mL) low-fat milk

$^{1}/_{2}$ cup (125 mL) fresh strawberries

2 tsp (10 mL) vanilla

Place all the ingredients in the blender and mix until smooth and fluffy.

From the kitchen of Jesse and Cole Bauer

Peanut Butter Yogurt Milkshake

Serves two

4 big scoops vanilla frozen yogurt   4 big scoops

1 cup (125 mL) low-fat milk

1–2 Tbs (15–25 mL) peanut butter

Mix all the ingredients in the blender until thick and smooth.

From the kitchen of Haley and Mike Simon

Food for Thought

Unfortunately enough, recent studies report that 25 percent of Canadian kids age 12 to 19 are obese.

For further reading, look for

The Can-Do Eating Plan for Overweight Kids and Teens
Michelle Daum, MS, RD
Avon Books, 1997

1-800-223-0690

What About Sweets?

Clearly, some foods are healthier than others, but there's room in every meal plan for all foods, even the junky stuff. Develop a positive attitude about food by emphasizing healthy choices and limiting—but not eliminating—the not-so-healthy cakes, cookies, and candy. In fact, forbidding your kids to eat certain foods doesn't work; it only makes the high-fat stuff that much more enticing.

Place a limit of one to two dessert-like foods each day—and keep the serving sizes relatively small (2 cookies, small slice of cake, 1 scoop of ice cream). You can also serve healthier dessert alternatives such as chocolate fondue (orange segments, banana slices, and berries dipped in chocolate syrup) or an angel-food cake topped with strawberries. Both can satisfy a sweet craving with a lot less fat and sugar than other desserts.

What about your teenagers? As your kids grow up, you tend to have much less control over what they eat. Continue to encourage healthy food choices and certainly downplay the unhealthy stuff—but be careful not to create an obsessive environment of "bad food/good food." It can backfire into a serious eating disorder.

Q & A

How can you get your finicky child to eat more healthily?

Education is an important tool. Children as young as age 2 can begin to understand the importance of certain food groups. Make it simple and fun by incorporating games, taste tests, and colour drawings. A great idea is to hang a sticker chart on the fridge and reward your child each time he or she tastes a new food at a meal or eats a vegetable at dinner. Don't get hung up on the portion sizes; remember, kids have a small capacity and the idea is to create a willingness toward new food (not a clean plate award).

The Sneaky Gourmet: 15 Ways to Disguise Vegetables

Your kid won't go near vegetables? See if you can sneak in a few here and there with some of these suggestions:

1. Add a mixed vegetable medley to your meatloaf recipe.

2. Scatter cooked vegetables throughout pasta and then cover with tomato sauce.

3. Grate carrots into tuna or chicken salad and stuff in a pita pocket.

4. Make homemade pizza. Toss on sliced mushrooms and chopped broccoli *before* spreading on the cheese.

5. Make vegetable lasagna. You can stick with a single vegetable such as spinach (see the recipe for Vegetarian Spinach Lasagna in Chapter 19, "Going Vegetarian") or mix in a variety of chopped, cooked vegetables such as zucchini, cauliflower, broccoli, carrots, mushrooms, green beans, and so on.

6. Add cooked peas, corn, and carrots to mashed potatoes.

7. Serve vegetable soup with crackers.

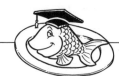

Food for Thought

Research has shown that vitamin C and omega-3 fats (fats found in oily fish) can reduce asthmatic symptoms in children.

8. Purée cooked squash and carrots, and then add small amounts to ground beef or ground turkey. Shape into hamburgers or turkey-burgers, and cook on the grill.

9. Top a baked potato with chopped broccoli and low-fat melted cheese.

10. Make low-fat zucchini and carrot muffins.

11. Serve "make-your-own tacos" and have different stations set up with lean ground beef (or ground turkey), sliced tomatoes, shredded lettuce, and carrots.

12. Make chicken-vegetable kabobs. Alternate chunks of grilled chicken, peppers, tomatoes, onions, zucchini, and mushrooms on metal skewers. Set up a variety of dips that your kids can have fun experimenting with, such as barbecue sauce, honey mustard sauce, sweet and sour sauce, and low-fat salad dressings. Of course, maybe you'll get lucky and your kids will simply like the original marinade.

13. Finely chop cooked broccoli and thoroughly mix into rice.

14. Turn your kids on to wok cooking and have them assist with washing and cutting up the vegetables. Try chicken-vegetable stir-fry, beef-vegetable stir-fry, or seafood-vegetable stir-fry. Pour them all over rice or linguine and hand out the chopsticks.

15. Make a spinach dip with low-fat plain yogurt, low-fat sour cream, and puréed cooked spinach, dip into which your kids can dip carrots, celery, peppers, and zucchini slices. If they don't want to dip with raw veggies, give them some crackers; at least they'll get the spinach from the dip.

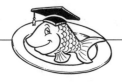

Food for Thought

Have your kids log their exercise for a week so that they understand the importance of regular physical activity and feel proud about their accomplishments.

Monday: Rode my bike for 1 hour

Tuesday: Danced at dance class for 45 minutes

Wednesday: Walked the dog for 20 minutes

Turn Off That Tube!

Too much television generally means too much sitting around. Put a two-hour limit on TV watching and encourage your kids to get up and move. Teach them about the importance of exercise and have them do something physical for at least 30 minutes every day. Have them walk the dog, jump rope, skate, throw a ball around, swim, play tag, play basketball, sign up for an after-school class, or join a sports team.

The Least You Need to Know

➤ Most health experts recommend breast milk over formula because breast milk is believed to pass protective substances from mother to baby.

➤ When your baby is between 4 and 6 months old, your pediatrician will probably give you the okay to start him or her on solid foods. Stick with one food at a time to rule out food allergies.

➤ All growing kids should eat a daily total of at least 6 servings of grain foods, 5 servings of veggies and fruit, 3 servings of milk products, and 2 servings of meat, poultry, dried beans, fish, eggs, or nuts. Expect younger kids to eat much smaller serving sizes than older children.

➤ Let kids be kids and occasionally eat junk food. Understand that an obsessive environment of denial can backfire.

➤ Put a two-hour limit on television watching and encourage your kids to become physically active.

Part 6
Weight Management 101

Weight control seems to be a full-time job for some people; they're on and off every diet on the planet. I have a friend, Cathy, who once told me her biggest fear of death is that they will print her weight in her obituary! Needless to say, she's alive and well and on another crazy diet.

It's finally time to stop going up and down like a yo-yo and stick with a sensible plan of attack. Whether you want to lose weight, gain weight, or most importantly, stop obsessing, this final section covers it all, so read on. I provide weight loss programs to help knock off (and keep off) those extra unwanted pounds, along with calorie-cramming strategies to help you skinny people beef up your bods. I also take a look at life-threatening eating disorders and where to find help when food and exercise go beyond health and get way out of control.

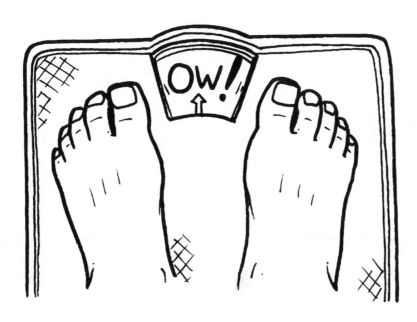

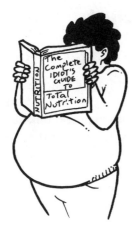

Chapter 25

Come On, Knock It Off

In This Chapter

➤ Why crash dieting *doesn't* work

➤ The scoop on some popular fad diets

➤ Identifying your ideal body weight

➤ Lose weight on a well-balanced program

➤ A meal plan to get you started

➤ Maintaining your new weight after you've lost weight

Let's take a walk down memory lane. We've had the Scarsdale Diet, the Grapefruit Diet, the Cabbage Soup Diet, the Food-Combining Diet, the High-Protein Diet, the High-Carb Diet, and even the "Lose 10 Pounds in a Week Eating All You Want" Diet (sure, tell me another one). And it seems we've come full circle—high protein is back, and not necessarily for the better.

Unfortunately, crash dieting is a North American sport that just won't go away. Diets are sort of like trick candles on a birthday cake: Every time you blow one out, another one pops up to taunt you. But with all these blubber-blasting gimmicks, the Canadian waistline continues to bulge! In fact, most people who lose weight on these crazy programs wind up gaining it all back—plus some extra pounds to boot. What's more, crash diets usually leave you feeling deprived and irritable. If you're thinking of jumping on the fad diet bandwagon, get the lowdown below before you do your body harm!

The Scoop on Some Popular Fad Diets

Before you rush off to the bookstore with your new resolve (I really want to do it this time!), here are the real facts about today's hyped weight loss diets.

➤ **High-Protein, No-Carb Diets** (Dr. Atkins, Protein Power, Scarsdale): These diets forbid virtually all carbs—sugar, fruit, grains, bread, milk—and you can forget the carrots, beets and squash! But for carnivores, this diet may seem like a dream since you can eat all the meat, cheese, and fat you like for the two or three weeks the diet lasts. Starving your body of all carbs deprives your brain and nervous system of it's only fuel source—glucose. Your body has a built-in survival mechanism though. In the process of burning fat, ketones are formed (a process called *ketosis*). Ketones then fill up your brain's fuel tank. Do you lose weight? You bet! You're eating fewer calories, for one thing. I mean, really, how much chicken breast and broccoli can you really eat at one sitting? The high-protein diet gurus claim that ketosis causes weight loss by suppressing your appetite (yet to be proven).

The list of cons is long—too little fibre (call the plumber), calcium, vitamin D, and, if you're not a veggie lover, vitamins A and C, folate, and beta-carotene. Worse yet, long-term ketosis may increase the risk of heart disease. What's more, once you go off this diet (and I promise you will), weight gain is inevitable, and fast! Keep in mind that 1 gram of carbohydrate stored in your muscles packs 3 grams of water away with it. Bottom line—this plan won't help you make a permanent lifestyle change. Keep on reading!

➤ **Moderate-Protein, Moderate-Carb Diets** (The Zone, SugarBusters!): Welcome back carbos! But if you're a pasta lover, don't get too excited. On these plans, portion sizes and the types of carbo-containing foods (dairy products, fruit, grains, bread, sweet vegetables) are limited. Choosing the right kinds of carbs and limiting your serving size makes your pancreas secrete less insulin (less sugar in the blood means less insulin is needed to carry that sugar into your cells). The theory here is that a lower insulin level causes your body to break down fat and the numbers on the scale to plummet. People do lose weight, most likely because they are simply eating less food.

When it comes to nutritional content, these types of diets can differ. The Zone, for instance, is relatively healthy. It promotes more whole grains, healthy oils, and lean protein foods. It loses points for it's lousy calcium content. SugarBusters, on the other hand, is not as nutrition conscious, offering its followers red meat, cheese, and pâté. If you're overeating carbs (and I see many clients who do), these diets get you eating more protein and veggies. Not a bad thing for the "cereal bar for breakfast," "bagel for lunch," and "pasta for dinner" folks. But if you work out and need your muscles primed with carbs, these diets are not for you!

➤ **Food-Combining Diets (Fit for Life, Suzanne Somers)** Don't eat toast with eggs...only eat meat with veggies...never eat fruit with a meal. Chances are you've heard this before, maybe even tried it yourself. Why is this diet so popular? According to the food-combining experts, your body cannot digest protein and starch at the same time. The meal sits in your stomach, ferments, and causes indigestion and weight gain. If you eat only starch with vegetables or protein with vegetables, your body breaks down your food properly. The net result—you feel better and you lose weight. And guess what? It's true (the weight loss part, that is). Just consider the calories you're saving when you eat this way. Say goodbye to meat sauce on pasta, ciao to cheese on pizza, adios chicken fajitas! There's no doubt that many people feel more energetic and less bloated following these diets. Eating less food makes most of us feel that way. But there's no secret potion behind combining protein and starch, other than the magic of cutting back on calories.

What's the Best Diet, Anyway?

Confused and frustrated? Well, if you're looking for a quick fix, the rest of this chapter is *not* going to help you. The bottom line is that people should lose weight eating the very same healthy foods that they will continue to eat *after* they have lost the weight—that is, plenty of complex carbs coming from whole grains, fruits and vegetables, low-fat dairy products, and lean sources of protein. Makes perfect sense, right? To lose weight *forever*, you must work on changing your eating behaviour forever. Read on and try my suggested meal plan. You've got nothing to lose except some unwanted weight—and perhaps a lifetime of professional dieting. It's time to change your eating habits for the long haul.

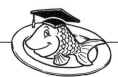

Food for Thought

For your personal nutrition profile, visit my Web site at www.lesliebeck.com. Simply fill out your food for a typical day (plus your height, weight, and age), and I'll show you how you measure up to your daily requirements for vitamins, minerals, calories, carbohydrate, protein, fat, sugar, fibre, and much more.

What Should You Weigh?

First, figure out a realistic weight to strive for. Here's a quick way to estimate your healthy weight range:

➤ **For men:** Start with 106 pounds (48 kg) for 5 feet (152.4 cm), and then add 6 pounds (2.7 kg) for every inch (2.2 cm) over 5 feet (152.4 cm) (or subtract 6 pounds [2.7 kg] for every inch [2.2 cm] under 5 feet [152.4 cm]).

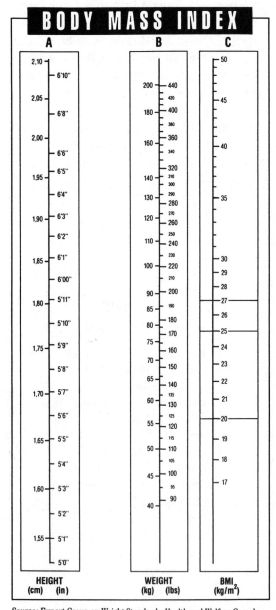

HOW TO FIND YOUR BMI – IT'S EASY

1. Mark an X at your height on line A.
2. Mark an X at your weight on line B.
3. Take a ruler and join the two X's.
4. To find your BMI, extend the line to line C.

FOR EXAMPLE:

- If Michael is 5'11'' (1.80 m) and weighs 188 lbs (85 kg), his BMI is about 26.
- If Irene is 5'4'' (1.60 m) and weighs 132 lbs (60 kg), her BMI is about 23.

Under 20 A BMI under 20 may be associated with health problems for some individuals. It may be a good idea to consult a dietitian and physician for advice.

20-25 This zone is associated with the lowest risk of illness for most people. This is the range you want to stay in.

25-27 A BMI over 25 may be associated with health problems for some people. Caution is suggested if your BMI is in this zone.

Over 27 A BMI over 27 is associated with increased risk of health problems such as heart disease, high blood pressure and diabetes. It may be a good idea to consult a dietitian and physician for advice.

Source: Expert Group on Weight Standards, Health and Welfare Canada

IF YOU FALL BELOW 20 OR ABOVE 27 ON THE BMI RANGE .....

It's time to reduce your chance of developing health problems. The first and most important thing is to determine why you are not within the healthy weight range and seek the assistance of your physician and dietitian/nutritionist.

Then, calculate the weight range for your frame by subtracting or adding 10 percent of the sum to your number.

Example: A man standing 5'10" will calculate 106 + 60 = 166 pounds. If he is small framed, he *subtracts* 10 percent of that from 166 pounds to get 150 pounds. If he is large framed, he *adds* 10 percent to 166 to get 182 pounds. Therefore, a man who is 5'10" has a healthy weight range of between 150 and 182 pounds.

➤ **For women:** Start with 100 pounds (45.4 kg) for 5 feet (152.4 cm), and then add 5 pounds (2.3 kg) for every inch (2.2 cm) over 5 feet (152,4 cm) (or subtract 5 pounds [2.3 kg] for every inch [2.2 cm] under 5 feet [152.4 cm]). Then, calculate your weight range by subtracting or adding 10 percent of that sum to your number.

Example: A woman standing 5'5" will calculate 100 + 25 = 125 pounds. If she is small framed, she *subtracts* 10 percent of that from 125 pounds to get 112 pounds. If she is large framed, she *adds* 10 percent to 125 to get 137 pounds. Therefore, a woman who is 5'5" has a healthy weight range of between 112 and 137 pounds.

Here's another quick way to get an idea of what a *healthy* weight range is for you. Use the table on the previous page to determine your body mass index (BMI). First, find out your current BMI by following the instructions below. Then to learn what a healthy weight range (BMI of 20 to 25) is, use a ruler to join the X at your height and the X at a BMI of 20. This is the lower end of your healthy weight range. To determine your upper limit, join the X at your height to a BMI of 25!

For the example shown, Michael's healthy weight range is 145 to 175 pounds. I know what you're thinking, "Wow, what a huge weight range!" You're right. Even though Michael's health is not in jeopardy within this range, he still might be carrying an extra layer of fat at 175 pounds. To figure out what's right for *you*, consider your weight history, the shapes and sizes of family members, your lifestyle, and what you're willing to change in your life. It may be unrealistic for Michael to reach a weight of 145 pounds, but it's reassuring to know that weighing in at 175 is still good for his health.

Testing Your Body Fat: Getting Pinched, Dunked, and Zapped

Although your weight indicates the total of *all* your body parts, it doesn't take into consideration your body composition (the amount of body fat versus lean body mass), which is important to know because muscle weighs more than fat. In fact, some people might appear a bit high on the weight chart *but* have very little body fat, indicating that the weight is coming from muscle mass and *not* blubber mass. (Of course, *you* know whether that extra weight is solid muscle or just extra weight.)

To get a more accurate idea about where you stand in terms of fat, check out your body fat percentage by getting pinched, dunked, or zapped—especially if you regularly work out. Compare your results with the normative ranges in the following chart:

289

Percent Body Fat for Women

Age	Good	Excellent
20–29	20.6–22.7	17.1–19.8
30–39	21.6–24.0	18.0–20.8
40–49	24.9–27.3	21.3–24.9
50–59	28.5–30.8	25.0–27.4
60–	29.3–31.8	25.1–28.5

Percent Body Fat for Men

Age	Good	Excellent
20–29	14.1–16.8	9.4–12.9
30–39	17.5–19.7	13.9–16.6
40–49	19.6–21.8	16.3–18.8
50–59	21.3–23.4	17.9–20.6
60–	22.0–24.3	18.4–21.1

Food for Thought

Take a trained athlete and a couch potato of the same height and weight: The athlete looks healthier and leaner and most likely wears a smaller clothing size than the couch spud. This is because muscle weighs more than fat, even though it takes up less space.

Skin-Fold Calipers

Getting "pinched" involves what are called *calipers*, a contraption that looks like a handgun with salad tongs. A tester positions the gun on certain parts of your body and grabs your fat so that it is pulled away from your muscle and bone. (Sounds painful, but it's not.) After gathering a few different measurements, typically from the back of your arm, your thigh, your abdomen, your shoulder, and your hip, the tester will plug each number into a formula to calibrate your overall body-fat percentage.

Although the caliper method is quick, simple, and convenient, the test results can sometimes be skewed if a tester pinches some muscle along with the fat or does not pinch enough of the fat. You will also need to have this type of test performed *before* a workout; during exercise, your skin slightly swells, which can make you appear fatter than you are.

Underwater Weighing

Getting "dunked" is actually the most accurate of the classic methods of testing body fat. Basically, you sit on a scale in a small pool of warm water. Next, you blow *all* the air out of your lungs and dunk underneath until you are completely submerged for about five seconds. Your underwater weight will then register on a digital scale; a tester plugs that number into a formula to determine the percentage of body fat.

Bio-Electrical Impedance

Getting "zapped" requires you to lie on your back with one electrode attached to your hand and another to your foot. A signal is then sent from one electrode to the other. The faster the signal travels, the more muscle you have. On the other hand, the slower the signal moves, the more fat you have because fat impedes or blocks the signal. This test measures your fat weight, muscle weight, and water weight, so you get the whole picture.

Food for Thought

If you decide to work with a nutritionist, remember this: You want a food partner, not a food dictator! Find a qualified registered dietitian (RD) who will move at your pace and make you feel completely comfortable. For a registered dietitian in your area, call the Consulting Dietitians of Canada at 1-888-901-7776 or visit the Dietitians of Canada Web site at www.dietitians.ca.

How Many Calories Should You Eat for Weight Loss and Weight Maintenance?

Counting the calories in each morsel of food that you eat is not the way to go. But you can get a general idea of how many total calories you should eat each day, to either maintain or lose weight, with the following formula:

1. First find your BMR (basal metabolic rate: the number of calories needed to perform your normal bodily functions at rest).

   BMR = your current weight in pounds × 10 (weight in kg × 2.2)

2. Next, multiply your BMR × an activity factor.

   BMR × 0.30 (for average daily activities)

3. Last, add your BMR to your activity factor.

Here's an example of a 130-pound (59 kg) woman:

   130 pounds × 10 = BMR of 1,300 calories

   1,300 calories × 0.30 = 390 activity factor

   1,300 + 390 = 1,690 calories per day

Food for Thought

People are different and lose weight at different speeds on different plans. For instance, you and your friend might do the math and come up with the same 1,400-calorie weight loss plan, but she might lose 1–2 pounds each week, and you might lose only half a pound each week. In this case, assume that you have a slower metabolism and need to step up your exercise and use the lower 1,200-calorie plan.

People who participate in regular physical activity more than three times a week will need to raise the activity factor to 0.40–0.60.

The example shows that an average 130-pound (59 kg) woman can maintain her weight on 1,690 calories per day. Now, let's say she wants to lose a few pounds. To lose weight, she needs to create a negative balance by reducing the number of daily calories and increasing her exercise to burn even more calories. For instance, she needs to get on a 1,400-calorie food plan and work out aerobically four to five days per week. She'd have no problem shedding some weight safely and efficiently.

Plug your own stats into the formula, and figure out what it will take calorically to melt away those unwanted pounds. Understand that no one should ever eat less than 1,200 calories per day; you will slow down your metabolism and set yourself up to gain all the weight back. Even if you are very petite, and the math works out to be less than 1,200, stick with 1,200 calories and jack up your exercise.

Your Personal Weight Loss Plan

Now that you've done the math, roll up your sleeves and get ready to learn what you need to eat to achieve your calorie target. On the following pages, you'll be provided with several plans that use bubbles (O O O) to represent servings sizes. Each plan is designed to provide a specific caloric level—1,200 calories, 1,400 calories, 1,600 calories, or 1,800 calories. You can select one of the balanced weight loss plans, experiment, and create an in-between plan of your own. Make it into a game and simply follow the food group sheets by focusing on the number of total daily servings from each of the five food groups (I've added "Fats and Oils" as the fifth food group). Notice that all the calculations have been done for you, so there's no need to count a single calorie. In fact, calorie counting from here on is off limits.

Understanding the Food Plans

At the bottom of each sample food plan in this chapter, you'll see checkmarks beside each food group. This is the number of servings in your plan each day. For example, if you are following the 1,200-calorie plan, you have 2 fruit servings and 3 grain/bread servings. Browse the various items under each food category and learn exactly what counts as 1 serving so that you know how to plan your foods for the day.

It's *not* necessary to weigh or measure; an eyeball guess-timation will work just fine. Here's how to guesstimate your serving sizes, and remember, this is only a general list; there are many other foods that can fit perfectly into each category, so go ahead and plug in your favourites.

One Grain/Bread Serving = Approximately 80 Calories

○ 1 medium slice of *any* type of bread

○ ¹/₂ small bagel or English muffin

○ Small pita bread (or ¹/₂ large)

○ ¹/₂ cup (125 mL) cereal (hot or cold)

○ ¹/₂ cup (125 mL) cooked pasta, rice, barley, or couscous

○ *Small* baked potato or sweet potato (size of your fist)

○ ¹/₂ cup (125 mL) peas or corn

○ 1 small snack-size bag pretzels

○ Low-fat granola bar

○ 2 fig cookies

Note: Some vegetables are included in this group because they are very starchy.

Here are some common grains and how they count:

➤ Pasta entrée = 4 grain servings

➤ Side of pasta or rice = 2 grain servings

➤ Large baked potato = 2 grain servings

➤ Large, hot pretzel = 3 grain servings

➤ Potato knish = 3 grain servings

➤ Large New York bagel = 3–4 grain servings

One Vegetable Serving = Approximately 25 Calories

Most vegetables are unlimited; just make sure to eat your minimal quota!

○ 1 cup (250 mL) green salad

○ ¹/₂ cup (125 mL) cooked vegetables

○ 1 cup (250 mL) vegetable juice

The only exceptions are the starchy vegetables (potatoes, peas, and corn) which get counted as grains.

One Fruit Serving = Approximately 60–90 Calories

○ Any medium piece of fruit (apple, small banana, pear, and so on)

○ ¹/₂ small cantaloupe

○ Large wedge of watermelon or honeydew

○ 1 cup (250 mL) fresh fruit salad or berries

○ Small glass of fruit juice (about ¹/₂ cup/ 125 mL)

○ Large scoop of fruit sorbet

○ Noncreamy frozen fruit bar

○ Small handful of dried fruit

Food for Thought

A sensible weight loss plan should let you shed pounds slowly but steadily—approximately 1–2 pounds (0.5–1.0 kg) per week.

One Milk Serving = Approximately 90–150 Calories

○ 1 cup (250 mL) low-fat milk (skim or 1%)

○ ³/₄ cup (175 mL) container of nonfat (flavoured) yogurt

○ Small low-fat frozen yogurt

○ 2–3 slices of low-fat hard cheese (or 1¹/₂ oz/45 g)

○ ³/₄ cup (175 mL) low-fat cottage cheese

○ 1 cup (250 mL) low-fat pudding

○ Skim-milk cappuccino, caffe latte, or hot cocoa

○ 3–4 Tbs (45–50 mL) Parmesan cheese

1 Milk Plus 1 Fat = Approximately 150–200 Calories

○ 1 cup (250 mL) whole milk

○ Regular cheese on anything

○ One scoop real ice cream

○ Regular hot chocolate, cappuccino, or caffe latte

○ 1 cup (250 mL) chocolate pudding

○ Anything else made with whole milk

One Protein Serving = Approximately 225 Calories per 3 Ounces

○ Approximately 3 ounces (90 g) lean meat, poultry, or fish (the size of a deck of cards), unless otherwise indicated

○ Chicken breast (3 oz/90 g)

○ Turkey breast (3 oz/90 g)

○ Lean red meats (3 oz/90 g)

○ Turkey burger or veggie burger (3 oz/90 g)

○ All seafood and fish (3 oz/90 g)

○ Tofu (6 oz/150 g)

○ Egg whites (approximately 4)

○ Whole eggs (2)

○ Beans ($^1/_2$–1 cup [125-250 mL] cooked)

One Fat Serving = Approximately 45 Calories

○ Any time you *think* something is prepared with fat, for example, sautéed vegetables, a sauce on your fish, fried chicken cutlet, and so on.

○ Any time you use 1 tsp (5 mL) butter, oil, margarine, or mayonnaise

○ 1 Tbs (15 mL) cream cheese, or salad dressing

○ 2 Tbs (25 mL) sour cream

For reduced-calorie spreads, double the serving size; you do not need to count fat-free spreads at all.

"Free Foods" That Don't Count as Anything!

○ Mustard

○ Ketchup

○ Soy sauce*

○ Teriyaki sauce*

○ Worcestershire sauce

○ All spices and seasonings

○ Jams and jellies

○ Pancake syrup (a drizzle only))

○ Coffee/tea

○ Sugar-free beverages

○ Cocktail sauce

○ Salsa

○ Tomato sauce

○ Bouillon*

○ Sugar

○ Sugar substitutes

○ Hard candies (3 per day)

○ Fat-free salad dressings and spreads (in moderation)

○ Horseradish

These foods are extremely high in salt; when they're available, choose the low-sodium versions.

Tracking Your Food on the Daily Plans

Make 20 or more copies of the food plan on the following pages that's right for you, and chart your daily food intake for the first few weeks, just to get the hang of it. After eating each meal or snack, check off the appropriate servings at the bottom. This will help you keep an eye on exactly how much food you've eaten and how much is left for the rest of the day.

Approximately
1,200–Calorie Food Plan

Breakfast

Lunch

Snack

Dinner

Snack

Grains and breads: ○ ○ ○

Vegetables: ○ ○ ○

Fruits: ○ ○

Milks: ○ ○

Protein foods: ○ ○

Fats: ○ ○

Water: ○ ○ ○ ○ ○ ○ ○

Sample Day of
1,200-Calorie Food Plan

Breakfast

1 serving of dry cereal

1 cup (250 mL) skim milk

Banana

Lunch

Large salad with 3 ounces (90 g) grilled chicken with 1 Tbs (15 mL) dressing (or 2 Tbs [25 mL] low-fat
   Italian salad dressing)

Small pita bread

Snack

Low-fat frozen yogurt

Dinner

Lean steak, 3 ounces (90 g)

A lots of steamed broccoli

Small baked potato with 1 tsp (5 mL) margarine

1 cup (250 mL) fresh strawberries

Grains and breads: ☑ ☑ ☑

Vegetables: ☑ ☑ ☑

Fruit: ☑ ☑

Milk: ☑ ☑

Protein foods: ☑ ☑

Fat: ☑ ☑

Water: ☑ ☑ ☑ ☑ ☑ ☑ ☑ ☑

Approximately
1,400-Calorie Food Plan

Breakfast

Lunch

Snack

Dinner

Snack

Grains and breads: ○ ○ ○ ○

Vegetables: ○ ○ ○

Fruits: ○ ○ ○

Milks: ○ ○

Protein foods: ○ ○

Fats: ○ ○

Water: ○ ○ ○ ○ ○ ○ ○ ○

Sample Day of
1,400-Calorie Food Plan

Breakfast

Toasted English muffin with 1 Tbs (15 mL) cream cheese

1 cup (250 mL) low-fat milk plus 1 cup (250 mL) blueberries blended with ice

Lunch

3 ounces (90 g) turkey breast on a plain tortilla wrap

Lettuce, tomato slices, and mustard

Apple

Snack

Pear

Dinner

Tossed green salad with 1 ounce (30 g) grated low-fat cheese and fat-free dressing

4 ounces (120 g) grilled fish in lemon

Medium baked potato with 2 Tbs (25 mL) sour cream

Steamed spinach

Grains and breads: ☑ ☑ ☑ ☑

Vegetables: ☑ ☑ ☑

Fruit: ☑ ☑ ☑

Milk: ☑ ☑

Protein foods: ☑ ☑

Fat: ☑ ☑

Water: ☑ ☑ ☑ ☑ ☑ ☑ ☑ ☑

Approximately
1,600–Calorie Food Plan

Breakfast

Lunch

Snack

Dinner

Snack

Grains and breads: ◯ ◯ ◯ ◯ ◯ ◯

Vegetables: ◯ ◯ ◯

Fruits: ◯ ◯ ◯

Milks: ◯ ◯

Protein foods: ◯ ◯

Fats: ◯ ◯ ◯

Water: ◯ ◯ ◯ ◯ ◯ ◯ ◯

Sample Day of
1,600-Calorie Food Plan

<u>Breakfast</u>

Bowl of oatmeal with some skim milk

6-ounce (175 mL) container nonfat flavoured yogurt

Small glass orange juice

<u>Lunch</u>

Hamburger on a bun

Side salad with 1 Tbs (15 mL) dressing

Fresh fruit salad

<u>Snack</u>

Frozen fruit bar

<u>Dinner</u>

Stir-fry of chicken and a lot of veggies (use only 1–2 tsp/5–10 mL oil and soy sauce)

1 cup (250 mL) brown rice

Small frozen yogurt

Grains and breads: ☑ ☑ ☑ ☑ ☑ ☑

Vegetables: ☑ ☑ ☑

Fruit: ☑ ☑ ☑

Milk: ☑ ☑

Protein foods: ☑ ☑

Fat: ☑ ☑ ☑

Water: ☑ ☑ ☑ ☑ ☑ ☑ ☑ ☑

Approximately
1,800-Calorie Food Plan

<u>Breakfast</u>

<u>Lunch</u>

<u>Snack</u>

<u>Dinner</u>

<u>Snack</u>

Grains and breads: ○ ○ ○ ○ ○ ○ ○

Vegetables: ○ ○ ○ ○ ○ ○

Fruits: ○ ○ ○ ○

Milks: ○ ○ ○

Protein foods: ○ ○

Fats: ○ ○ ○

Water: ○ ○ ○ ○ ○ ○ ○

Sample Day of 1,800-Calorie Food Plan

Breakfast

Egg-white omelet with veggies (use 1 whole egg plus 2 egg whites and nonstick cooking spray)

2 slices whole-wheat toast with 2 tsp (10 mL) reduced-fat margarine

1/2 cup (125 mL) sliced bananas and strawberries

1 cup (250 mL) skim milk

Lunch

1 slice of vegetable cheese pizza

Tossed salad with low-fat dressing

Snack

Peach

2 fig cookies

Dinner

Grilled swordfish (about 3–4 ounces/90–120 g) marinated in lemon and 1 tsp (5 mL) olive oil

1 1/2 cups (375 mL) pasta with tomato sauce

Grated low-fat mozzarella cheese (1 1/2 oz/45 g)

Cooked carrots and green beans

A baked apple

Grains and breads: ☑ ☑ ☑ ☑ ☑ ☑ ☑

Vegetables: ☑ ☑ ☑ ☑ ☑ ☑

Fruit: ☑ ☑ ☑ ☑

Milk: ☑ ☑ ☑

Protein foods: ☑ ☑

Fat: ☑ ☑ ☑

Water: ☑ ☑ ☑ ☑ ☑ ☑ ☑ ☑

No More "I've Blown It" Syndrome; All Foods Are Allowed

Are you guilty of the "all-or-nothing" mentality? Do you place all your favourites "off limits" when you diet, and then, the second you eat anything on the "bad list," you go whole hog and eat the house? (*"I've already blown it—might as well polish off the rest of the chips and cookies. I'll start fresh on Monday."*)

Diets fail when you're deprived of your favourite foods—even if they aren't healthy. You *don't* gain weight from occasionally eating moderate amounts of high-fat foods. In fact,

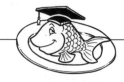

Food for Thought

Did you know that *six pieces* of broken cookie equals an entire cookie that you could have enjoyed?

you *lose* weight because in the end, you don't feel deprived, and you're not tempted to abandon your whole weight loss program.

The following list shows you that almost *anything* can fit in: You just have to check off the appropriate servings and account for the food item during that day. Try your best to stick with healthier choices most of the time, but go ahead and occasionally splurge on pizza, cookies, cake, or anything else that tempts you; I encourage you to do so! Simply stay within your daily serving limit by shifting other meals around to compensate, and you'll still lose weight.

Fat-Combo Foods

Fat-combo foods have fat built in. In other words, they are not straight oil, dressing, or butter, but fat combos such as pizza, chocolate, and so on.

- ➤ Cookies (2 medium) = 1 grain, 1 fat
- ➤ Cake (medium slice, *any* type) = 2 grains, 2 fats
- ➤ Doughnut = 2 grains, 2 fats
- ➤ Large bakery cookie = 2 grains, 2 fats
- ➤ Scone (medium) = 2 grains, 2 fats
- ➤ Danish/pastry = 2 grains, 2 fats
- ➤ Bakery muffin (large) = 3 grains, 2 fats
- ➤ Potato chips (small bag) = 1 grain, 1 fat
- ➤ Corn chips (small bag) = 1 grain, 1 fat
- ➤ Chocolate bar (Kit-Kat, Snickers, and so on) = 1 grain, 3 fats
- ➤ Coleslaw ($^1/_2$ cup/125 mL) = 1 vegetable, 1 fat
- ➤ Potato salad ($^1/_2$ cup/125 mL) = 1 grain, 1 fat
- ➤ Real ice cream (2 scoops) = 2 milks, 2 fats
- ➤ French fries (about 20) = 2 grains, 2 fats
- ➤ Chinese lo mein (1 cup/250 mL) = 2 grains, 2 fats

➤ Cornbread (medium piece) = 1 grain, 1 fat
➤ Cream soups (1 cup/250 mL) = 1 grain, 1 vegetable, 1 fat
➤ Macaroni and cheese (1 cup/250 mL) = 2 grains, 1 milk (or protein), 1 fat
➤ Pizza (1 medium slice) = 2 grains, 1 milk (or protein), 1 vegetable, 1 fat

Notice that for macaroni and cheese and pizza, the cheese can either be counted as milk or protein.

Q & A

Where do you carry your excess padding, on your belly or your butt?

Studies have shown that people carrying excess fat on the upper body and stomach have *more* health risks than people carrying fat on the hips and buttocks. Weight that is carried in the abdominal region is closer to the heart and the larger coronary arteries, unlike weight on the hips. Therefore, excess weight on your belly poses a greater risk of heart disease.

Setting Realistic Goals

Don't overwhelm yourself trying to lose a tremendous amount of weight. Instead, break it into smaller, more achievable short-term goals. For example, if you have your heart set on losing, say, 40 pounds (18 kg), aim for 10 pounds (4.5 kg) at a time. Even with a mere 8 pounds (3.6 kg) to lose, strive for knocking off 2 pounds (0.9 kg) at a time.

Also, understand that genetics plays a key role in determining your body makeup, so don't dream about that Cindy Crawford body; it isn't gonna happen. Take a look at your mom, dad, and other relatives; biology isn't destiny, but heredity does play an integral part in shaping your shape.

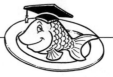

Food for Thought

Don't obsess about what the scale says; it can drive you nuts! Limit weighing yourself to once a week. In fact, avoid hopping on the scale each time you hit the bathroom; pack that scale away in the closet between weigh-ins, *or* simply weigh yourself outside your home (at the gym, at your nutritionist's office, and so on).

The most important thing is to learn to love the body you have and keep your focus on ways to make it healthy. You might never be a size 6 or have bulging muscles, but you can learn to be happy with the body you have by taking care of it.

Get Moving and Keep Moving

Following a healthy food plan is only half of the weight loss equation: You've got to move to lose! Numerous studies have shown that exercise helps promote weight loss *and* weight maintenance by revving up your metabolism (that is, burning more calories). What's more, exercise relieves stress and can even psych you up so that you're motivated to make smart food choices during the day.

Maintaining Your New Weight After You've Lost Weight

So you have reached your goal—now what? "Hooray!" on one hand, "Eek!" on the other! Maintaining your weight is actually harder than losing weight because there's no goal to strive for; you're already there. Hang tight and read the following tips. This time, your shapely physique is here to stay.

➤ The trick is to loosen the diet reins, but not too much. Continue with a *modified* version of your food plan (in your head only) because it's well balanced and encourages you to eat healthily.

➤ Figure out a 5-pound (2.3 kg) weight range with your present weight in the middle. For example, if your weight is 130 pounds (59 kg), give yourself a range of 128–133 pounds (58–60 kg). Continue to weigh in once every week or so, and if you go over the range, get back on the food plan.

➤ Plan one meal "off" each week—in other words, a meal that doesn't fit or calculate into your plan (anything you'd like). If your weight continues to stay put, add a second meal off, or possibly a dessert. Experiment and see what your body can handle; everyone is different.

➤ You might prefer to simply add a few more grains to your plan (or a fruit and milk). See what your weekly weigh-ins reveal (or if your clothes seem to "shrink" or "grow") and never panic if you think you've gained. Just take away some of the additions the following week. Remember, the key to maintaining your new weight is to find out how much food your body can handle.

➤ Absolutely continue with your regular exercise program. Exercise allows you to eat more food because it burns plenty of calories and keeps you tight and toned by zapping body fat and increasing your lean body mass.

The Least You Need to Know

➤ Fad diets don't work. People should lose weight eating the very same healthy foods they will continue to eat after the weight is lost.

➤ Your weight on the scale is the total of all your body parts (fat mass and lean mass); therefore, it's also helpful to test your body-fat percentage because it identifies how much of your body is actually fat.

➤ Don't set your heart on a supermodel body. Plan realistic weight loss goals by understanding that genetics plays a key role in body makeup.

➤ Learn to love the body you have, and focus on making it healthy, not perfect.

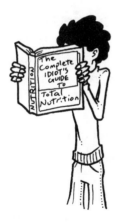

Chapter 26

Adding Some Padding

In This Chapter

➤ Strategies to help you gain weight

➤ High-calorie meals and snacks

➤ Refreshing shakes to boost your calories

Is your metabolism so speedy that you burn calories quicker than you can pack 'em in? Maybe you're one of those "uninterested in food" people, who look down at their watches and think, "Oops, I forgot to eat lunch." Whatever the reasons for your thin physique, fear not: With some attention and determination, you can start an upward trend on your bathroom scale.

Is Being Underweight a Health Concern?

For some people—specifically for people that are underweight because they undereat—being too thin can be a health concern. When your body does not receive adequate food energy (calories), it basically runs out of gas and leaves you feeling fatigued, irritable, and with decreased concentration. Furthermore, with an inadequate food intake you run the risk of developing vitamin and mineral deficiencies that may cause serious long-term problems (e.g., too little calcium and Vitamin D = bone loss).

On the other hand, being underweight may *not* pose a health risk and gaining weight may merely be about improving appearance. Some people are born with fast metabolisms that burn calories quicker than they can eat them. In this case, your caloric intake is most probably providing your daily requirements for nutrition, and you'll have to learn to eat more calorie-dense foods, more often, to try to defy your genetics.

To check if you are underweight, flip back to Chapter 25, "Come On, Knock It Off," and look at the BMI charts provided (or follow the equation provided).

Six Tips to Help You Pack in the Calories

Gaining weight requires devouring more calories than you burn. In fact, to gain 1 pound (0.5 kg), you need an extra 3,500 calories coming from food. Naturally, that's not at one sitting, but by simply eating an extra 500 calories a day, you can gain 1 pound (0.5 kg) per week—because 500 calories × 7 = 3,500 calories. Some people are "hard gainers" and require an extra 1,000 calories each day.

Stick with the basic food principles and concentrate on the following tips:

➤ Eat larger portions at your three main meals; even consider adding an extra meal to your day.

➤ Snacks are important! Plan at least three snacks a day. Snack 1 can fit between breakfast and lunch; snack 2, between lunch and dinner; snack 3, before bedtime. Tote along some trail mix, dried fruits, crackers, sports bars, fig bars, and nuts, or keep them in your desk at work.

➤ Add calorie-dense foods to your meals. For example, toss beans, seeds, nuts, peas, avocado, cheese, and dressings into salads. Add shrimp, fish, chunks of chicken, and a lot of Parmesan cheese to pastas. Add crackers, rice, corn, noodles, and beans to your soups. Don't forget the bread basket; spread on the margarine and dig in!

➤ Drink plenty of pure fruit juice or milk (preferably 1% or 2%) with and between your meals; it's a great way to painlessly add calories.

➤ Add powdered skim milk to your soups and casseroles.

➤ Try a calorie-dense supplement, such as Ensure Plus, Boost, Essentials, and Carnation Instant Breakfast. Just make sure you drink them between meals or with meals—not instead of meals—or you won't be getting extra calories at all.

➤ Consult a certified personal trainer about embarking on a weight lifting program. It can help you build muscles and put on some weight.

Nutri-Speak

Calorically dense foods provide a lot of calories and fat in a relatively small portion size. (Nuts, seeds, and avocado are examples.)

Adding More of the Good Stuff

Although the idea is to increase your calorie intake, you also want to keep your diet well balanced and nutritious. The last thing you want to do is to chow down on chocolate bars, donuts, cakes, cookies, and other high-fat junk foods that will pad you with fat and supply little in the nutrition department. Instead, eat more of the good stuff and stick with foods that are calorie dense. Here are some examples:

Basic, Healthy Meal	To Add Some Calories
Vegetable omelet	Add cheese and a bagel with margarine.
Salads	Add shredded cheese, avocado, olives, and plenty of dressing.
Pizza	Add extra cheese and vegetables.
Pasta	Add olive oil, olives, and parmesan cheese.
Chicken stir-fry	Add peanuts or cashews.
Burritos	Add guacamole or sour cream.

Here are some high-calorie and nutritional snack ideas:

➤ Frozen-yogurt milkshake (anything goes)

➤ Bowl of low-fat granola with fruit and 1% milk

➤ Tortilla chips with salsa and guacamole

➤ Peanut butter and jelly on whole wheat toast

➤ Bran, corn, or blueberry muffins

➤ Peanut butter on apple slices or bananas

➤ Cheese and whole-grain crackers

➤ Cereal mixed with yogurt

➤ Dried fruit and nut mixture

➤ Fruit bars and granola bars

Shake It Up Baby

Shakes can be a refreshing, filling alternative to snacks and can add a significant number of calories to your day. Try these ideas:

➤ Process in a blender: 4 ice cubes, $1/2$ cup (125 mL) orange juice, $1/2$ cup (125 mL) of melon chunks, 1 banana or $1/2$ cup (125 mL) strawberries, and wheat germ (optional). Add more or less juice and fruit to achieve the desired consistency.

➤ Mix Carnation Instant Breakfast or Ovaltine with 1 cup (250 mL) of low-fat milk; drink it with your breakfast or have it for a mid-morning or bedtime snack.

➤ Purée 10 oz (300 g) silken tofu, $3/4$ cup (175 mL) apple juice, 1 banana, or $1/2$ cup (125 mL) blueberries in a blender and top with walnuts or almonds.

➤ For a thick smoothie, purée 1 cup (250 mL) yogurt, 2 tsp (10 mL) honey, 1 banana, and $3/4$ cup (175 mL) fruit juice. (Pineapple or orange juice works well.) Mix in wheat germ if desired.

Want to gain some weight? Try this sample menu:

Sample Menu

Breakfast
Bran flakes (large bowl) with low-fat milk
2 handfuls of raisins
Large glass of orange juice
Bagel with margarine

Snack 1
8 ounces (250 mL) low-fat milk with Carnation Instant Breakfast
Large blueberry muffin

Lunch
Chicken-salad sandwich on whole-wheat bread
Bowl of vegetable soup with crackers
Apple
Large glass of fruit juice (try cranberry, grape, or fruit nectar)

Snack 2
Peanut butter on crackers with low-fat milk
Dried fruit and nuts
Glass of juice

Dinner
Vegetable cheese pizza
A lot of Italian bread
Salad with olive oil and vinegar
Flavoured fruit drink

Bedtime snack
Frozen yogurt cone with peanuts

By following these tips and becoming consistent about eating larger meals and frequent snacks, you should be able to gain some weight. Remember to focus on more servings of the four major food groups—grains, vegetables and fruits, meats and other protein foods, and dairy foods—and not try to gain weight by overdoing foods from the "Other Foods" section of the Canada Food Guide..

The Least You Need to Know

➤ To gain weight, you must take in more calories than your body burns.

➤ Increase your daily calories by eating bigger portions with your meals and by snacking on calorically dense foods that also offer nutrition.

➤ Guzzle tons of fruit juice, make creative shakes, or drink the popular supplements that are on the market.

➤ Embark on a weight-lifting program. It can help beef up your muscles and your weight.

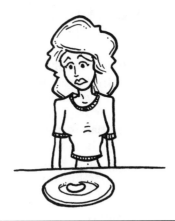

Chapter 27

Understanding Eating Disorders

In This Chapter

➤ All about anorexia nervosa and bulimia

➤ What is compulsive overeating?

➤ Real-life stories from people with eating issues

➤ How to help a friend with an eating disorder

The ideal of beauty has become more and more slender—a bone-thin slenderness, in fact, that most people are not capable of achieving through healthy, normal eating. Surrounded by skinny-minnies on TV and in movies and magazines, it's no wonder that so many Canadians each year suffer from serious eating disorders. More than 90 percent of those afflicted with eating disorders are adolescents and young adult women, who are at a time in their life when the quest for that "ideal body" is overwhelming.

Many psychological theories about eating disorders have been proposed, and today, there are numerous comprehensive treatment centres to help people struggling with anorexia nervosa, bulimia, and compulsive overeating. As a society, we need to overcome this obsession with unreasonably low body weight and learn to accept and love the healthy genetic shapes we were given. This chapter provides you with the basics on eating disorders so that you can better understand the world of dieting gone haywire—and perhaps help a friend, a relative, or even yourself.

I would also like to extend a very special thanks to three of my clients, who have allowed me to share their struggles with food.

Anorexia Nervosa: The Relentless Pursuit of Thinness

Anorexia nervosa is a complex psychological disorder that literally involves self-starvation. People who suffer from this illness eat next to nothing, refuse to maintain a healthy body weight corresponding to their height, and frequently claim to "feel fat" even though they are obviously emaciated. Because anorexics are severely malnourished, they often experience symptoms of starvation: brittle nails and hair; dry skin; extreme sensitivity to the cold; anemia (low iron); lanugo (fine hair growth on the body); loss of bone; swollen joints; and dangerously low blood pressure, heart rates, and potassium levels. If anorexia nervosa is not caught and treated in time, its victims can literally diet themselves to death.

The prevalence of anorexia nervosa is estimated at 0.1–0.6 percent of the general population, with 90 percent of the sufferers being women and roughly 6 percent boys and young men. Although any personality can fall victim to this life-threatening illness, most anorexics tend to be perfectionists who keep their feelings bottled up inside, straight-A students, good athletes, and people who always do the right thing. For anorexics, restricting and controlling food becomes a way to cope with just about anything.

Here are some of the warning signs of anorexia nervosa:

➤ Abnormal loss of 15 percent (or more) of normal body weight with no medical reason for the loss. Another sign among younger children and adolescents is a failure to gain the expected amount of weight during a period of growth.

➤ An intense fear of becoming fat or gaining weight, along with strict dieting and severe caloric restriction—-despite a rail-thin appearance.

➤ In females, absence of at least three consecutive menstrual cycles that otherwise would be expected to be normal.

➤ Always moving the diet "finish line" (*"Just five more pounds and then I'll stop"*).

➤ Constant preoccupation with food. Anorexics will often cook and prepare food for others but refuse to eat anything themselves.

➤ Distorted body image. For example, an anorexic will claim to "have fat hips" even though scales and mirrors show that the person is severely emaciated.

➤ Strange eating rituals such as cutting food into tiny pieces, taking an unusually long time to eat a meal, and constantly preferring to eat alone.

➤ Obsessively overexercising despite fatigue and weakness.

➤ Becoming socially withdrawn, isolated, and depressed.

"Weighting to Be Normal"

At 13 years of age and 172 pounds, I wasn't very involved in the world around me. Sure, I saw the fried chicken, mashed potatoes, cakes, and cookies, but boys, clothing, and beaches eluded me. Don't get me wrong, I wasn't miserable all the time; I just wasn't particularly happy. In fact, most of the time I was nothing; I was just FAT!

Nutri-Speak

Anorexia nervosa means "appetite loss of nervous origins." **Bulimia** means "ox-like hunger."

Like most perfectionists, I seemed to do everything to extremes. Initially, I ate to the fullest, and later, when my doctor told me I needed to lose weight, I dieted to the skinniest. Three hundred and sixty-five days later and 52 pounds lighter, the new Jane emerged. I had exercised and dieted my way to health. Burgers and taxis were out, low-fat foods and biking were in.

Not surprisingly, my doctor was ecstatic with my success, and my family was beaming with pride. My friends, on the other hand, were filled with that strange combination of jealousy and admiration, and finally for the first time in my life, guys noticed me. They whistled when I walked down the street and approached me at school. "Wow," I thought. "If I can get this much attention at 120 pounds, imagine how great life could be at 110."

At 100 pounds, I thought I had found bliss: I could count my ribs, pull down my pants without unbuttoning them, and most importantly, I could go an entire day on just a small fat-free frozen yogurt.

The months flew by, and my weight continued to plummet. Exhausted, freezing, and wearing size 0 clothing, I had propelled myself into a lonely abyss. Summer nights felt like the dead of winter, and the urge to sleep was unstoppable. I knew I was sick—everyone knew I was sick—and I was ultimately diagnosed with anorexia nervosa.

Although I rejected the notion of having a disease, I struggled both mentally and physically with solid foods and decreasing my amount of exercise. Gradually over the course of a year, I regained both my body and my life. I admit, low-fat foods and exercising are still entrenched in my life, but this time in a healthy manner, not as a destructive disaster. I must push myself to eat a risky meal (a "scary" meal with fat) every other day and allow myself to indulge in a dessert treat twice a week. Although I still obsess about my weight, it's no longer about losing; instead, it's about maintaining. I have been at my current healthy, thin weight of 112 pounds for the last year, and I guess you can say I have finally found an ideal way to exercise my "control." I "control" what I eat and how much I exercise, not in a freezing abyss, but in a hot, sweaty gym.

—Jane Stern, a 20-year-old recovered anorexic

Bulimia Nervosa

The eating disorder termed *bulimia* is at least two or three times more prevalent than anorexia nervosa. In fact, recent surveys report that about 1 percent of the general population and 4 percent of women age 18 to 30 suffer from this troublesome disease. People with bulimia have repeated episodes of *binge eating*—rapidly consuming large quantities of food and then ridding their bodies of the excess calories by vomiting, abusing laxatives or diuretics, and/or exercising obsessively. In most cases, this binge/purge syndrome is an outlet for anxiety, frustration, depression, loneliness, boredom, or sadness. Because most bulimics are typically of normal weight, they can keep their bulimia a secret and go undetected for years. Although some researchers think the problem is getting worse, others believe that people are just more willing to seek help, and therefore, bulimia is noticed and treated more often.

Here are some of the warning signs of bulimia:

➤ Dissatisfaction with body shape and constant preoccupation with becoming thin.

➤ Recurrent mood swings and depression.

Food for Thought

For further reading, order newsletters from the National Eating Disorder Information Centre (NEDIC). Call 416-340-4156 or visit the Web site at www.nedic.on.ca. Newsletters include *Eating Disorders and Weight Preoccupation; Treatments, Prevention and Self-care; Body Image and Self-esteem;* and *Family and Eating Disorders.* NEDIC is a Toronto-based, nonprofit organization established in 1985 to provide information and resources on eating disorders and preoccupation with weight.

➤ Frequent episodes of rapidly consuming large amounts of food (binge eating), followed by attempts to purge (get rid of food) through self-induced vomiting, use of laxatives or diuretics, prolonged exercise, or by following severe low-calorie diets between binges.

➤ Serious physical complications from chronic vomiting, including erosion of dental enamel from acidic vomit, scars on the hands from sticking fingers down the throat, swollen glands, sore throat, irritation of the esophagus, and poor digestion (heartburn, gas, diarrhea, constipation, bloating). The more serious physical dangers include severe dehydration, loss of potassium (potassium controls the heart beat), and rupture of the esophagus.

➤ Awareness that eating pattern is abnormal.

➤ Fear of not being able to control eating voluntarily.

➤ Light-headedness and dizziness or fainting.

➤ Frequent weight fluctuations of 10 pounds (4.5 kg) in either direction from the constant bingeing and purging.

"My Vicious Cycle of Starving and Stuffing"

Food for Thought

Many people aren't diagnosed as suffering from anorexia or bulimia but suffer from less serious "food issues" that nonetheless control and hinder their lives.

Remember, you only have one life to live. Get help and live it to the fullest!

It all started when I was preparing to go off to college. My anxiety stemmed from separating from my family and manifested itself in a body-image and eating problem. Up until this time, I was a "normal" eater, eating when I was hungry, stopping when I was full, and occasionally overeating during special occasions. I ate chocolate bars, pizza, and movie popcorn without as much as a blink. What was it like then?

Suddenly, it was as if my body wasn't mine anymore. It became this "thing" separate from myself. I became hyper-aware and mentally obsessed with how to control my shape through obsessive exercise and restrictive eating patterns. Skipping two meals in a row and exercising two hours a day became normal to me. I used to stand in front of my dorm room mirror naked, poking and scrutinizing myself out loud. My self-esteem was so low that I actually needed someone to validate all of my insecurities. My overweight roommate would look on in disgust, reassuring me that I wasn't fat. A lot of people in my life got tired of reassuring me of this.

I did not allow myself to enjoy "forbidden foods" for a long time through college. I felt proud of this control but ironically continued with my dissatisfaction over my "chunky body" (which has always been very thin, so I'm told). But after a while of rigid restriction, my body rebelled and my disordered eating took on a new twist: a few days of restricting (sometimes as low as 500 calories a day) and then bam-I would "sabotage" all of my efforts by stuffing myself until I was uncomfortably full! Feeling disgusted, depressed, and ENORMOUS, I would get rid of the calories by making myself vomit, and then struggle back to my extremely low-cal, restrictive diet, and the vicious cycle continued. My weight could fluctuate 10 pounds depending upon the day of the week, but to the outside world, I still remained a "normal" little person.

I also developed strange idiosyncrasies. Certain colours had to be eaten together, and certain foods had to "match" each other, for no particular reason except that they made sense to me. I would also weigh myself up to 25 times each day. There was no room for error, spontaneity, or change.

Finally, coming to terms with the fact that this obsession with food and exercise was ruining my life, I started to see a psychotherapist. For the first time, I realized that my "food thing" was only a symptom of unlimited emotions that I had bottled up inside. I needed to work hard to break free from my extremist attitudes and my belief that being less than perfect was not worth being. (What is "perfect" anyway?)

Today, I allow myself to feel entitled to my words and actions and realize that a middle ground is healthier in relation to feeling, thinking, and eating. I've also worked with a nutritionist for the past year. She has taught me that restricting inevitably leads to bingeing, and I'm desperately trying to do away with black/white days (restricting or bingeing) and instead focus on the "grey."

I no longer let one M&M dictate my self-esteem, and I have learned that normal eating is flexible and always changing. It's okay to eat a big piece of cake on my birthday, chocolate when I have PMS, and movie popcorn once in a while. "Normal eating" means eating healthy most of the time, while allowing yourself to indulge when you feel like it. It's feeding yourself when you're hungry and sometimes when you're not-even just for the fun of it! It's feeding your mind as well as your body and realizing that weight fluctuations are normal. It is seeing life as more than what you put in your mouth and enjoying social situations for the conversation and laughter. It is learning to accept our bodies, our strengths, and our limitations as well. I admit, every day is a struggle right now, but at least I finally believe that I am worth it.

—A 27-year-old recovering bulimic

Compulsive Overeating

People who compulsively overeat repeatedly consume excessive amounts of food, sometimes to the point of abdominal discomfort. However, unlike bulimics, they do not get rid of the food with any of the methods mentioned earlier. In fact, most people with this type of eating disorder are overweight from the constant bingeing and have a long history of weight fluctuations.

Food for Thought

Eating disorders can sometimes run in families. In fact, the rate of anorexia among sisters has been estimated at 2–10 percent.

Because compulsive overeaters feel out of control with their food (and often eat in secret), there seems to be a high incidence of depression, in addition to the serious medical complications that go hand in hand with being overweight.

"Dieting My Way to Obesity"

The cycle began when I was 11 or 12. I wore a size 7 and thought I looked fat. I dieted, starved, exercised, overate, and ended up a size 9. I did the size 7-9 dance several times until I finally graduated to the 9-11 routine. This continued until I ultimately reached size 13.

The turning point from "eating problem" to "life-threatening disorder" happened in my adult years after the break-up of a serious relationship. I just couldn't face the anxiety of the dating world again! It was also right after my grandmother passed away and my father had a heart attack. Starting a high-powered, senior-level job, my binges became out of control. Suddenly, walking home from work, I felt an urgent need to eat; I stopped at a grocery store, a deli, and a restaurant, buying chips, cakes, ice cream, and cookies. I reached my apartment and rushed into the kitchen, still wearing my heavy winter coat and hat, and started shovelling cake into my mouth. My hands were shaking and not able to get the cake in fast enough. I finished the entire cake, a pint of ice cream, and 20 Oreos before I was finally calm enough to take off my coat and order Chinese take-out.

This routine went on night after night for months. Within six months, I was up 85 pounds, and for the first time in my life, I topped 200 pounds on the scale. I was depressed, desperate, and terrified. I cried on and off all day long-in the shower, on the train, and in my office, frantically searching for help from diet centres, obesity researchers, and hospital programs. I frequently and seriously contemplated suicide. I was humiliated and weighed 250 pounds. I felt like a heroin addict, only I was addicted to food.

With the understanding, support, and guidance from trusting, caring, and knowledgeable practitioners, a psychiatrist, a nutritionist, group therapy, and anti-depression medication, I am presently working my way out of this perpetual hell. I now follow a non-deprivational approach-all foods in moderation. Believe me, it took a lot for me to be willing to try this because all I've ever known is either 750-calorie diets or 20,000-calorie binges. Today, I allow myself a chocolate bar if I really crave one, and if I need to overeat (not binge) because of a heavy, stressful workload-I give myself permission.

I presently weigh 185 pounds, eat normally, and, at 45, have a rebirth of hope.

—A 45-year-old compulsive overeater

How to Help a Friend or Relative with an Eating Disorder

Combating an eating disorder is a huge undertaking and generally involves a collaborative team of specialists, including a psychiatrist (or psychologist) to work through the psychological dynamics, a physician to monitor physical status, and a nutritionist (or dietitian) to reintroduce food as an ally-not an enemy. Here are some things you can do if you suspect a friend or family member has an eating disorder:

➤ Call your local hospital (or some of the treatment centres listed later in this chapter) and gather information on the various programs in your area. Ask about individual therapists, group therapy sessions, and nutritionists that specialize in food issues.

➤ In a very caring and gentle way, discuss your concerns with your friend or relative,

Food for Thought

Many women, and a growing number of men, struggle with food and weight issues. In fact, 90 percent of women experience body–image dissatisfaction, 80 percent have dieted by the age of 18 years, and up to 15 percent have many of the symptoms of an eating disorder.

and provide some of the professional resources and phone numbers that you've found. Be very supportive and patient; even offer to go along for any initial consults.

➤ If the person is a minor and refuses to get help, you might need to speak with a family member.

Where to Go for Help

The following organizations can provide information, literature, and qualified referrals for the treatment of eating disorders:

National Eating Disorder Information Centre
The Toronto Hospital
200 Elizabeth Street
College Wing, 1–211
Toronto, Ontario M5G 2C4
Tel: 416-340-4156 Fax: 416-340-4736
nedic@uhn.on.ca

Anorexia Nervosa and Bulimia Association
767 Bayridge Drive
PO Box 20058
Kingston, Ontario K7P 1C0
www.phe.queensu.ca/anab

Something Fishy Website on Eating Disorders
An extensive resource on eating disorders by a recovering sufferer of anorexia nervosa.
www.something-fishy.org

These are some of the comprehensive treatment centres:

Eating Disorders Clinic
St. Paul's Hospital
1081 Burrard Street
Vancouver, BC V6Z 1Y6
604-682-2344

Pickhaven Centre
Calgary, Alberta
403-251-5228

BridgePoint Centre for Eating Disorders
PO Box 190
Milden, Saskatchewan S0L 2L0
306-935-2240

Westwind Eating Disorder Recovery Centre
458-14th Street
Brandon, Manitoba R7A 4T3
204-728-2499
1-888-353-3372

National Eating Disorder Information Centre
The Toronto Hospital
200 Elizabeth Street
College Wing, 1-304
Toronto, Ontario M5G 2C4
416-340-3041

Eating Disorder Unit
Douglas Hospital
6875 LaSalle Boulevard
Montreal, Quebec H4H 1R3
514-761-6131 ext. 2895

Eating Disorder Clinic
Queen Elizabeth II Health Sciences Centre
5909 Jubilee Road
Halifax, Nova Scotia B3H 2E1
902-473-6288

The Least You Need to Know

➤ Anorexia nervosa is a life-threatening eating disorder that involves self-induced starvation and refusal to maintain a normal healthy weight.

➤ Bulimia nervosa is a serious eating disorder that involves repeated episodes of rapidly consuming large quantities of food and then ridding the body of the excess calories by self-induced vomiting, abuse of laxatives or diuretics, and/or prolonged exercising.

➤ Compulsive overeating is repeatedly eating excessive amounts of food. Unlike bulimics, compulsive overeaters do not purge and therefore tend to be extremely overweight.

➤ Treating an eating disorder generally requires a collaborative approach that includes a psychiatrist or psychologist, a physician, and a nutritionist.

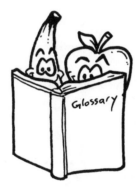

Recipes for Your Health

Jam in Popovers

Serves eight

Nonstick vegetable spray	1 Tbs (15 mL) canola oil
1 egg	1 tsp (5 mL) baking powder
1 cup (250 mL) 1% milk	$1/4$ tsp (1 mL) salt
1 cup (250 mL) flour	Jam or preserves

Preheat oven to 425°F (220°C). Use nonstick vegetable spray on muffin tin (or popover tin). Measure out all ingredients (except jam) and pour into a blender. Blend well. Next, pour mixture into prepared muffin tray, filling each tin only $1/2$ to $2/3$ of the way. Bake 25–35 minutes until sides are rigid and top is puffed.

Each popover with an additional teaspoon of jam (optional) is the equivalent of 1 serving. Serve with plenty of fresh fruit.

<u>Nutrition Analysis</u>
Calories: 112
Total fat: 3 grams
Saturated fat: 0.5 grams
Dietary fibre: 0.5 grams
Protein: 3 grams
Sodium: 136 mg
Cholesterol: 28 mg

From the kitchen of Meg Fein

Breakfast Berry Crêpes

Serves four

2 cups (500 mL) whole grain flour

1 egg, beaten

2$\frac{1}{2}$ cups (625 mL) low-fat milk

Nonstick vegetable spray

$\frac{1}{2}$ cup (125 mL) blueberries

$\frac{1}{2}$ cup (125 mL) raspberries

$\frac{1}{2}$ cup (125 mL) sliced strawberries

Place flour in a bowl and add egg plus 1$\frac{1}{2}$ cups (375 mL) of the milk. Beat with a wire whisk until all lumps are gone and the mixture is completely smooth. Gradually add the remaining $\frac{1}{2}$ cup (125 mL) milk to make a thin batter. Use nonstick cooking spray on hot skillet on medium-high, and pour enough batter into the pan just to make a large circle. Sprinkle desired amount of fruit on top and press down into the crêpe. Cook for approximately 2–3 more minutes, and then flip the crêpe and cook the other side. Carefully lift onto a plate and roll crêpe up.

<u>Nutrition Analysis</u>

Calories: 325

Total fat: 4 grams

Saturated fat: 1.6 grams

Dietary fibre: 5 grams

Protein: 15 grams

Sodium: 95 mg

Cholesterol: 59 mg

From the kitchen of Andrea Mendonca and Jesse and Cole Bauer

Greek "Village" Salad

Serves six

4 large tomatoes, cut into chunks

2 green peppers, cut into rings

1 large cucumber, peeled and sliced

1 large red onion, cut into rings

$\frac{1}{2}$ lb (250 g) feta cheese, $\frac{1}{2}$ sliced, $\frac{1}{2}$ crumbled

$\frac{1}{2}$ cup (125 mL) light Greek salad dressing

Black pepper to taste

Dried oregano to taste

Place the cut tomatoes in a salad bowl with the peppers, cucumber, onions, and the crumbled feta cheese. Mix in the salad dressing and some black pepper to taste. On top, arrange the feta slices neatly and sprinkle with the oregano and a bit more dressing.

<u>Nutrition Analysis</u>

Calories: 180

Total fat: 13 grams

Saturated fat: 6 grams

Dietary fibre: 2 grams

Protein: 7 grams

Sodium: 509 mg

Cholesterol: 33 mg

From the kitchen of Olympia Dukakis

Garden Tostada

Serves four

Salad

2 ripe tomatoes, chopped medium

1 Anaheim chile pepper, seeded and chopped medium

$^1/_2$ red bell pepper, chopped medium

3 cups (750 mL) shredded dark green lettuce

2 cups (500 mL) black beans, drained

$^1/_4$ cup (50 mL) chopped scallions

4 Tbs (50 mL) prepared salsa

2 Tbs (25 mL) vinegar

Tortillas

8 corn tortillas

Topping

$^1/_4$ cup (50 mL) grated nonfat mozzarella

$^1/_4$ cup (50 mL) nonfat sour cream

Preheat oven to 375° (190°C). Place corn tortillas on cookie trays; do not overlap. Bake for 5 minutes and turn. Bake for 10 more minutes or until curled and golden brown. Combine salad ingredients in large mixing bowl. To serve: Place 2 corn tortillas on each plate. Place salad mixture on top of each tortilla. Place $^1/_2$ Tbs (7 mL) mozzarella and $^1/_2$ Tbs (7 mL) sour cream on each tortilla.

Nutrition Analysis
Calories: 300
Total fat: 2 grams
Saturated fat: 0 grams
Dietary fibre: 9 grams

Protein: 15 grams
Sodium: 200 mg
Cholesterol: 0 mg

Curried Chicken and Rice

Serves four

1 1/2 cups (375 mL) water

1 1/4 cups (300 mL) uncooked basmati rice

1 cup (250 mL) canned crushed tomatoes

1 cup (250 mL) chicken broth

1/4 cup (50 mL) dark, seedless raisins

1 tsp (5 mL) curry powder

1/2 tsp (2 mL) cumin

12 oz (420 g) boneless, skinless chicken breasts, cut into 1/2-inch (1 cm) cubes

2 cups (500 mL) broccoli florets

4 Tbs (50 mL) nonfat plain yogurt

In a large saucepan, combine all ingredients except for chicken, broccoli, and yogurt. Bring to a boil, reduce to a simmer (turn stove to medium or medium-low), and cook covered for 8 minutes or until liquid is almost absorbed. Add chicken breast and broccoli florets and cook an additional 5 minutes or until chicken is done and rice is tender. It might be necessary to add more water. Serve with nonfat yogurt spooned over the top of each portion.

<u>Nutrition Analysis</u>
Calories: 370
Total fat: 1 grams
Saturated fat: 0 grams
Dietary fibre: 4 grams

Protein: 28 grams
Sodium: 230 mg
Cholesterol: 50 mg

Eggplant Parmigiana

Serves four

1 large eggplant

2 cups (500 mL) cornflake crumbs

1/4 tsp (1 mL) garlic powder

Pinch cayenne pepper

1 cup (250 mL) nonfat plain yogurt

Olive oil cooking spray

1 cup (250 mL) grated nonfat mozzarella cheese

2 cups (500 mL) pasta sauce

Preheat oven to 350° (180°C). Slice eggplant lengthwise into 1/4-inch (0.5 cm) thick slices. (It is optimal to get 6 or 8 slices; that way, you have 1 1/2 to 2 slices per person.) Combine cornflake crumbs, garlic powder, and cayenne pepper in large mixing bowl. Coat eggplant slices with yogurt on both sides, and then press both sides into corn-flake crumb mixture.

Set coated eggplant on cookie tray sprayed with olive oil cooking spray, and spray top of eggplant lightly with cooking spray. Bake for 15 minutes or until crisp and golden brown. Top with grated mozzarella and bake an additional 3–5 minutes until cheese melts. Serve each portion over 1/4 cup (50 mL) hot pasta sauce.

<u>Nutrition Analysis</u>
Calories: 160
Total fat: 0 grams
Saturated fat: 0 grams
Dietary fibre: 4 grams

Protein: 11 grams
Sodium: 500 mg
Cholesterol: 5 mg

Chicken Teriyaki over Linguine

Serves four

Pasta

8 oz (250 g) dried linguine noodles

Sauce

Vegetable oil cooking spray

12 oz (375 g) chicken breast strips (skinless)

1 1/4 cups (300 mL) water

2 Tbs (25 mL) orange juice

1 Tbs (15 mL) low-sodium soy sauce

3 cups (750 mL) fresh mixed stir-fry vegetables

1 cup (250 mL) snow peas

1/2 cup (125 mL) sliced green onion (scallions)

1 Tbs (15 mL) cornstarch

Cook linguine in 2 quarts (2 L) rapidly boiling water. Follow package directions for cooking time. Pasta is done when tender but slightly firm in centre. Drain in colander.

Make the sauce: Heat a large nonstick skillet and spray with vegetable oil cooking spray. Cook chicken strips just until done, approximately 5–7 minutes; set chicken aside. In the same skillet, add 1 cup of the water, the orange juice, and the soy sauce. Bring to a simmer. Add all the vegetables and cook until tender, approximately 6 minutes. Dilute the cornstarch in remaining water and stir into the vegetable mixture. Broth should form a light glaze. Add chicken and serve over pasta.

<u>Nutrition Analysis</u>

Calories: 220

Total fat: 1 gram

Saturated fat: 0 grams

Dietary fibre: 9 grams

Protein: 25 grams

Sodium: 260 mg

Cholesterol: 50 mg

Copyright Food for Health *newsletter, 1996. Reprinted with permission.*

Asparagus with Dijon Sauce

Serves four

³/₄ lb (375 g) fresh asparagus spears
¹/₄ cup (50 mL) reduced-sodium chicken
  broth

2 tsp (10 mL) Dijon mustard or tarragon
  Dijon mustard
1 Tbs (15 mL) grated Romano or Asiago cheese

Break woody ends off asparagus and place spears in skillet. Pour broth over asparagus, and then cover and steam over medium heat until crisp-tender (about 4 minutes). Remove asparagus to warm serving plate with slotted spatula and keep warm. Add mustard to skillet; increase heat to high and bring to a boil, stirring constantly. Pour over asparagus and sprinkle with cheese.

Microwave Method

Break woody ends off asparagus and place spears in 2-quart (2 L) rectangular microwave-safe dish. Pour broth over asparagus; cover with vented plastic wrap and cook on high power 3–4 minutes or until crisp-tender. Remove asparagus, and pour off liquid into 1-cup (250 mL) glass measure. Keep asparagus covered. Whisk mustard into liquid. Cook uncovered at high power until boiling, about 30 seconds. Pour over asparagus; sprinkle with cheese.

Nutrition Analysis
Calories: 20
Total fat: 0.7 grams
Saturated fat: 0.4 grams
Dietary fibre: 1.4 grams

Protein: 3 grams
Sodium: 51 mg
Cholesterol: 1 mg

Copyright 1995, The American Dietetic Association. "Skim the Fat: A Practical and Up-to-Date Food Guide."
Used with permission.

Traditional Tapioca

Serves four

1 egg, beaten
2 cups (500 mL) skim milk
3 Tbs (45 mL) sugar

2 Tbs (25 mL) quick-cooking tapioca
¹/₈ tsp (0.5 mL) salt
¹/₂ tsp (2 mL) vanilla

Mix all ingredients except vanilla in a saucepan. Let stand 5 minutes. Bring to a full boil, stirring constantly. Remove from heat. Stir in vanilla. Stir again after 20 minutes. Chill.

Nutrition Analysis
Calories: 115
Total fat: 1.5 grams
Saturated fat: 0.5 grams
Dietary fibre: 0 grams

Protein: 1.4 grams
Sodium: 172 grams
Cholesterol: 55 mg

Copyright 1995, The American Dietetic Association. "Skim the Fat: A Practical and Up-to-Date Food Guide."
Used with permission.

Cinnamon Apple Phyllo Rolls

Serves six

1 Tbs (15 mL) margarine

3–4 medium-sized apples (cleaned, peeled, seeded, coarsely chopped, and rinsed in water and lemon juice)

$1/4$ cup (50 mL) brown sugar

$1/4$ cup (50 mL) sugar

$1/2$ tsp (2 mL) cinnamon

$1/4$ tsp (1 mL) cloves (optional)

$1/2$ tsp (2 mL) vanilla

1 box phyllo dough, room temperature (you need 3 strips)

Nonstick vegetable spray

Melt margarine in a skillet and add apples, sugar, spices, and vanilla, stirring often. Cook until tender. Remove from heat and let cool to room temperature. Preheat oven to 400°F (200°C). Take 3 sheets of phyllo dough and cut them into $1/2$- or $1/3$-sheet strips. Lightly spray over each group of strips with nonstick vegetable spray, spoon apple mixture onto the strips, and roll up. Place rolls on a cookie sheet seam-side down, and again lightly gloss the outer phyllo with nonstick cooking spray. Bake 20–30 minutes, or until lightly browned.

Nutrition Analysis

Calories: 274

Total fat: 4 grams

Saturated fat: .5 grams

Dietary fibre: 2 grams

Protein: 2 grams

Sodium: 175 mg

Cholesterol: 0 mg

From the kitchen of Meg Fein

Caribbean Rice Salad

Serves four

Rice

1^1/$_2$ cups (375 mL) white long-grain rice

2^1/$_4$ cups (550 mL) water

Dressing

4 Tbs (50 mL) nonfat Italian salad dressing

2 Tbs (25 mL) cider vinegar

2 Tbs (25 mL) orange juice

Salad

1 can (15^1/$_4$ oz/430 mL) black beans, drained and rinsed

1 fresh tomato, diced into ^{1}/$_2$-inch (1 cm) cubes

1 mango, peeled, pit removed, chopped into ^{1}/$_2$-inch (1 cm) cubes

1 orange, peeled, seeds removed, chopped into ^{1}/$_2$-inch (1 cm) cubes

^{1}/$_2$ jalapeño pepper, seeds and veins removed, minced fine

^{1}/$_2$ red bell pepper, seeds removed, sliced into thin strips

6 cups (1.5 L) shredded dark green lettuce

^{1}/$_4$ cup (50 mL) sliced green onions

Prepare long-grain rice according to package directions. If you are in a hurry, use instant rice instead. Allow to cool to room temperature. (This process can be hurried by putting the cooked rice in your freezer in a shallow pan.)

Combine dressing ingredients and toss with salad ingredients; toss with rice and serve. You can use additional orange segments and pepper strips for garnish if you want. Divide entire tossed salad between 4 plates and serve.

<u>Nutrition Analysis</u>

Calories: 340

Total fat: 1 gram

Saturated fat: 0 grams

Dietary fibre: 8 grams

Protein: 11 grams

Sodium: 230 mg

Cholesterol: 0 mg

Copyright Food for Health *newsletter, 1996. Reprinted with permission.*

Sweet Potato Stew

Serves six

$^1/_2$ Tbs (7 mL) margarine

2 cups (500 mL) cooked, sliced fresh sweet potatoes

1 can (8 oz/250 g) crushed pineapple in natural juice

$^1/_4$ tsp (1 mL) ground cinnamon

$^1/_8$ tsp (0.5 mL) salt

Heat margarine in a large frying pan. Add potato slices and pineapple. Sprinkle with cinnamon and salt. Simmer uncovered until most of the juice has evaporated (about 10–15 minutes), turning potato slices several times.

Nutrition Analysis ($^1/_2$ cup serving)

Calories: 135

Total fat: 1.6 grams

Saturated fat: 0.3 grams

Dietary fibre: 2.3 grams

Protein: 1.3 grams

Sodium: 78 mg

Cholesterol: 0 mgf

Papaya Sorbet

Serves four

1 ripe papaya (1$^1/_4$ lb/570 g), peeled and diced

$^1/_2$ cup (125 mL) light corn syrup

$^1/_4$ cup (50 mL) plain low-fat yogurt

1 tsp (5 mL) fresh lime juice

Place papaya in a 9-inch (2.5 L) square baking pan and freeze for about 1 hour. Place frozen papaya in food processor with corn syrup, yogurt, and lime juice. Process until smooth. Freeze for at least 1 hour. Makes 2 cups.

Nutrition Analysis

Calories: 160

Total fat: 0 grams

Saturated fat: 0 grams

Dietary fibre: 0.3 grams

Protein: 1.4 grams

Sodium: 60 mg

Cholesterol: 1 mg

Spicy Poached Pears

Serves four

1 cup (250 mL) apple juice

$^1/_2$ cup (125 mL) cranberry juice cocktail

1 Tbs (15 mL) orange juice

$^1/_3$ cup (75 mL) water

$^1/_4$ tsp (1 mL) cinnamon

$^1/_4$ tsp (1 mL) ground cloves

$^1/_8$ tsp (0.5 mL) ground ginger

4 ripe Bosc pears, peeled

Pour juice, water, and spices into a deep saucepan; cover and bring to a boil. Trim the bottom off pears, if necessary, so they stand up straight. Remove core. Add pears and simmer uncovered until tender (15–25 minutes, depending on how ripe the pears are). Remove pears and set aside. Cook the remaining liquid over medium–high heat, stirring periodically, until mixture has reduced by half. Drizzle this juice–syrup over pears, and serve while warm, or chill and serve later.

Nutrition Analysis

Calories: 165

Total fat: 0.7 grams

Saturated fat: 0.1 grams

Dietary fibre: 3.8 grams

Protein: 1 gram

Sodium: <5 mg

Cholesterol: 0 mg

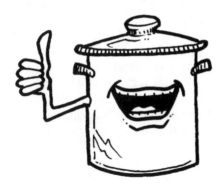

Glossary

active lifestyle—The lifestyle of folks who are constantly on the go. They do a lot of walking, take the stairs, play sports, or regularly work out.

anaphylactic shock—A life-threatening whole-body allergic reaction to an offending substance. Symptoms include swelling of the mouth and throat, difficulty breathing, a drop in blood pressure, and loss of consciousness. In other words, get help fast!

anorexia nervosa—A complex psychological disorder characterized by self-induced starvation. People who suffer from anorexia nervosa, meaning "appetite loss of nervous origin," believe they are overweight, often despite the fact that they are skinny to an unhealthy degree.

antibodies—Large protein molecules that are produced by the body's immune system in response to foreign substances.

bulimia—Another psychological disorder characterized by abnormal eating habits. People who suffer from bulimia, meaning "ox-like hunger," are in a vicious cycle of gorging on massive amounts of food and inducing vomiting, taking laxatives, or exercising excessively to purge the food from their systems.

calorie—The amount of energy food provides. The number of calories a food provides is determined by burning it in a device called a calorimeter and measuring the amount of heat produced. One calorie is equal to the amount of energy needed to raise the temperature of 1 L of water 1°C. Carbohydrates and protein contain 4 calories per gram, fat contains 9 calories per gram, and alcohol contains 7 calories per gram.

calorie-dense foods—Foods that provide a lot of calories and fat in a relatively small portion size.

CATA—Canadian Athletic Therapists' Association

complementary proteins—Incomplete proteins in foods that, when combined, compensate for one another's shortfalls.

complex carbohydrates (complex sugars)—Compounds composed of long strands of many simple sugars linked together.

CPTN—Canadian Personal Trainers' Network

cross conditioner/cross-country ski machine—This is a great aerobic exercise machine that uses the entire body and burns tons of calories without any jarring impact. These machines are also good for quick warm-ups because they get the whole body going. There is, however, one catch: Learning the required movement can be a bit tricky for some people; let's just say the term "poetry in motion" takes on a whole new meaning.

CSEP—Canadian Society for Exercise Physiology

diastolic pressure—This number, the smaller number of a blood pressure measurement, represents the pressure in your arteries while your heart is relaxing between beats. During this relaxation period, your heart is filling up with blood for the next squeeze. Although both systolic and diastolic numbers are critically important, your doctor might be more concerned with an elevated diastolic number because it indicates there is increased pressure on the artery walls even when your heart is resting.

diverticulosis—An illness or condition in which tiny pouches (called diverticula) form in the wall of the colon. The condition is often without symptoms, but when the pouches become infected or inflamed, it can be painful. When this happens, the condition is known as diverticulitis, which can cause fever, abdominal pain, and diarrhea.

empty calories—Calories with no nutritional value.

essential amino acids—Amino acids that cannot be synthesized by the body. We must get these from outside food sources.

fat-soluble nutrients—Nutrients that dissolve in fat. Some essential nutrients, such as the vitamins A, D, E, and K, require fat for circulation and absorption.

food allergy—An overreaction by the body's immune system, usually triggered by protein-containing foods (such as cow's milk, nuts, soybeans, shellfish, eggs, and wheat).

food intolerance—An adverse reaction to foods (such as in the case of lactose intolerance) that generally does *not* involve the immune system.

food poisoning—An adverse reaction caused by contaminated food (microorganisms, parasites, or other toxins).

food sensitivity—A general term used to describe *any* abnormal response to food or a food additive.

free radicals—Unstable, hyperactive atoms that circulate in your body damaging healthy cells and tissue.

glucose (also called dextrose)—A simple sugar found in fruits, honey, and vegetables. It is also the substance measured in blood. (Blood sugar equals blood glucose.)

hemorrhoid—A painful swelling of a vein in the rectal area.

homogenized milk—Milk that has been processed to reduce the size of milkfat globules so the cream does not separate and the milk stays consistently smooth and uniform.

hypertension—The medical term for sustained high blood pressure. Contrary to what this term sounds like it means, it does not refer to being tense, nervous, or hyperactive.

hyponatremia—Excessive loss of sodium and water due to persistent vomiting, diarrhea, or profuse sweating. Both water and salt must be replenished to maintain the correct balance for your body.

incontinence—The inability to control excretory functions.

iron toxicity—Although not very common, iron toxicity is a serious problem that occurs from either a genetic abnormality causing the body to store excessive amounts or the unnecessary oversupplementation of iron. The result can be liver and other organ damage.

lacto-vegetarians—This group of vegetarians eliminates meat and eggs from its diet but includes all dairy products.

lacto-ovo vegetarians—This group of vegetarians eliminates all meat from its diet (red meat, poultry, fish, and seafood); however, it does include dairy products and eggs.

legumes—Vegetables, borne in pods, of the bean and pea family that are especially rich in complex carbohydrates, protein, and fibre. They supply iron, zinc, magnesium, phosphorous, potassium, and several B-vitamins, including folic acid. Because foods in this category provide ample amounts of both complex carbs and protein, they can fit into either the meat and beans group *or* the vegetable group. Legumes you might know by a more common name include black beans, pinto beans, kidney beans, lima beans, navy beans, soybeans (tofu), black-eyed peas, chickpeas (garbanzos), split peas, lentils, nuts, and seeds.

pasteurized milk—Milk that has been briefly heated to kill harmful bacteria and then rapidly chilled.

pesco-vegetarians—This group of vegetarians has chosen to say good-bye to meat and poultry but eats fish and seafood.

PFLC—Professional Fitness and Lifestyle Consultant

proteins—Compounds composed of carbon, hydrogen, oxygen, and nitrogen and arranged as strands of amino acids.

RD, RDN, PDt, RDt—Registered Dietitian, Registered Professional Dietitian, Professional Dietitian

rowing machine—Another good machine for a total-body workout (and warm-up) that involves no impact. Be sure to get some pointers on technique; there is an easy way and the *right* way to use this machine. Obviously, the right way requires a lot more energy, concentration, and muscular effort.

scurvy—A disease resulting from a deficiency of vitamin C, characterized by bleeding and swollen gums, joint pain, muscle wasting, and bruises. Scurvy is now rare, except among alcoholics, and can be cured by as little as 5 to 7 milligrams of vitamin C.

sedentary lifestyle—The lifestyle of folks who generally have desk jobs, watch a lot of TV, and tend to sit around most of the time.

semi-vegetarians—This group does not eat red meat but eats most poultry and fish, as well as dairy products and eggs.

simple carbohydrates (simple sugars)—Molecules of single sugar units or pairs of small sugar units bonded together.

stairclimber—This equipment provides a very challenging cardiovascular workout with some potential stress to your knees and lower back. (Listen carefully to your body.) This is a more advanced piece of machinery due to the importance of technique, and therefore, you need a base level of stamina and strength to use this machine even at lower levels.

stationary bike—Stationary bikes come in two types: the upright bike (which is like a regular outdoors bicycle) and the recumbent bike (which you ride with your legs out in front while sitting in a high bucket seat that gives you more support, especially if you have lower back problems). Both types of stationary bikes provide effective aerobic workouts that can give your joints a break because they involve a non-weight-bearing activity. Make sure that the tension is not too high and that the seat is not too low. If you are a beginning biker, ask a trainer to help you get into the proper position for an effective workout. When you are ready to pump up the intensity, play around with increasing your speed before increasing the tension.

systolic pressure—The top, larger number of a blood pressure measurement. This represents the amount of pressure in your arteries while your heart contracts (or beats). During this contraction, blood is ejected from the heart and into the blood vessels that extend throughout your body.

tofu, firm—This tofu is stiff, dense, and perfect for stir-fry dishes, soups, or any dish in which you want the tofu to maintain its shape. A 4-ounce (120 g) serving of firm tofu supplies 13 grams of protein, 120 milligrams of calcium, and about 40 percent of your daily iron.

tofu, silken—This tofu is creamy and custard-like and therefore works well in puréed or blended recipes such as dips, soups, and pies. Silken tofu doesn't provide as much calcium as the more solid tofu varieties (only 40 mg/4 oz [120 g] serving), but it is the lowest in fat and is packed with $9^{1}/2$ grams of protein per 4-ounce (120 g) serving.

tofu, soft—This tofu provides 9 grams of protein, 130 milligrams of calcium, and a little less than 40 percent of your daily iron from a 4-ounce (120 g) serving. Soft tofu is good for dishes that require blended tofu (commonly used in soups).

treadmill—A machine for cardiovascular exercise that presents light to moderate impact on your joints, depending on whether you are running or walking. Walking on a flat grade is a good starting place for beginning exercisers. As your fitness and confidence levels build, you can experiment with increasing the incline and speed.

vegans—These are the strictest type of vegetarian (sort of the granddaddy of all vegetarians). Vegans do not eat or use *any* animal products; they avoid eating meat, dairy products, and eggs and wearing wool, silk, or leather. If you're a vegan, you'll need to be extra responsible about getting adequate protein, iron, calcium, vitamin D, vitamin B-12, and zinc.

vegetarians—People who substitute vegetables, nuts, and seeds for meat in a diet. Vegetarians vary in strictness from those who avoid all animal products to those who avoid only meat. Vegetarian groups include vegans and lacto-vegetarians, ovolacto-vegetarians, pesco-vegetarians, and semi-vegetarians.

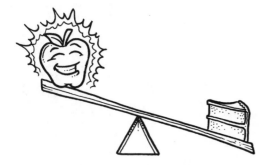

Food Values

A Closer Look at the Foods We Eat

This section provides a comprehensive nutrition profile for a wide variety of foods. It lists the nutrient values for calories, carbohydrate, protein, fat, saturated fat, dietary fibre, sugar, sodium, and cholesterol, plus seven other vitamins and minerals found in the foods and beverages we consume. Keep in mind that this chart provides you with the nutrient facts based on standard items—the nutritional content of packaged foods can vary from brand to brand. All information was derived from Nutritionist Five © First Databank 1999 and Nutrient Values for Common Foods © Health Canada, 1999.

The items for this table have been organized into several categories:

Breads and Grains

Fruit

Vegetables

Dairy: Cheese, Milk, Yogurt

Meats: Beef, Veal, Pork, Lamb

Poultry: Chicken, Turkey, Duck

Seafood

Eggs

Nuts and Seeds

Combination Foods

Fats: Oils, Salad Dressings, Spreads

Beverages

Sweets

Condiments

GRAINS	Amount	Portion	Kcal	Protein	Carb	Fat	Chol	Sat Fat	Mono Fat	Poly Fat	Sodium	Potas
BREADS:												
White Bread	1	SLICE	66.75	2.05	12.38	0.90	0.25	0.20	0.40	0.19	134.50	29.75
Wheat Bread	1	SLICE	65.00	2.28	11.80	1.03	0.00	0.22	0.43	0.23	132.50	50.25
Cracked Wheat Bread	1	SLICE	65.00	2.18	12.38	0.98	0.00	0.23	0.48	0.17	134.50	44.25
Mixed Grain Bread	1	SLICE	65.00	2.60	12.06	0.99	0.00	0.21	0.40	0.24	126.62	53.04
100% Whole Wheat Bread	1	SLICE	118.80	3.68	21.55	2.72	0.49	0.58	1.05	0.85	295.24	165.64
Italian Bread	1	SLICE	81.30	2.64	15.00	1.05	0.00	0.26	0.24	0.42	175.20	33.00
Rye Bread	1	SLICE	82.88	2.72	15.46	1.06	0.00	0.20	0.42	0.26	211.20	53.12
Plain Hamburger Roll/Bun	1	ITEM	122.98	3.66	21.63	2.19	0.00	0.52	0.36	1.08	240.80	60.63
Hard Roll	1	ITEM	167.01	5.64	30.04	2.45	0.00	0.35	0.65	0.98	310.08	61.56
Submarine/Hoagie Roll	1	ITEM	400.00	11.00	72.00	8.00	0.00	1.80	3.00	2.20	683.00	128.00
Pita Bread	1	ITEM	165.00	5.46	33.42	0.72	0.00	0.10	0.06	0.32	321.60	72.00
English Muffin, Toasted	1	ITEM	127.50	4.20	25.00	1.00	0.00	0.14	0.16	0.48	252.00	71.50
Plain Bagel	1	ITEM	195.25	7.46	37.91	1.14	0.00	0.16	0.09	0.49	379.14	71.71
Plain Biscuit, Ready to Eat	1	ITEM	127.40	2.17	16.98	5.78	0.35	0.87	2.42	2.17	368.20	78.40
Plain Waffle, Prepared	1	ITEM	218.25	5.93	24.68	10.58	51.75	2.15	2.64	5.09	383.25	119.25
Plain Pancakes, Prepared	3	ITEM	258.78	7.30	32.26	11.06	67.26	2.42	2.82	5.07	500.46	150.48
Taco Shell	1.00	ITEM	60.84	0.94	8.11	2.94	0.00	0.42	1.16	1.10	47.71	23.27
Corn Tortilla	1.00	ITEM	55.50	1.43	11.65	0.63	0.00	0.08	0.16	0.28	40.25	38.50
Flour Tortilla	1.00	ITEM	113.75	3.05	19.46	2.49	0.00	0.61	1.32	0.37	167.30	45.85
CRACKERS:												
Saltine Crackers	10	ITEM	130.20	2.76	21.45	3.54	0.00	0.88	1.93	0.50	390.60	38.40
Wheat Crackers	10	ITEM	141.90	2.58	19.47	6.18	0.00	1.55	3.43	0.84	238.50	54.90
Plain Rice Cakes (Brown Rice)	3.00	ITEM	104.49	2.21	22.01	0.76	0.00	0.15	0.28	0.27	88.02	78.30
Animal Cracker	14	ITEM	124.88	1.93	20.75	3.86	0.00	0.97	2.17	0.51	110.04	28.00
Plain Graham Crackers	4	ITEM	118.44	1.93	21.50	2.83	0.00	0.43	1.14	1.07	169.40	37.80
Cheese Crackers	30	ITEM	150.90	3.03	17.46	7.59	3.90	2.81	3.63	0.74	298.50	43.50
Plain Bread Sticks	2	ITEM	49.44	1.44	8.21	1.14	0.00	0.17	0.43	0.44	78.84	14.88
Seasoned Croutons, Ready to Eat	1	SERVING	32.55	0.76	4.45	1.28	0.49	0.37	0.37	0.17	86.66	12.67
CEREALS:												
Oatmeal Cereal, Made with Milk	1.00	CUP	237.78	12.34	32.76	6.51	17.34	3.03	1.96	0.95	350.08	434.00
Shredded Wheat Cereal, Large Biscuit	1.00	ITEM	84.96	2.57	19.19	0.39	0.00	0.07	0.06	0.21	0.47	77.17
Shredded Wheat Cereal, Small Biscuit	1.00	CUP	107.10	3.30	24.12	0.50	0.00	0.08	0.08	0.26	3.00	108.30
Granola Cereal, Prepared	1.00	CUP	569.74	17.93	64.66	30.01	0.00	5.80	9.60	12.90	29.28	656.36
KELLOGG'S FROSTED FLAKES Cereal	0.75	CUP	120.00	1.00	27.98	0.00	0.00	0.00	0.00	0.00	200.25	20.03
KELLOGG'S ALL-BRAN Cereal	0.50	CUP	80.00	4.00	22.00	1.00	0.00	0.00	0.00	0.50	280.00	340.00
KELLOGG'S CORN FLAKES Cereal	1.00	CUP	110.00	2.00	26.00	0.00	0.00	0.00	0.00	0.00	330.00	35.00
KELLOGG'S FROOT LOOPS Cereal	1.00	CUP	120.00	1.00	26.00	1.00	0.00	0.50	0.00	0.00	150.00	30.00
KELLOGG'S Raisin Bran Cereal	1.00	CUP	170.00	5.00	43.00	1.00	0.00	0.00	0.00	0.50	310.00	400.00
KELLOGG'S RICE KRISPIES Cereal	1.25	CUP	110.00	2.00	26.00	0.00	0.00	0.00	0.00	0.00	320.00	35.00
KELLOGG'S SPECIAL K Cereal	1.00	CUP	110.00	6.00	21.00	0.00	0.00	0.00	0.00	0.00	250.00	55.00
KELLOGG'S FROSTED MINI-WHEATS Cereal	1.00	CUP	190.00	5.00	45.00	1.00	0.00	0.00	0.00	0.50	0.00	160.00
GENERAL MILLS MULTI-BRAN CHEX Cereal	1.00	CUP	200.00	4.00	49.00	1.50	0.00	0.00	0.00	0.00	360.00	230.00
GENERAL MILLS CORN CHEX Cereal	1.00	CUP	110.00	2.00	26.00	0.00	0.00	0.00	0.00	0.00	300.00	30.00
GENERAL MILLS CHEERIOS Cereal	1.00	CUP	110.00	3.00	22.00	2.00	0.00	0.00	0.50	0.50	280.00	95.00
GENERAL MILLS HONEY NUT CHEERIOS Cereal	1.00	CUP	120.00	3.00	24.00	1.50	0.00	0.00	0.50	0.00	270.00	95.00
GENERAL MILLS WHEATIES Cereal	1.00	CUP	110.00	3.00	24.00	1.00	0.00	0.00	0.00	0.00	220.00	110.00
GENERAL MILLS FIBER ONE Cereal	0.50	CUP	60.00	2.00	24.00	1.00	0.00	0.00	0.00	0.00	140.00	250.00
GENERAL MILLS TOTAL Raisin Bran Cereal	1.00	CUP	180.00	4.00	43.00	1.00	0.00	0.00	0.00	0.00	240.00	280.00
QUAKER OATS CAP'N CRUNCH Cereal	0.75	CUP	110.00	1.00	23.00	1.50	0.00	0.00	0.32	0.39	210.00	35.00
CREAM OF WHEAT Cereal, Regular, Prepared	1.00	CUP	123.00	3.58	26.00	0.20	0.00	0.03	0.02	0.09	2.68	34.00
POST GRAPE NUTS Cereal	0.50	CUP	200.00	6.00	47.00	1.00	0.00	0.00	0.13	0.45	350.00	160.00
POST Bran Flakes Cereal	0.75	CUP	100.00	3.00	24.00	0.50	0.00	0.00	0.00	0.54	220.00	190.00
POST Fruity PEBBLES Cereal	0.75	CUP	110.00	0.50	24.00	1.00	0.00	0.00	0.25	0.25	160.00	30.00

Vit A (IU)	Beta-C	Vit C	Calcium	Iron	Vit D (IU)	Vit E (IU)	Thiamin	Ribo	Niacin	Vit B6	Folate	Vit B12	Phosp	Magn	Zinc	Diet Fiber	Sugar
0.00	0.00	0.00	27.00	0.76			0.12	0.09	0.99	0.02	23.75	0.01	23.50	6.00	0.16	0.58	0.98
0.00	0.00	0.00	26.25	0.83			0.11	0.07	1.03	0.02	19.25	0.00	37.50	11.50	0.26	1.08	1.12
0.00	0.00	0.00	10.75	0.70			0.09	0.06	0.92	0.08	15.25	0.01	38.25	13.00	0.31	1.38	1.00
0.00	0.00	0.08	23.66	0.90			0.11	0.09	1.14	0.09	20.80	0.02	45.76	13.78	0.33	1.66	1.01
9.95		0.04	22.81	1.18			0.10	0.08	1.58	0.11	14.84	0.01	96.09	43.01	0.78	3.05	
0.00	0.00	0.00	23.40	0.88			0.14	0.09	1.31	0.01	28.50	0.00	30.90	8.10	0.26	0.81	0.98
2.24	0.00	0.13	23.36	0.91			0.14	0.11	1.22	0.02	27.52	0.00	40.00	12.80	0.37	1.86	3.07
0.00	0.00	0.04	59.77	1.36			0.21	0.13	1.69	0.02	40.85	0.03	37.84	8.60	0.27	1.16	3.18
0.00	0.00	0.00	54.15	1.87			0.27	0.19	2.42	0.02	54.15	0.00	57.00	15.39	0.54	1.31	2.22
0.00	0.00	0.00	100.00	3.80			0.54	0.33	4.50	0.05			115.00			3.75	10.00
0.00	0.00	0.00	51.60	1.57			0.36	0.20	2.78	0.02	57.00	0.00	58.20	15.60	0.50	1.32	3.24
0.00	0.00	0.05	94.50	1.36			0.19	0.14	1.90	0.02	14.50	0.02	72.50	11.00	0.38	1.45	
0.00	0.00	0.00	52.54	2.53			0.38	0.22	3.24	0.04	62.48	0.04	68.16	20.59	0.63	1.63	2.34
0.70		0.00	17.15	1.16			0.15	0.10	1.17	0.02	20.65	0.05	150.50	5.95	0.17	0.46	1.54
171.00		0.30	191.25	1.73			0.20	0.26	1.56	0.04	34.50	0.19	142.50	14.25	0.51	1.68	4.12
223.44		0.34	249.66	2.05			0.23	0.32	1.79	0.05	43.32	0.25	181.26	18.24	0.64	1.13	5.46
0.00	0.00	0.00	20.80	0.33			0.03	0.01	0.18	0.04	13.65	0.00	32.24	13.65	0.18	0.98	
0.00	0.00	0.00	43.75	0.35			0.03	0.02	0.38	0.06	28.50	0.00	78.50	16.25	0.24	1.30	
0.00	0.00	0.00	43.75	1.16			0.19	0.10	1.25	0.02	43.05	0.00	43.40	9.10	0.25	1.16	
0.00	0.00	0.00	35.70	1.62			0.17	0.14	1.58	0.01	37.20	0.00	31.50	8.10	0.23	0.90	0.00
0.00	0.00	0.00	14.70	1.32			0.15	0.10	1.49	0.04	13.20	0.00	66.00	18.60	0.48	1.35	
12.42	0.00	0.00	2.97	0.40			0.02	0.05	2.11	0.04	5.67	0.00	97.20	35.37	0.81	1.13	
0.00	0.00	0.00	12.04	0.77			0.10	0.09	0.97	0.01	3.92	0.01	31.92	5.04	0.18	0.31	
0.00	0.00	0.00	6.72	1.04			0.06	0.09	1.15	0.02	16.80	0.00	29.12	8.40	0.23	0.78	5.18
48.60	0.00	0.00	45.30	1.43			0.17	0.13	1.40	0.17	24.00	0.14	65.40	10.80	0.34	0.72	0.48
0.00	0.00	0.00	2.64	0.51			0.07	0.07	0.63	0.01	14.64	0.00	14.52	3.84	0.11	0.36	
2.73		0.00	6.72	0.20			0.04	0.03	0.33	0.01	6.16	0.01	9.80	2.94	0.07	0.35	0.00
392.89		1.67	267.91	1.47			0.27	0.37	0.42	0.12	16.57	0.60	351.40	77.99	1.85	3.63	
0.00	0.00	0.00	9.68	0.74			0.07	0.07	1.08	0.06	11.80	0.00	85.67	40.12	0.59	2.31	
0.00	0.00	0.00	11.40	1.27			0.08	0.08	1.58	0.08	15.00	0.00	105.90	39.60	0.99	2.94	
45.14		1.71	98.82	1.47			0.90	0.34	2.50	0.39	104.92	0.00	563.64	217.16	4.95	12.81	33.40
750.00		15.00	0.00	4.50	50.12		0.38	0.43	5.00	0.50	99.75	0.00	0.00	0.00	0.00	0.00	12.98
750.00	0.00	15.00	100.00	4.50	50.00		0.38	0.43	5.00	0.50	100.00	1.50	294.00	120.00	3.75	10.00	5.00
750.00	0.00	15.00	0.00	8.40	50.00		0.38	0.43	5.00	0.50	100.00	0.00	0.00	0.00	0.00	1.00	2.01
750.00		15.00	0.00	4.50	50.00		0.38	0.43	5.00	0.50	100.00	0.00	20.50	8.00	3.75	1.00	14.00
750.00		0.00	40.00	4.50	50.00		0.38	0.43	5.00	0.50	100.00	1.50	191.00	80.00	3.75	7.00	18.00
750.00		15.00	0.00	1.80	50.00		0.38	0.43	5.00	0.50	100.00	0.00	35.75	8.00	0.60	1.00	3.00
750.00		15.00	0.00	8.40	50.00		0.53	0.60	7.00	0.70	100.00	0.00	60.70	16.00	3.75	1.00	3.00
0.00	0.00	0.00	0.00	16.20	0.00		0.38	0.43	5.00	0.50	100.00	1.50	160.00	60.00	1.50	6.00	12.00
0.00	0.00	6.00	0.00	16.20	0.00		0.38	0.00	5.00	0.50	100.00	1.50	200.00	60.00	3.75	7.00	12.00
0.00	0.00	6.00	0.00	9.00	0.00		0.38	0.07	5.00	0.50	100.00	1.50	11.70	4.20	0.11	0.54	3.00
500.00	0.00	6.00	40.00	8.10	40.00		0.38	0.43	5.00	0.50	100.00	1.50	100.00	32.00	3.75	3.00	1.00
500.00	0.00	6.00	0.00	4.50	40.00		0.38	0.43	5.00	0.50	100.00	1.50	100.00	24.00	3.75	2.00	11.00
500.00	0.00	6.00	0.00	8.10	40.00		0.38	0.43	5.00	0.50	100.00	1.50	100.00	32.00	3.75	3.00	4.00
0.00	0.00	6.00	20.00	4.50	0.00		0.38	0.43	5.00	0.50	100.00	1.50	150.00	60.00	1.20	13.00	0.00
500.00	0.00	0.00	200.00	18.00	40.00	30.00	1.50	1.70	20.00	2.00	400.00	6.00	100.00	40.00	15.00	5.00	19.00
0.00	0.00	0.00	4.38	4.50			0.38	0.43	5.00	0.50	174.00	1.71	34.30	10.90	2.93	1.00	12.00
0.00	0.00	0.00	55.60	10.80	0.00		0.15	0.08	1.20	0.02	0.01	0.00	38.00	5.13	0.22	0.94	0.00
750.00	0.00	0.00	20.00	8.10	40.00		0.38	0.43	5.00	0.50	100.00	1.50	150.00	60.00	1.20	5.00	7.00
750.00		0.00	0.00	8.10	40.00		0.38	0.43	5.00	0.50	100.00	1.50	150.00	60.00	1.50	5.00	6.00
750.00		0.00	0.00	1.80	39.90		0.38	0.43	5.00	0.50	99.75	1.50	0.00	0.00	1.50	0.00	12.00

GRAINS	Amount	Portion	Kcal	Protein	Carb	Fat	Chol	Sat Fat	Mono Fat	Poly Fat	Sodium	Potas
PASTA:												
Spaghetti, Enriched, Cooked	0.50	CUP	98.70	3.34	19.84	0.47	0.00	0.07	0.06	0.19	0.70	21.70
Egg Noodles, Enriched, Cooked	0.50	CUP	106.40	3.80	19.87	1.18	26.40	0.25	0.34	0.33	5.60	22.40
Ramen Noodles, Prepared	0.50	CUP	103.50	2.95	15.35	4.30	17.75	0.19	0.22	0.21	414.50	34.45
Japanese Somen Noodles, Wheat, Cooked	0.50	CUP	115.28	3.52	24.24	0.16	0.00	0.02	0.02	0.06	141.68	25.52
Chinese Cellophane Noodles (rice or mung bean), Dehydrated	2.00	OUNCE	199.37	0.09	48.91	0.03	0.00	0.01	0.01	0.01	5.68	5.68
Chow Fun Rice Noodles, Cooked, Fat Added	0.50	CUP	69.54	1.13	15.23	0.27	0.00	0.07	0.08	0.07	1.71	14.44
Cheese Gnocchi, Cooked	0.50	CUP	63.89	3.38	2.99	4.23	24.29	1.64	1.65	0.67	102.88	25.49
Potato Gnocchi, Cooked	0.50	CUP	132.84	2.35	16.40	6.51	17.50	3.98	1.84	0.31	314.96	121.34
PURE GRAINS:												
Rice	1.00	SERVING	99.34	1.94	21.76	0.18	0.00	0.05	0.06	0.05	92.06	31.32
Brown Rice	1.00	SERVING	257.94	5.34	54.28	1.91	0.00	0.38	0.69	0.68	8.18	190.97
Short Grain White Rice, Cooked	0.50	CUP	120.90	2.20	26.72	0.18	0.00	0.05	0.05	0.05	0.00	24.18
Medium Grain White Rice, Cooked	0.50	CUP	120.90	2.21	26.59	0.20	0.00	0.05	0.06	0.05	0.00	26.97
Long Grain White Rice, Instant, Enriched, Boiled	0.50	CUP	80.85	1.70	17.55	0.13	0.00	0.04	0.04	0.04	2.48	3.30
Wild Brown Rice, Cooked	0.50	CUP	82.82	3.27	17.50	0.28	0.00	0.04	0.04	0.18	2.46	82.82
Medium Grain Brown Rice, Cooked	0.50	CUP	109.20	2.26	22.92	0.81	0.00	0.16	0.29	0.29	0.98	77.03
Long Grain Brown Rice, Cooked	0.50	CUP	108.23	2.52	22.39	0.88	0.00	0.18	0.32	0.32	4.88	41.93
Spanish Rice	1.00	CUP	217.18	4.94	41.53	3.84	0.00	0.61	1.48	1.44	765.69	535.57
Bulgur, Cooked	0.50	CUP	75.53	2.80	16.91	0.22	0.00	0.04	0.03	0.09	4.55	61.88
Barley	2.00	OUNCE	200.72	7.08	41.66	1.30	0.00	0.27	0.17	0.63	6.80	256.28
Buckwheat	2.00	OUNCE	194.48	7.51	40.54	1.93	0.00	0.42	0.59	0.59	0.57	260.82
Millet, Cooked	0.50	CUP	142.80	4.21	28.40	1.20	0.00	0.21	0.22	0.61	2.40	74.40
Oats	2.00	OUNCE	220.56	9.58	37.58	3.91	0.00	0.69	1.24	1.44	1.13	243.24
Quinoa	2.00	OUNCE	212.06	7.43	39.07	3.29	0.00	0.34	0.87	1.33	11.91	419.58
Rice Bran, Crude	2.00	OUNCE	179.17	7.57	28.17	11.82	0.00	2.37	4.28	4.23	2.84	842.00
Rye	2.00	OUNCE	189.95	8.37	39.55	1.42	0.00	0.16	0.17	0.63	3.40	149.69
Durum Wheat	2.00	OUNCE	192.21	7.76	40.33	1.40	0.00	0.26	0.20	0.56	1.13	244.38
Wheat Germ, Crude	0.50	CUP	207.00	13.31	29.79	5.59	0.00	0.96	0.79	3.46	6.90	512.90
Amaranth, Dry	2.00	OUNCE	212.06	8.19	37.52	3.69	0.00	0.94	0.81	1.64	11.91	207.52
FLOUR:												
All Purpose Wheat Flour, White, Bleached, Enriched	1.00	CUP	455.00	12.91	95.39	1.23	0.00	0.19	0.11	0.52	2.50	133.75
Wheat Flour, White, Bread, Enriched	1.00	CUP	494.57	16.41	99.37	2.27	0.00	0.33	0.19	1.00	2.74	137.00
Whole Grain Wheat Flour	1.00	CUP	406.80	16.44	87.08	2.24	0.00	0.39	0.28	0.94	6.00	486.00
Barley Flour	1.00	CUP	396.48	8.40	89.38	1.57	0.00	0.33	0.20	0.76	8.96	371.84
White Rice Flour	1.00	CUP	578.28	9.40	126.61	2.24	0.00	0.61	0.70	0.60	0.00	120.08
Whole Grain Corn Flour	1.00	CUP	422.37	8.11	89.91	4.52	0.00	0.64	1.19	2.06	5.85	368.55
Brown Rice Flour	1.00	CUP	573.54	11.42	120.84	4.39	0.00	0.88	1.59	1.57	12.64	456.62
Dark Rye Flour	1.00	CUP	414.72	17.96	87.99	3.44	0.00	0.40	0.42	1.54	1.28	934.40
Semolina, Enriched	1.00	CUP	601.20	21.18	121.63	1.75	0.00	0.25	0.21	0.72	1.67	310.62
Oat Bran, Raw	2.00	OUNCE	139.48	9.81	37.55	3.99	0.00	0.75	1.35	1.57	2.27	320.92
Wheat Bran, Crude	1.00	CUP	125.28	9.02	37.42	2.47	0.00	0.37	0.37	1.28	1.16	685.56
White Bread Crumbs, Enriched	1	CUP	93.45	2.87	17.33	1.26	0.35	0.28	0.56	0.26	188.30	41.65
Plain Bread Crumbs	1	CUP	426.60	13.50	78.30	5.83	0.00	1.31	2.58	1.20	930.96	238.68
Seasoned Bread Crumbs	1	CUP	440.40	17.04	84.48	3.12	1.20	0.87	1.16	0.79	3180.00	324.00
SNACKS:												
Plain Popcorn	3.00	CUP	91.68	2.88	18.70	1.01	0.00	0.14	0.26	0.46	0.96	72.24
Popcorn, with Oil and Salt, Popped	3.00	CUP	165.00	2.97	18.88	9.27	0.00	1.61	2.70	4.43	291.72	74.25
Popcorn, Buttered, Popped in Oil	1.00	CUP	72.95	1.15	7.23	4.65	2.97	1.30	1.35	1.74	122.97	28.80
Pretzels, Twisted, Thin	5.00	ITEM	114.30	2.73	23.76	1.05	0.00	0.23	0.41	0.37	514.50	43.80
Soft Pretzel	1.00	ITEM	214.52	5.08	43.28	1.92	1.86	0.43	0.66	0.59	870.48	54.56
Plain Corn Chips	1.00	OUNCE	153.08	1.87	16.16	9.49	0.00	1.29	2.74	4.68	178.92	40.33
Plain Tortilla Chip	1.00	OUNCE	142.28	1.99	17.86	7.44	0.00	1.43	4.39	1.03	149.95	55.95

Vit A (IU)	Beta-C	Vit C	Calcium	Iron	Vit D (IU)	Vit E (IU)	Thiamin	Ribo	Niacin	Vit B6	Folate	Vit B12	Phosp	Magn	Zinc	Diet Fiber	Sugar
0.00	0.00	0.00	4.90	0.98			0.14	0.07	1.17	0.02	49.00	0.00	37.80	12.60	0.37	1.19	0.90
16.00		0.00	9.60	1.27			0.15	0.07	1.19	0.03	51.20	0.07	55.20	15.20	0.50	0.88	1.03
552.50	98.50	0.09	8.75	0.89			0.08	0.05	0.71	0.03	4.00	0.01	35.00	8.50	0.31	1.02	
0.00	0.00	0.00	7.04	0.46			0.02	0.03	0.09	0.01	1.76	0.00	23.76	1.76	0.19		
0.00	0.00	0.00	14.20	1.23			0.09	0.00	0.11	0.03	1.14	0.00	18.18	1.70	0.23	0.28	
0.00	0.00	0.00	3.04	0.07			0.02	0.00	0.44	0.07	0.53	0.00	18.62	7.22	0.17	0.46	
260.18		0.01	75.87	0.28			0.02	0.07	0.18	0.01	3.60	0.11	56.30	4.43	0.31	0.08	
658.84		1.72	21.76	0.73			0.11	0.09	1.08	0.09	5.14	0.05	39.22	10.27	0.22	0.88	
0.00	0.00	0.00	7.68	1.17	0.00		0.16	0.01	1.14	0.05	62.87	0.00	31.30	6.81	0.30	0.35	0.15
0.00	0.00	0.00	27.08	1.30	0.00		0.29	0.03	3.07	0.36	14.25	0.00	188.11	103.67	1.49	2.42	0.51
0.00	0.00	0.00	0.93	1.36			0.15	0.02	1.39	0.06	54.87	0.00	30.69	7.44	0.37	0.28	0.19
0.00	0.00	0.00	2.79	1.39			0.16	0.02	1.71	0.05	53.94	0.00	34.41	12.09	0.39	0.28	0.19
0.00	0.00	0.00	6.60	0.52			0.06	0.04	0.73	0.01	33.83	0.00	11.55	4.13	0.20	0.50	0.17
0.00	0.00	0.00	2.46	0.49			0.04	0.07	1.06	0.11	21.32	0.00	67.24	26.24	1.10	1.48	0.58
0.00	0.00	0.00	9.75	0.52			0.10	0.01	1.30	0.15	3.90	0.00	75.08	42.90	0.60	1.76	0.30
0.00	0.00	0.00	9.75	0.41			0.09	0.02	1.49	0.14	3.90	0.00	80.93	41.93	0.61	1.76	0.29
1145.12		38.77	69.28	2.52			0.24	0.08	2.98	0.31	20.10	0.00	89.22	39.18	0.88	3.00	5.91
0.00	0.00	0.00	9.10	0.87			0.05	0.03	0.91	0.08	16.38	0.00	36.40	29.12	0.52	4.10	
12.47		0.00	18.71	2.04			0.37	0.16	2.61	0.18	10.77	0.00	149.69	75.41	1.57	9.81	
0.00	0.00	0.00	10.21	1.25			0.06	0.24	3.98	0.12	17.01	0.00	196.75	130.98	1.36	5.67	1.47
0.00	0.00	0.00	3.60	0.76			0.13	0.10	1.60	0.13	22.80	0.00	120.00	52.80	1.09	1.56	0.35
0.00	0.00	0.00	30.62	2.68			0.43	0.08	0.55	0.07	31.75	0.00	296.54	100.36	2.25	6.01	1.02
0.00	0.00	0.00	34.02	5.25			0.11	0.23	1.66	0.13	27.78	0.00	232.47	119.07	1.87	3.35	
0.00	0.00	0.00	32.32	10.51			1.56	0.16	19.28	2.31	35.72	0.00	950.86	442.83	3.43	11.91	0.51
0.00	0.00	0.00	18.71	1.51			0.18	0.14	2.42	0.17	34.02	0.00	212.06	68.61	2.12	8.28	
0.00	0.00	0.00	19.28	2.00			0.24	0.07	3.82	0.24	24.55	0.00	288.04	81.65	2.36	6.91	1.04
0.00	0.00	0.00	22.43	3.60			1.08	0.29	3.92	0.75	161.58	0.00	484.15	137.43	7.07	7.59	7.00
0.00	0.00	2.38	86.75	4.30			0.05	0.12	0.73	0.13	27.78	0.00	257.99	150.82	1.80	8.62	1.11
0.00	0.00	0.00	18.75	5.80	0.98	0.62	7.38	0.06	32.50	0.00	135.00	27.50	0.88		3.38	2.13	
0.00	0.00	0.00	20.55	6.04			1.11	0.70	10.35	0.05	210.98	0.00	132.89	34.25	1.16	3.29	2.33
0.00	0.00	0.00	40.80	4.66			0.54	0.26	7.64	0.41	52.80	0.00	415.20	165.60	3.52	14.64	2.40
0.00	0.00	0.00	32.48	1.41			0.13	0.06	5.14	0.31	25.76	0.00	252.00	90.72	2.09	4.26	
0.00	0.00	0.00	15.80	0.55			0.22	0.03	4.09	0.69	6.32	0.00	154.84	55.30	1.26	3.79	1.58
548.73		0.00	8.19	2.79			0.29	0.09	2.22	0.43	29.25	0.00	318.24	108.81	2.02	15.68	
0.00	0.00	0.00	17.38	3.13			0.70	0.13	10.02	1.16	25.28	0.00	532.46	176.96	3.87	7.27	1.60
0.00	0.00	0.00	71.68	8.26			0.40	0.32	5.47	0.57	76.80	0.00	808.96	317.44	7.19	28.93	5.92
0.00	0.00	0.00	28.39	7.28			1.35	0.95	10.00	0.17	257.18	0.00	227.12	78.49	1.75	6.51	3.07
0.00	0.00	0.00	32.89	3.07			0.66	0.13	0.53	0.09	29.48	0.00	416.18	133.25	1.76	8.73	1.47
0.00	0.00	0.00	42.34	6.13			0.30	0.34	7.88	0.76	45.82	0.00	587.54	354.38	4.22	24.82	2.50
0.00	0.00	0.00	37.80	1.06			0.17	0.12	1.39	0.02	11.90	0.01	32.90	8.40	0.22	0.81	1.37
0.00	0.00	0.00	245.16	6.61			0.83	0.47	7.40	0.11	117.72	0.02	158.76	49.68	1.32	2.59	4.10
15.60		0.48	118.80	3.82			0.19	0.20	3.28	0.18	130.80	0.05	159.60	45.60	1.09	5.04	4.44
47.04		0.00	2.40	0.64			0.05	0.07	0.47	0.06	5.52	0.00	72.00	31.44	0.83	3.62	0.10
50.82		0.10	3.30	0.92			0.04	0.05	0.51	0.07	5.61	0.00	82.50	35.64	0.87	3.30	0.33
61.01		0.04	1.59	0.35			0.02	0.02	0.20	0.03	2.19	0.00	31.92	13.68	0.33	1.26	
0.00	0.00	0.00	10.80	1.30			0.14	0.19	1.58	0.04	24.90	0.00	33.90	10.50	0.26	0.96	
0.00	0.00	0.00	14.26	2.43			0.26	0.18	2.65	0.01	8.68	0.00	48.98	13.02	0.58	1.05	
26.70	12.20	0.00	36.07	0.38			0.01	0.04	0.34	0.07	5.68	0.00	52.54	21.58	0.36	1.39	
55.66	12.20	0.00	43.74	0.43			0.02	0.05	0.36	0.08	2.84	0.00	58.22	24.99	0.44	1.85	

FRUITS	Amount	Portion	Kcal	Protein	Carb	Fat	Chol	Sat Fat
Apple	1.00	ITEM	81.42	0.26	21.05	0.50	0.00	0.08
Applesauce	1.00	SERVING	102.90	0.29	26.43	0.47	0.00	0.08
Avocado, California	0.25	ITEM	76.55	0.91	2.99	7.50	0.00	1.12
Banana, Peeled	1.00	ITEM	108.56	1.22	27.65	0.57	0.00	0.22
Grapes, European Type (Adherent Skin)	1.00	CUP	113.60	1.06	28.43	0.93	0.00	0.30
Lemon	1.00	ITEM	21.60	1.30	11.56	0.32	0.00	0.04
Cantaloupe	1.00	CUP	56.00	1.41	13.38	0.45	0.00	0.11
Honeydew	1.00	CUP	61.95	0.81	16.25	0.18	0.00	0.04
Watermelon	1.00	CUP	48.64	0.94	10.91	0.65	0.00	0.07
Casaba Melon	0.75	CUP	33.15	1.15	7.91	0.13	0.00	0.03
Orange	1.00	ITEM	61.57	1.23	15.39	0.16	0.00	0.02
Tangerine	2.00	ITEM	73.92	1.06	18.80	0.32	0.00	0.04
Grapefruit	0.50	CUP	36.80	0.73	9.29	0.12	0.00	0.02
Peach	1.00	ITEM	42.14	0.69	10.88	0.09	0.00	0.01
Pear	1.00	CUP	97.35	0.64	24.93	0.66	0.00	0.04
Nectarine	1.00	CUP	67.62	1.30	16.26	0.64	0.00	0.07
Apricots	4.00	ITEM	67.20	1.96	15.57	0.55	0.00	0.04
Papaya	0.50	CUP	27.30	0.43	6.87	0.10	0.00	0.03
Pineapple	0.50	CUP	37.98	0.30	9.60	0.33	0.00	0.03
Cherries	24.00	ITEM	85.44	1.58	19.01	0.38	0.00	0.00
Raspberries	0.50	CUP	30.14	0.56	7.12	0.34	0.00	0.01
Strawberries	0.50	CUP	21.60	0.44	5.05	0.27	0.00	0.01
Blackberries	0.50	CUP	37.44	0.52	9.19	0.28	0.00	0.01
Blueberries	0.50	CUP	35.23	0.51	7.79	0.24	0.00	0.00
Cranberries, Chopped	0.50	CUP	26.95	0.21	6.97	0.11	0.00	0.01
Figs	3.00	ITEM	111.00	1.13	28.77	0.45	0.00	0.09
Fruit Cocktail, Canned in Light Syrup	0.50	CUP	68.97	0.48	18.07	0.09	0.00	0.01
Fruit Cocktail, Canned in Heavy Syrup	0.50	CUP	90.52	0.48	23.45	0.09	0.00	0.01
Guava	1.00	ITEM	45.90	0.74	10.69	0.54	0.00	0.16
Kiwi Fruit	1.00	ITEM	46.36	0.75	11.31	0.33	0.00	0.02
Kumquats	3.00	ITEM	35.91	0.51	9.37	0.06	0.00	0.01
Lychee	0.75	CUP	94.05	1.18	23.56	0.63	0.00	0.14
Mango	0.50	ITEM	67.28	0.53	17.60	0.28	0.00	0.07
Passion Fruit (Granadilla)	0.50	CUP	114.46	2.60	27.59	0.83	0.00	0.07
Persimmon	5.00	ITEM	158.75	1.00	41.88	0.50	0.00	0.05
Pomegranate	1.00	ITEM	104.72	1.46	26.44	0.46	0.00	0.06
DRIED FRUITS:								
Dried Apples, Sulfured	0.25	CUP	52.25	0.20	14.17	0.07	0.00	0.01
Raisins, Seedless	0.25	CUP	108.75	1.17	28.69	0.17	0.00	0.05
Dried Apricot Halves, Sulfured	0.25	CUP	77.35	1.19	20.07	0.15	0.00	0.01
Dates	1.00	OUNCE	71.75	0.66	19.13	0.07	0.00	0.00
Prunes, Dried	0.25	CUP	101.58	1.11	26.66	0.22	0.00	0.02
Dried Figs	0.25	CUP	126.86	1.52	32.51	0.58	0.00	0.12

Sodium	Potas	Beta-C	Vit C	Calcium	Iron	Vit E (IU)	Zinc	Diet Fiber	Sugar
0.00	158.70		7.87	9.66	0.25		0.06	3.73	18.40
5.80	224.84	6.40	5.57	13.06	0.36		0.09	2.66	16.00
5.19	274.21		3.42	4.76	0.51		0.18	2.12	0.39
1.18	467.28	50.93	10.74	7.08	0.37		0.19	2.83	18.43
3.20	296.00		17.28	17.60	0.42		0.08	1.60	29.00
3.24	156.60	3.24	83.16	65.88	0.76		0.11	5.08	2.70
14.40	494.40	3100.00	67.52	17.60	0.34		0.26	1.28	13.90
17.70	479.67		43.90	10.62	0.12		0.12	1.06	14.58
3.04	176.32		14.59	12.16	0.26		0.11	0.76	13.68
15.30	267.75	3.83	20.40	6.38	0.51		0.20	1.02	6.00
0.00	237.11		69.69	52.40	0.13		0.09	3.14	12.10
1.68	263.76		51.74	23.52	0.17		0.40	3.86	12.90
0.00	159.85	13.80	39.56	13.80	0.10		0.08	1.27	7.10
0.00	193.06		6.47	4.90	0.11		0.14	1.96	8.56
0.00	206.25		6.60	18.15	0.41		0.20	3.96	17.40
0.00	292.56	102.49	7.45	6.90	0.21		0.12	2.21	11.77
1.40	414.40		14.00	19.60	0.76		0.36	3.36	13.01
2.10	179.90	69.50	43.26	16.80	0.07		0.05	1.26	4.15
0.78	87.58		11.94	5.43	0.29		0.06	0.93	9.20
1.22	295.20	0.05	11.18	16.68	0.72		0.10	3.19	20.26
0.00	93.48		15.38	13.53	0.35		0.28	4.18	5.85
0.72	119.52		40.82	10.08	0.27		0.09	1.66	4.16
0.00	141.12		15.12	23.04	0.41		0.19	3.82	5.85
0.78	59.99	0.03	7.02	6.13	0.20		0.10	3.29	5.23
0.55	39.05	2.75	7.43	3.85	0.11		0.07	2.31	
1.50	348.00	21.00	3.00	52.50	0.56		0.23	4.95	10.35
7.26	107.69	25.40	2.30	7.26	0.35		0.11	1.21	
7.44	109.12		2.36	7.44	0.36		0.10	1.24	
2.70	255.60	71.10	165.15	18.00	0.28		0.21	4.86	5.40
3.80	252.32	13.70	74.48	19.76	0.31		0.13	2.58	7.98
3.42	111.15	17.10	21.32	25.08	0.22		0.05	3.76	5.70
1.43	243.68	0.00	101.89	7.13	0.44		0.10	1.85	
2.07	161.46	402.50	28.67	10.35	0.14		0.04	1.86	15.30
33.04	410.64	82.60	35.40	14.16	1.89		0.12	12.27	13.24
1.25	387.50		82.50	33.75	3.13				
4.62	398.86	0.00	9.39	4.62	0.46		0.19	0.92	15.50
18.71	96.75	0.00	0.84	3.01	0.30		0.04	1.87	
4.35	272.24		1.20	17.76	0.75		0.10	1.45	23.55
3.25	447.85		0.78	14.63	1.53		0.24	2.93	12.65
0.25	186.54			11.75	0.28		0.10	2.11	18.24
1.70	316.63		1.40	21.68	1.05		0.23	3.02	18.69
5.47	354.22	6.48	0.40	71.64	1.11		0.25	6.07	31.00

VEGGIES	Amount	Portion	Kcal	Protein	Carb	Fat	Chol	Sat Fat
LEGUMES:								
Black Beans, Boiled	0.50	CUP	113.52	7.62	20.39	0.46	0.00	0.12
Split Peas, Boiled	0.50	CUP	115.64	8.17	20.69	0.38	0.00	0.05
Pinto Beans, Boiled	0.50	CUP	117.14	7.02	21.93	0.45	0.00	0.09
White Beans, Boiled	0.50	CUP	124.41	8.71	22.47	0.31	0.00	0.08
Lima Beans, Boiled, Drained	0.50	CUP	104.55	5.79	20.09	0.27	0.00	0.06
Kidney Beans, Boiled	0.50	CUP	112.40	7.67	20.19	0.44	0.00	0.06
Red Kidney Beans, Canned with Liquid	0.50	CUP	108.80	6.72	19.97	0.44	0.00	0.06
Lentils, Boiled	0.50	CUP	114.84	8.93	19.94	0.38	0.00	0.05
Garbanzo Beans, Boiled	0.50	CUP	134.48	7.27	22.48	2.12	0.00	0.22
Boston Baked Beans	0.50	CUP	193.45	7.70	27.33	6.42	6.41	2.27
Navy Beans, Boiled	0.50	CUP	129.22	7.92	23.94	0.52	0.00	0.14
Refried Beans, Canned	0.50	CUP	118.91	6.95	19.65	1.59	10.12	0.60
Hummus	0.50	CUP	210.33	6.03	24.81	10.39	0.00	1.56
SOY:								
Soybeans, Boiled	0.50	CUP	148.78	14.31	8.53	7.71	0.00	1.12
Tofu, Raw, Soft, with Calcium Sulfate	1.00	PIECE	73.20	7.86	2.16	4.43	0.00	0.64
Tofu, Raw, Firm, with Calcium Sulfate	0.50	CUP	182.70	19.88	5.39	10.99	0.00	1.59
Miso (Fermented Soybeans), Paste	1.00	TBSP	35.41	2.03	4.81	1.04	0.00	0.15
Tempeh	0.50	CUP	165.17	15.73	14.14	6.37	0.00	0.92
STARCHY VEGETABLES:								
Sweet Corn, Frozen, Boiled, Drained	0.50	CUP	65.60	2.26	16.04	0.35	0.00	0.05
Sweet Corn, Cream Style, Canned	0.50	CUP	92.16	2.23	23.21	0.54	0.00	0.08
Green Peas, Boiled, Drained	0.50	CUP	67.20	4.29	12.51	0.18	0.00	0.03
Blackeye Peas	1.00	SERVING	102.39	6.82	18.33	0.47	0.00	0.12
Cowpeas (Black-Eyed, Croweder, Southern), Common, Boiled	0.50	CUP	99.18	6.61	17.76	0.45	0.00	0.12
Potatoes, Baked	1.00	ITEM	220.18	4.65	50.97	0.20	0.00	0.05
Potatoes, Mashed, Dehydrated Granules, Dry	1.00	CUP	744.00	16.44	171.02	1.08	0.00	0.28
Baked Sweet Potatoes	1.00	SERVING	60.96	0.58	12.18	1.36	0.00	0.24
Sweet Potato, Candied	1.00	PIECE	143.85	0.91	29.25	3.41	8.40	1.42
ALL OTHERS:								
Broccoli	1.00	CUP	24.64	2.62	4.61	0.31	0.00	0.05
Cabbage, Shredded	1.00	CUP	17.50	1.01	3.80	0.19	0.00	0.02
Carrots	1.00	CUP	52.46	1.26	12.37	0.23	0.00	0.04
Peas and Carrots, Frozen, Boiled, Drained	0.50	CUP	38.40	2.47	8.10	0.34	0.00	0.06
Cauliflower, Boiled, Drained	0.50	CUP	14.26	1.14	2.55	0.28	0.00	0.04
Celery, Stalk	1.00	ITEM	6.40	0.30	1.46	0.06	0.00	0.02
Collards, Boiled, Drained	0.50	CUP	24.70	2.00	4.66	0.34	0.00	0.05
Cucumber	1.00	ITEM	39.13	2.08	8.31	0.39	0.00	0.10
Green Beans, Frozen, Boiled, Drained	0.50	CUP	18.90	1.01	4.35	0.12	0.00	0.03
Iceberg Lettuce	1.00	CUP	6.60	0.56	1.15	0.11	0.00	0.01
Onions, Red, Sliced	1.00	CUP	43.70	1.33	9.92	0.18	0.00	0.03
Sweet (Bell) Pepper	1.00	CUP	21.56	1.36	4.72	0.18	0.00	0.00
Hot Chili Peppers, Green	1.00	ITEM	18.00	0.90	4.26	0.09	0.00	0.01
Pumpkin, Canned	0.50	CUP	41.65	1.35	9.90	0.34	0.00	0.18
Spinach, Trimmed Leaves	1.00	CUP	3.16	0.90	0.05	0.10	0.00	0.00
Tomato, Red	1.00	ITEM	25.83	1.05	5.71	0.41	0.00	0.06
Romaine Lettuce, Shredded	1.00	CUP	7.84	0.91	1.33	0.11	0.00	0.02
Mushrooms	1.00	CUP	26.60	3.12	2.65	1.77	0.00	0.24
Summer Squash, All Varieties	0.50	CUP	18.00	0.82	3.88	0.28	0.00	0.06
Winter Squash, All Varieties	1.00	CUP	42.92	1.68	10.21	0.27	0.00	0.05
Vegetable Combinations (Broccoli, Carrots, Corn, Cauliflower, etc.), Cooked	0.50	CUP	27.65	1.57	6.18	0.14	0.00	0.02
Mixed Vegetables, Frozen, Boiled, Drained	0.50	CUP	53.69	2.60	11.91	0.14	0.00	0.03

Sodium	Potas	Beta-C	Vit C	Calcium	Iron	Vit E (IU)	Zinc	Diet Fiber	Sugar
0.86	305.30		0.00	23.22	1.81		0.96	7.48	0.95
1.96	354.76	0.96	0.39	13.72	1.26		0.98	8.13	2.83
1.71	400.14	0.00	1.80	41.04	2.23		0.92	7.35	1.88
5.37	502.10	0.00	0.00	80.55	3.31		1.24	5.64	1.97
14.45	484.50	25.50	8.59	27.20	2.08		0.67	4.51	2.50
1.77	356.66	0.00	1.06	24.78	2.60		0.95	5.66	1.95
436.48	328.96	0.00	1.41	30.72	1.61		0.70	8.19	2.82
1.98	365.31	0.99	1.49	18.81	3.30		1.26	7.82	1.80
5.74	238.62		1.07	40.18	2.37		1.26	6.23	3.94
575.19	536.78		1.06	87.61	3.12		1.16	4.99	
0.91	334.88	0.00	0.82	63.70	2.26		0.97	5.82	2.00
378.24	337.76	0.00	7.59	44.28	2.10		1.48	6.71	
300.12	214.02	2.46	9.72	61.50	1.93		1.35	6.27	
0.86	442.90	0.86	1.46	87.72	4.42		0.99	5.16	2.60
9.60	144.00	9.62	0.24	133.20	1.33		0.77	0.24	0.84
17.64	298.62		0.25	860.58	13.19		1.98	2.90	0.17
626.85	28.19		0.00	11.34	0.47		0.57	0.93	
4.98	304.61		0.00	77.19	1.88		1.50		
4.10	120.54		2.54	3.28	0.29		0.33	1.97	1.48
364.80	171.52	12.80	5.89	3.84	0.49		0.68	1.54	
2.40	216.80	51.00	11.36	21.60	1.23		0.95	4.40	4.64
3.53	245.39	1.62	0.35	21.19	2.22		1.14	5.74	2.92
3.42	237.69	1.57	0.34	20.52	2.15		1.10	5.56	2.83
16.16	844.36	0.00	26.06	20.20	2.75		0.65	4.85	3.23
134.00	1406.00		74.00	82.00	2.18		1.82	14.20	
32.24	122.36	240.78	8.04	11.65	0.39		0.07	0.98	7.60
73.50	198.45	592.00	7.04	27.30	1.19		0.16	2.52	
23.76	286.00	136.00	82.02	42.24	0.77		0.35	2.64	1.75
12.60	172.20	9.10	22.54	32.90	0.41		0.13	1.61	2.52
42.70	394.06	3431.25	11.35	32.94	0.61		0.24	3.66	8.05
54.40	126.40	617.00	6.48	18.40	0.75		0.36	2.48	4.00
9.30	88.04		27.47	9.92	0.21		0.11	1.67	2.36
34.80	114.80	5.20	2.80	16.00	0.16		0.05	0.68	0.44
8.55	247.00	316.17	17.29	113.05	0.44		0.40	2.66	
6.02	433.44		15.95	42.14	0.78		0.60	2.41	6.92
6.08	85.05		2.77	33.08	0.59		0.32	2.03	1.76
4.95	86.90	18.16	2.15	10.45	0.28		0.12	0.77	0.99
3.45	180.55	0.00	7.36	23.00	0.26		0.22	2.07	7.13
2.07	269.08	0.24	113.07	12.45	0.52		0.15	2.43	3.58
3.15	153.00	483.60	109.13	8.10	0.54		0.14	0.68	1.13
6.13	252.35	175.50	5.15	31.85	1.70		0.21	3.55	4.05
37.97	134.09	1.01	7.50	25.01	2.13		0.18	2.77	0.00
11.07	273.06	139.00	23.49	6.15	0.55		0.11	1.35	3.40
4.48	162.40	18.50	13.44	20.16	0.62		0.14	0.95	1.12
4.06	341.41	0.00	0.00	2.69	0.55			0.68	1.89
0.90	172.80	25.95	4.95	24.30	0.32		0.35	1.26	1.89
4.64	406.00		14.27	35.96	0.67		0.15	1.74	2.55
183.85	112.62		14.15	20.85	0.34		0.19	2.09	
31.85	153.79		2.91	22.75	0.75		0.45	4.00	3.93

DAIRY	Amount	Portion	Kcal	Protein	Carb	Fat	Chol	Sat Fat	Sodium
CHEESE:									
American Cheese	1.00	OUNCE	106.44	6.28	0.45	8.86	26.76	5.58	405.52
Cheddar Cheese, Shredded	0.25	CUP	113.73	7.03	0.36	9.36	29.63	5.96	175.29
Cottage Cheese, 1% Fat	0.50	CUP	81.81	14.00	3.07	1.15	4.97	0.73	458.78
Cottage Cheese, 4% Fat, Creamed	0.50	CUP	108.51	13.12	2.81	4.74	15.65	3.00	425.04
Fat Free Cream Cheese	2.00	TBSP	28.80	4.32	1.74	0.41	2.40	0.27	163.50
Lowfat Cream Cheese	2.00	TBSP	69.30	3.18	2.10	5.28	16.80	3.33	88.80
Cream Cheese	2.00	TBSP	101.22	2.19	0.77	10.11	31.81	6.37	85.70
Mozzarella Cheese, Part Skim Milk	1.00	OUNCE	71.19	6.79	0.78	4.46	16.18	2.83	130.48
Mozzarella Cheese, Whole Milk	1.00	OUNCE	78.79	5.44	0.62	6.05	21.95	3.68	104.47
Monterey Jack Cheese	1.00	OUNCE	104.53	6.85	0.19	8.48	24.92	5.34	150.16
Parmesan Cheese, Grated	1.00	TBSP	22.79	2.08	0.19	1.50	3.94	0.95	93.08
Provolone Cheese	1.00	OUNCE	98.42	7.16	0.60	7.45	19.29	4.78	245.14
Ricotta Cheese, Whole Milk	0.50	CUP	213.95	13.85	3.74	15.97	62.24	10.20	103.44
Ricotta Cheese, Part Skim Milk	0.50	CUP	169.81	14.01	6.32	9.73	37.88	6.06	153.38
Swiss Cheese	1.00	OUNCE	105.21	7.96	0.95	7.69	25.68	4.98	72.80
Romano Cheese	1.00	OUNCE	108.26	8.90	1.02	7.54	29.12	4.79	336.00
Brie Cheese	1.00	OUNCE	93.42	5.81	0.13	7.75	28.00	4.88	176.23
Muenster Cheese	1.00	OUNCE	103.14	6.56	0.31	8.41	26.77	5.35	175.76
Blue Cheese, Crumbled	0.50	CUP	238.31	14.45	1.58	19.40	50.76	12.60	941.83
Goat Cheese, Hard	1.00	OUNCE	128.37	8.67	0.62	10.11	29.82	6.99	98.26
Goat Cheese, Soft	1.00	OUNCE	76.11	5.26	0.25	5.99	13.06	4.14	104.51
MILK:									
Whole Milk, 3.3%	8.00	FL OZ	149.92	8.03	11.37	8.15	33.18	5.07	119.56
Reduced Fat Milk, 2%	8.00	FL OZ	121.20	8.13	11.71	4.69	18.30	2.92	121.76
Lowfat Milk, 1%	8.00	FL OZ	102.15	8.03	11.66	2.59	9.76	1.61	123.22
Nonfat/Skim/Fat Free Milk	8.00	FL OZ	85.53	8.35	11.88	0.44	4.41	0.29	126.18
Chocolate Milk, Whole	8	FL OZ	208.38	7.93	25.85	8.48	30.50	5.26	149.00
Reduced Fat Chocolate Milk, 2%	8	FL OZ	178.84	8.03	26.00	5.00	17.00	3.10	150.50
Chocolate Flavored Milk, Powder	2.5	TSP	75.38	0.71	19.51	0.67	0.00	0.40	45.36
YOGURT:									
Lowfat Fruit Yogurt, with Nonfat Milk Solids	1.00	CUP	257.56	11.91	45.57	3.45	13.48	2.23	159.01
Lowfat Plain Yogurt, with Nonfat Milk Solids	1.00	CUP	155.05	12.86	17.25	3.80	14.95	2.45	171.99
Nonfat Plain Yogurt, with Nonfat Milk Solids	1.00	CUP	136.64	14.04	18.82	0.44	4.41	0.28	187.43
Nonfat Fruit Yogurt, Sweetened with Low-Calorie Sweetener	1.00	CUP	121.89	10.62	19.38	0.39	3.25	0.21	139.48
CREAM:									
Half and Half Cream	2.00	TBSP	39.11	0.89	1.29	3.45	11.07	2.15	12.21
Heavy Whipping Cream, Liquid	2.00	TBSP	103.43	0.62	0.84	11.10	41.13	6.91	11.28
Sour Cream	2.00	TBSP	51.42	0.76	1.03	5.03	10.66	3.13	12.79
Cream Substitute, Liquid	1.00	TBSP	20.35	0.15	1.71	1.50	0.00	0.29	11.88
Cream Substitute, Powder	1.00	TSP	10.93	0.10	1.10	0.71	0.00	0.65	3.62

Potas	Beta-C	Vit C	Calcium	Iron	Vit E (IU)	Zinc	Diet Fiber	Sugar
45.93		0.00	174.49	0.11		0.85	0.00	0.45
27.80		0.00	203.77	0.19		0.88	0.00	0.51
96.62		0.00	68.82	0.16		0.43	0.00	3.08
88.52		0.00	63.00	0.15		0.39	0.00	0.63
48.90		0.00	55.50	0.05		0.26	0.00	
50.10		0.00	33.60	0.50		0.23	0.00	
34.63		0.00	23.17	0.35		0.16	0.00	0.50
23.44		0.00	180.80	0.06		0.77	0.00	0.11
18.79		0.00	144.76	0.05		0.62	0.00	0.11
22.60	6.86	0.00	208.99	0.20		0.84	0.00	0.00
5.36		0.00	68.79	0.05		0.16	0.00	
38.72		0.00	211.65	0.15		0.90	0.00	
128.66		0.00	254.61	0.47		1.43	0.00	1.85
153.75		0.00	334.56	0.54		1.65	0.00	1.72
31.00		0.00	269.05	0.05		1.09	0.00	0.19
24.16		0.00	297.86	0.22		0.72	0.00	
42.56	2.52	0.00	51.52	0.14		0.67	0.00	
37.63	3.64	0.00	200.84	0.12		0.79	0.00	
173.00	5.40	0.00	356.13	0.21		1.80	0.00	
13.63		0.00	254.18	0.53		0.45	0.00	
7.38		0.00	39.76	0.54		0.26	0.00	
369.66		2.29	291.34	0.12		0.93	0.00	12.00
376.74		2.32	296.70	0.12		0.95	0.00	11.20
380.88		2.37	300.12	0.12		0.95	0.00	11.20
405.72		2.40	302.33	0.10		0.98	0.00	10.80
417.25		2.28	280.25	0.60		1.03	2.00	
422.00		2.30	284.00	0.60		1.03	1.25	
127.66	0.43	0.15	7.99	0.68		0.34	1.25	8.67
529.94		1.81	413.81	0.17		2.01	0.00	37.78
572.81		1.96	447.37	0.20		2.18	0.00	12.52
624.51		2.13	487.80	0.22		2.38	0.00	12.52
549.90		26.40	369.51	0.62		1.83	1.27	
38.88		0.26	31.47	0.02		0.15	0.00	
22.62	0.00	0.17	19.38	0.01		0.07	0.00	0.84
34.56		0.21	27.94	0.01		0.07	0.00	
28.58		0.00	1.40	0.00		0.00	0.00	
16.24		0.00	0.45	0.02		0.01	0.00	

MEAT	Amount	Weight/g or Portion	Kcal	Protein/g	Carb/g	Total Fat/g	Chol/mg	Sat Fat/g
BEEF:								
Eye of round roast, lean, roasted (11 cm x 6 cm x 0.6 cm)	2 slices	88	155	24	0.00	6	50	2.3
Eye of round steak, lean, broiled (11 cm x 6 cm x 1.2 cm)	1 piece	86	176	27	0.00	7	49	2.8
Flank steak, lean, broiled (11 cm x 6 cm x 1.2 cm)	1 piece	86	197	27	0.00	9	47	3.8
Ground, lean, broiled well done	1 patty	70	174	20	0.00	10	57	3.4
Ground lean, medium broiled	1 patty	84	201	21	0.00	12	58	4.0
Ground, regular, medium broiled	1 patty	76	220	18	0.00	16	56	4.4
Inside (top) round steak, lean, broiled (11 cm x 6 cm x 1.2 cm)	1 piece	86	141	26	0.00	3	56	1.2
Rib eye steak, lean, broiled (11 cm x 6 cm x 1.2 cm)	1 piece	86	174	25	0.00	7	56	2.8
Sirloin tip roast, lean, roasted (11 cm x 6 cm x 0.6 cm)	2 slices	88	184	27	0.00	8	58	2.8
Standing rib roast, lean, roasted (11 cm x 6 cm x 0.6 cm)	2 slices	88	194	25	0.00	10	59	4.0
Strip loin (New York) steak, lean, broiled (11 cm x 6 cm x 1.2 cm)	1 piece	86	179	25	0.00	8	53	3.1
Tenderloin, lean, broiled (11 cm x 6 cm x 1.2 cm)	1 piece	86	172	24	0.00	8	59	2.8
VEAL:								
Cutlets, grain-fed veal, pan-fried (7 cm x 6 cm x 2 cm)	1 cutlet	84	127	26	0.00	2	116	
Ground, broiled	1 patty	75	129	18	0.00	6	77	
Leg, lean + fat, roasted	1 steak	93	148	26	0.00	4	95	
Loin, lean, roasted (11 cm x 6 cm x 0.6 cm)	2 slices	88	154	23	0.00	6	93	
PORK:								
Centre cut, lean, pan-fried	1 chop	69	160	22	0.00	7	63	2.5
Centre cut, lean, roasted (11 cm x 6 cm x 0.6 cm)	2 slices	88	162	25	0.00	6	70	3.0
Ground, cooked	250 mL	125	371	32	0.00	26	118	9.6
Loin, rib end, lean, roasted (11 cm x 6 cm x 0.6 cm)	2 slices	88	199	25	0.00	10	67	3.8
Shoulder, butt, lean braised	½ chop	79	216	25	0.00	12	92	4.4
Spareribs, lean + fat, braised	3 ribs	75	238	21	0.00	16	80	6.1
Tenderloin, lean, roasted (11 cm x 6 cm x 0.6 cm)	2 slices	88	143	27	0.00	3	60	1.1
LAMB:								
Domestic, rib, lean + fat, broiled	2 chops	92	332	20	0.00	27	91	
New Zealand, leg, whole, lean, roasted (11 cm x 6 cm x 0.6 cm)	2 slices	88	160	24	0.00	6	88	
New Zealand, loin, lean + fat, broiled (11 cm x 6 cm x 1.2 cm)	1 piece	85	266	20	0.00	20	95	

Sodium/mg	Potas/mg	Beta-C	Vit C/ mg	Calcium/mg	Iron/mg	Vit E (IU)	Zinc/mg	Total Dietary Fibre/g	Sugar
49	373	0.00	0.00	4	1.6		3.8	0.00	0.00
47	350	0.00	0.00	5	2.6		4.3	0.00	0.00
58	372	0.00	0.00	5	1.8		6.2	0.00	0.00
58	260	0.00	0.00	6	2.0		4.5	0.00	0.00
59	264	0.00	0.00	6	2.0		4.6	0.00	0.00
63	223	0.00	0.00	8	1.9		3.9	0.00	0.00
44	346	0.00	0.00	5	2.4		4.4	0.00	0.00
55	352	0.00	0.00	6	1.9		5.4	0.00	0.00
53	363	0.00	0.00	5	2.3		6.7	0.00	0.00
63	332	0.00	0.00	8	2.0		6.2	0.00	0.00
51	328	0.00	0.00	7	2.0		4.6	0.00	0.00
54	362	0.00	0.00	6	3.1		4.8	0.00	0.00
37	299	0.00	0.00	4	1.7		2.5	0.00	0.00
62	252	0.00	0.00	13	0.7		2.9	0.00	0.00
63	361	0.00	0.00	6	0.8		2.8	0.00	0.00
85	300	0.00	0.00	19	0.7		2.9	0.00	0.00
59	310	0.00	0.00	16	0.7		1.7	0.00	0.00
58	319	0.00	0.00	22	0.9		1.8	0.00	0.00
91	452	0.00	0.00	28	1.6		4.0	0.00	0.00
26	308	0.00	0.00	26	1.1		3.4	0.00	0.00
59	325	0.00	0.00	23	1.6		4.4	0.00	0.00
70	240	0.00	0.00	35	1.4		3.5	0.00	0.00
49	385	0.00	0.00	5	1.3		2.3	0.00	0.00
70	248	0.00	0.00	17	1.7		3.7	0.00	0.00
40	161	0.00	0.00	6	2.0		3.6	0.00	0.00
41	135	0.00	0.00	19	1.7		2.2	0.00	0.00
69	370	0.00	0.00	5	0.6		1.2	0.00	0.00

POULTRY	Amount	Weight/g or Portion	Kcal	Protein/g	Carb/g	Total Fat/g	Chol/mg	Sat Fat/g
Chicken, broiler, breast, meat + skin, roasted	½ breast	115	218	30	0.00	10	97	
Chicken, broiler, breast, meat, roasted	½ breast	98	156	32	0.00	2	84	
Chicken, broiler, thigh, meat, roasted	1 thigh	50	85	12	0.00	3	48	
Chicken, broiler, wing, meat + skin, roasted	1 wing	34	99	9	0.00	7	29	
Chicken, roasting, dark meat, roasted	1 leg + back	171	282	41	0.00	12	128	
Chicken, roasting, light meat, roasted	½ chicken	177	271	48	0.00	7	133	
Chicken, ground, lean, cooked	1 patty	82	168	18	0.00	10	N/A	
Cornish game hens, meat + skin, roasted	½ bird	115	298	25	0.00	21	150	
Duck, domesticated, light and dark meat, roasted	¼ duck	111	222	26	0.00	12	98	
Turkey, dark meat, roasted (8 cm x 5 cm x 0.6 cm)	3 slices	84	155	24	0.00	6	74	
Turkey, light meat (breast), roasted (8 cm x 5 cm x 0.6 cm)	3 slices	84	129	25	0.00	2	58	
Turkey, ground, cooked	1 patty	82	194	23	0.00	11	84	
PROCESSED MEATS:								
Pork sausage, patty, cooked	2 items	199.26	10.61	0.56	16.83	44.82	5.84	
Pork sausage, link, cooked	2 items	95.94	5.11	0.27	8.10	21.58	2.81	
Beef frankfurter	1 item	141.75	5.40	0.81	12.83	27.45	5.42	
Chicken frankfurter	1 item	115.65	5.82	3.06	8.77	45.45	2.49	
Turkey frankfurter	1 item	101.70	6.43	0.67	7.97	48.15	2.65	
Ham luncheon meat, sliced, prepackaged or deli	1 slice	34.02	3.84	0.48	1.76	11.13	0.57	
Turkey or chicken breast luncheon meat, prepackaged or deli	2 ounces	61.60	12.60	0.00	0.88	22.96	0.27	
Turkey loaf, breast meat	2 slices	46.75	9.56	0.00	0.67	17.43	0.20	
Pepperoni with beef and pork	10 slices	273.35	11.53	1.56	24.18	43.45	8.87	
Bologna, beef and pork, sliced	1 slice	89.59	3.31	0.79	8.01	15.59	3.03	
Pork and beef salami, dry	6 slice	250.80	13.72	1.55	20.63	47.40	7.32	

Sodium/mg	Potas/mg	Beta-C	Vit C/ mg	Calcium/mg	Iron/mg	Vit E (IU)	Zinc/mg	Total Dietary Fibre/g	Sugar
73	395	0.00	0.00	5	0.6		1.0	0.00	0.00
44	119	0.00	0.00	6	0.7		1.3	0.00	0.00
28	63	0.00	0.00	5	0.4		0.6	0.00	0.00
162	382	0.00	0.00	19	2.3		3.6	0.00	0.00
90	418	0.00	0.00	23	1.9		1.4	0.00	0.00
56	233	0.00	0.00	20	1.3		N/A	0.00	0.00
73	281	0.00	0.00	15	1.0		1.7	0.00	0.00
72	278	0.00	0.00	13	3.0		2.9	0.00	0.00
69	246	0.00	0.00	29	2.0		3.8	0.00	0.00
57	259	0.00	0.00	15	1.1		1.8	0.00	0.00
88	222	0.00	0.00	21	1.6		2.4	0.00	0.00
698.76	194.94	0.00	0.00	1.08	17.28		0.93	0.00	0.39
336.44	93.86	0.00	0.00	0.52	8.32		0.45	0.00	0.19
461.70	74.70	0.00	0.00	0.00	9.00		0.69	0.00	0.13
616.50	37.80	58.50	0.00	0.00	42.75		0.11	0.00	0.37
641.70	80.55	0.00	0.00	0.00	47.70		0.13	0.00	0.32
268.38	62.37	0.00	0.00	0.00	1.47		0.17	0.00	
801.36	155.68	0.00	0.00	0.00	3.92		1.13	0.00	
608.18	118.15	0.00	0.00	0.00	2.98	0.20	0.86	0.00	0.25
1122.00	190.85	0.00	0.00	0.00	5.50		1.38	0.00	1.03
288.89	51.03	0.00	0.00	0.00	3.40		0.38	0.00	0.08
1116.00	226.80	0.00	0.00	0.00	4.80		1.14	0.00	0.64

SEAFOOD	Amount	Portion	Kcal	Protein	Carb	Fat	Chol	Sat Fat	Sodium
SHELLFISH:									
Clams, Mixed Species, Cooked, Moist Heat	3.00	OUNCE	125.80	21.72	4.36	1.66	56.95	0.16	0.47
Shrimp, Mixed Species, Cooked, Moist Heat	3.00	OUNCE	84.15	17.77	0.00	0.92	165.75	0.25	0.37
Bay and Sea Scallops, Steamed	3.00	OUNCE	90.39	13.77	1.95	2.67	27.03		
Alaska King Crab, Cooked, Moist Heat	3.00	OUNCE	82.45	16.45	0.00	1.31	45.05	0.11	0.46
Imperial Crab	3.00	OUNCE	127.30	13.17	2.78	6.78	106.38	1.60	1.69
Northern Lobster, Cooked, Moist Heat	3.00	OUNCE	83.30	17.43	1.09	0.50	61.20	0.09	0.08
ALL OTHERS:									
Tuna, White, Canned in Water, Drained	3.00	OUNCE	108.80	20.08	0.00	2.52	35.70	0.67	320.45
Tuna, White, Canned in Oil, Drained	3.00	OUNCE	158.10	22.55	0.00	6.87	26.35	1.40	2.87
Light Tuna, Canned in Oil, Drained	1.00	OUNCE	168.30	24.76	0.00	6.98	15.30	1.30	300.90
Bluefin Tuna, Cooked, Dry Heat	3.00	OUNCE	156.40	25.42	0.00	5.34	41.65	1.37	1.57
Yellowtail, Mixed Species, Cooked, Dry Heat	3.00	OUNCE	158.95	25.22	0.00	5.71	60.35	1.45	1.53
Atlantic Cod, Cooked, Dry Heat	3.00	OUNCE	89.25	19.41	0.00	0.73	46.75	0.14	0.25
Haddock, Cooked, Dry Heat	3.00	OUNCE	95.20	20.60	0.00	0.79	62.90	0.14	0.26
Sea Trout, Mixed Species, Cooked, Dry Heat	3.00	OUNCE	113.05	18.24	0.00	3.94	90.10	1.10	0.79
Rainbow Trout, Farmed, Cooked, Dry Heat	3.00	OUNCE	143.65	20.63	0.00	6.12	57.80	1.79	1.98
Striped Bass, Cooked, Dry Heat	3.00	OUNCE	105.40	19.32	0.00	2.54	87.55	0.55	0.85
Sea Bass, Mixed Species, Cooked, Dry Heat	3.00	OUNCE	105.40	20.09	0.00	2.18	45.05	0.56	0.81
Bluefish, Cooked, Dry Heat	3.00	OUNCE	135.15	21.84	0.00	4.62	64.60	1.00	1.15
Halibut, Cooked, Dry Heat	3.00	OUNCE	119.00	22.69	0.00	2.50	34.85	0.35	0.80
Atlantic Herring, Pickled	1.00	PIECE	39.30	2.13	1.45	2.70	1.95	0.36	0.25
Atlantic Mackerel, Cooked, Dry Heat	3.00	OUNCE	222.70	20.27	0.00	15.14	63.75	3.55	3.66
Pacific/Jack Mackerel, Mixed Species, Cooked, Dry Heat	3.00	OUNCE	170.85	21.87	0.00	8.60	51.00	2.45	2.12
Snapper, Mixed Species, Cooked, Dry Heat	3.00	OUNCE	108.80	22.36	0.00	1.46	39.95	0.31	0.50
Atlantic Salmon, Wild, Cooked, Dry Heat	3.00	OUNCE	154.70	21.62	0.00	6.91	60.35	1.07	2.77
Atlantic Salmon, Farmed, Cooked, Dry Heat	3.00	OUNCE	175.10	18.79	0.00	10.50	53.55	2.13	3.76
Pink Salmon, Cooked, Dry Heat	3.00	OUNCE	126.65	21.73	0.00	3.76	56.95	0.61	1.47
Sturgeon, Steamed	3.00	OUNCE	110.63	17.01	0.00	4.26	63.22	0.97	0.73
Sturgeon, Mixed Species, Cooked, Dry Heat	3.00	OUNCE	114.75	17.60	0.00	4.40	65.45	1.00	0.75
Swordfish, Cooked, Dry Heat	3.00	OUNCE	131.75	21.58	0.00	4.37	42.50	1.20	1.01
Swordfish, Broiled, with Margarine	3.00	OUNCE	151.03	20.26	0.38	7.06	39.81	1.69	1.77
Gelfilte Fish, Sweet Recipe	2.00	PIECE	70.56	7.62	6.22	1.45	25.20	0.35	0.24
Sablefish, Cooked, Dry Heat	3.00	OUNCE	212.50	14.61	0.00	16.68	53.55	3.48	2.23
Sablefish, Smoked	3.00	OUNCE	218.45	15.00	0.00	17.12	54.40	3.58	2.29
Whitefish, Mixed Species, Cooked, Dry Heat	3.00	OUNCE	146.20	20.80	0.00	6.38	65.45	0.99	2.34
Perch, Mixed Species, Cooked, Dry Heat	3.00	OUNCE	99.45	21.13	0.00	1.00	97.75	0.20	0.40
Atlantic Sardine, Solids with Bone, Canned in	2.00	ITEM	49.92	5.91	0.00	2.75	34.08	0.37	1.24
Anchovy, Canned in Oil, Drained	14.00	ITEM	117.60	16.18	0.00	5.44	47.60	1.23	1.44
Octopus, Common, Cooked, Moist Heat	3.00	OUNCE	139.40	25.35	3.74	1.77	81.60	0.39	0.41
Atlantic Smelt, Canned	3.00	OUNCE	170.00	15.64	0.00	11.48			
Rainbow Smelt, Cooked, Dry Heat	3.00	OUNCE	105.40	19.21	0.00	2.64	76.50	0.49	0.97
Caviar, Red and Black, Granular	1.00	TBSP	40.32	3.94	0.64	2.86	94.08	0.65	1.19
Eel, Steamed or Poached	3.00	OUNCE	197.97	19.84	0.00	12.55	135.57	2.54	1.02

354

Potas	Beta-C	Vit C	Calcium	Iron	Vit E (IU)	Zinc	Diet Fiber	Sugar
95.20	484.50	0.05	18.79	78.20	0.00	15.30	2.32	0.00
190.40	186.15	0.00	1.87	33.15	0.00	28.90	1.33	0.00
365.86	128.59		1.97	20.55				0.00
911.20	24.65	0.00	6.46	50.15	0.00	53.55	6.48	0.00
358.37	271.10		4.58	82.07		22.08	2.48	0.14
323.00	73.95	0.00	0.00	51.85	0.00	29.75	2.48	0.00
201.45		0.00	11.90	0.83		0.41	0.00	0.00
336.60	68.00	0.00	0.00	3.40	0.00	28.90	0.40	0.00
175.95		0.00	11.05	1.18		0.77	0.00	0.00
42.50	2142.00	2.83	0.00	8.50	0.00	54.40	0.66	0.00
42.50	88.40		2.47	24.65		32.30	0.57	0.00
66.30	39.10	36.60	0.85	11.90	0.00	35.70	0.49	0.00
73.95	53.55	9.45	0.00	35.70	0.00	42.50	0.41	0.00
62.90	97.75		0.00	18.70		34.00	0.49	0.00
35.70	243.95		2.81	73.10		27.20	0.42	0.00
74.80	88.40		0.00	16.15		43.35	0.43	0.00
73.95	181.05	3.39	0.00	11.05	0.84	45.05	0.44	0.00
65.45	390.15		0.00	7.65		35.70	0.88	0.00
58.65	152.15		0.00	51.00	0.00	90.95	0.45	0.00
130.50	129.15	0.00	0.00	11.55	0.00	1.20	0.08	0.00
70.55	153.00	2.83	0.34	12.75	0.00	82.45	0.80	0.00
93.50	39.95		1.79	24.65		30.60	0.73	0.00
48.45	97.75		1.36	34.00	0.00	31.45	0.37	0.00
47.60	37.40		0.00	12.75		31.45	0.70	0.00
51.85	42.50		3.15	12.75		25.50	0.37	0.00
73.10	115.60		0.00	14.45		28.05	0.60	0.00
388.55	663.73		0.00	11.17		29.51	0.36	0.00
58.65	686.80	0.00	0.00	14.45	0.00	38.25	0.46	0.00
97.75	116.45	3.39	0.94	5.10	0.00	28.90	1.25	0.00
430.92	365.16		2.74	5.66		27.92	1.18	0.02
440.16	74.76	0.00	0.67	19.32	0.00	7.56	0.69	0.00
61.20	287.30		0.00	38.25		60.35	0.35	0.00
626.45	346.80		0.00	42.50		62.90	0.37	0.00
55.25	111.35		0.00	28.05		35.70	1.08	0.00
67.15	27.20	0.07	1.45	86.70	0.00	32.30	1.22	0.00
121.20	53.76		0.00	91.68	0.00	9.36	0.31	0.00
2054.08	39.20	0.00	0.00	129.92	168.00	38.64	1.37	0.00
391.00	229.50		6.80	90.10		51.00	2.86	0.00
	81.59		0.00	304.30	255.00			0.00
65.45	49.30	0.06	0.00	65.45	0.00	32.30	1.80	0.00
240.00	298.88	0.00	0.00	44.00	0.00	48.00	0.15	0.00
49.39	3179.29		1.45	21.52		19.37	1.74	0.00

EGGS

EGGS	Amount	Portion	kCal	Protein	Carb	Fat	Chol	Sat Fat	Sodium	Potas
Egg, Raw	1.00	ITEM	74.50	6.25	0.61	5.01	212.50	1.55	63.00	60.50
Egg Yolk, Raw	1.00	ITEM	59.43	2.78	0.30	5.12	212.65	1.59	7.14	15.60
Egg White, Raw	1.00	ITEM	16.70	3.51	0.34	0.00	0.00	0.00	54.78	47.76
Egg Substitute, Liquid	0.50	CUP	105.58	15.07	0.80	4.16	1.26	0.83	222.31	414.48
PREPARED:										
Hard Boiled Egg	1.00	ITEM	77.50	6.29	0.56	5.31	212.00	1.63	62.00	414.48
Fried Egg	1.00	ITEM	91.54	6.23	0.63	6.90	211.14	1.92	162.38	414.48
Scrambled Eggs	1.00	SERVING	81.12	6.50	0.97	5.48	1.26	1.63	211.64	414.48
Scrambled Egg or Omelet, Fat Added in Cooking	1.00	SERVING	189.94	12.94	2.98	13.69	399.49	4.07	222.31	466.76
Poached Egg	1.00	ITEM	74.50	6.22	0.61	4.99	211.50	1.54	222.31	140.00

NUTS & SEEDS
NUTS:

	Amount	Portion	kCal	Protein	Carb	Fat	Chol	Sat Fat	Sodium	Potas
Peanuts, All Types, Oil Roasted, with Salt	0.50	CUP	418.32	18.97	13.63	35.50	0.00	4.93	311.76	491.04
Peanut Butter, Smooth, with Salt	2	TBSP	189.76	8.07	6.17	16.33	0.00	3.31	149.44	214.08
Black Walnut, Chopped, Dried	0.50	CUP	379.38	15.22	7.56	35.36	0.00	2.27	0.63	327.50
Almonds, Dry Roasted, Unblanched, Salted	0.25	CUP	202.52	5.63	8.34	17.80	0.00	1.69	269.10	265.65
Almonds, Oil Roasted, Unblanched, Salted	0.25	CUP	242.57	8.00	6.23	22.64	0.00	2.15	305.76	268.08
Brazil Nuts, Whole, Unblanched, Dried	0.50	CUP	459.20	10.04	8.96	46.35	0.00	11.31	1.40	420.00
Cashew Nut, Oil Roasted	0.50	CUP	374.40	10.50	18.54	31.34	0.00	6.19	11.05	344.50
Coconut, Shredded	2.00	TBSP	35.40	0.33	1.52	3.35	0.00	2.97	2.00	35.60
Pecan Halves, Dried	0.50	CUP	360.18	4.19	9.85	36.53	0.00	2.93	0.54	211.68
Cashews, Dry Roasted	0.50	CUP	393.19	10.49	22.39	31.75	0.00	6.27	10.96	387.03
Macadamia Nut, Oil Roasted	0.50	CUP	481.06	4.86	8.64	51.27	0.00	7.68	4.69	220.43
Mixed Nuts with Peanuts, Dry Roasted	0.50	CUP	406.89	11.85	17.37	35.24	0.00	4.73	8.22	408.95
Pistachio Nuts, Dry Roasted	0.50	CUP	387.84	9.56	17.62	33.81	0.00	4.28	3.84	620.80
Pine Nut (Pingolia), Dried	1.00	TBSP	48.68	2.06	1.22	4.36	0.00	0.67	0.34	51.51

SEEDS:

	Amount	Portion	kCal	Protein	Carb	Fat	Chol	Sat Fat	Sodium	Potas
Pumpkin Seed	0.25	CUP	187.08	8.81	4.56	18.95	0.00	2.99	6.21	278.19
Sesame Seeds, Dried	1.00	TBSP	51.57	1.60	2.11	4.47	0.00	0.63	0.99	42.12
Sesame Seeds, Roasted, Toasted	1.00	TBSP	50.85	1.53	2.32	4.32	0.00	0.61	0.99	42.75
Psyllium Seed, Ground	1.00	TBSP	4.19	0.24	6.77	0.04	0.00	0.00	2.93	14.99
Sunflower Seed Kernels, Dry Roasted	0.25	CUP	186.24	6.19	7.70	15.94	0.00	1.67	0.96	272.00
Sunflower Seed Kernels, Oil Roasted	0.25	CUP	207.56	7.21	4.97	19.39	0.00	2.03	1.01	163.01

Beta-C	Vit C	Calcium	Iron	VitE (IU)	Zinc	Diet Fiber	Sugar
0.00	0.00	24.50	0.72		0.55	0.00	0.00
0.00	0.00	22.74	0.59		0.52	0.00	0.00
0.00	0.00	2.00	0.01		0.00	0.00	0.00
308.25	0.00	66.57	2.64		1.63	0.00	0.00
0.00	0.00	25.00	0.60		0.53	0.00	0.00
	0.00	25.30	0.72		0.55	0.00	0.00
0.00	0.07	33.83	0.72		0.58	0.00	0.00
	0.32	93.14	1.37		1.17	0.00	0.00
0.00	0.00	24.50	0.72		0.55	0.00	0.00
0.00	0.00	63.36	1.32		4.77	6.62	2.67
0.00	0.00	12.16	0.59		0.93	1.89	2.67
7.50	2.00	36.25	1.92		2.14	3.13	1.32
0.00	0.24	97.29	1.31		1.69	4.73	
0.00	0.28	91.85	1.50		1.92	4.40	
0.00	0.49	123.20	2.38		3.21	3.78	1.82
0.00	0.00	26.65	2.67		3.09	2.47	4.03
0.00	0.33	1.40	0.24		0.11	0.90	0.35
	1.08	19.44	1.15		2.95	4.10	2.32
0.00	0.00	30.83	4.11		3.84	2.06	4.25
0.67	0.00	30.15	1.21		0.74	6.23	4.15
0.69	0.27	47.95	2.53		2.60	6.17	2.74
15.35	4.67	44.80	2.03		0.87	6.91	4.23
	0.16	2.24	0.79		0.37	0.39	
13.12	0.66	15.55	3.40		2.58	0.58	0.35
0.09	0.00	87.75	1.31		0.70	1.06	0.10
0.09	0.00	89.01	1.33		0.64	1.26	0.10
	0.03	17.00	0.29		0.22	6.03	
0.00	0.45	22.40	1.22		1.69	3.55	
1.69	0.47	18.90	2.26		1.76	2.30	1.96

COMBINATION FOODS	Amount	Portion	Kcal	Protein	Carb	Fat	Chol	Sat Fat
BREAKFAST ITEMS:								
Grilled Cheese Sandwich	1	ITEM	291.51	9.79	27.07	15.94	19.45	6.22
Scrambled Egg, No Added Fat	2	ITEM	158.41	12.9	2.94	10.16	399.51	3.4
Cheese Omelet	1	ITEM	425.13	27.8	7.1	31.24	638.09	12.7
Egg, Ham and Cheese Sandwich on English Muffin	1	ITEM	299.31	19.33	24.66	13.15	212.46	5.28
French Toast, Prepared with 2% Lowfat Milk	1	SLICE	148.85	5.01	16.25	7.02	75.4	1.77
SOUPS:								
Chili con Carne	0.5	CUP	160.36	11.20	13.56	7.05	29.80	2.50
Vegetable Soup	1	CUP	100.25	4.30	12.29	4.51	0.00	0.89
Tomato Soup, Condensed, Prepared with Water	1	CUP	85.40	2.05	16.59	1.93	0.00	0.37
Chicken Broth, Condensed, Prepared with Water	1	CUP	39.04	4.93	0.93	1.39	0.00	0.39
Chicken Noodle Soup	1	CUP	127.11	17.83	6.97	2.71	60.13	0.68
Chunky Beef Soup, Canned, Ready to Eat	1	CUP	170.40	11.74	19.56	5.14	14.40	2.54
Chunky Chicken Soup, Canned, Ready to Eat	1	CUP	178.21	12.70	17.27	6.63	30.12	1.98
Green Pea Soup, Condensed, Prepared with Water	1	CUP	165.00	8.60	26.50	2.93	0.00	1.40
Cream of Mushroom Soup, Condensed, Canned	0.5	CUP	129.27	2.02	9.29	9.50	1.26	2.57
PIZZA, PASTA & RICE:								
Fried Rice, with Meat and/or Poultry	1	CUP	329.49	11.91	41.34	12.44	102.44	2.27
Ravioli, Canned, Meat-Filled with Tomato or Meat Sauce	1	CUP	219.76	8.75	37.90	4.10	16.56	1.58
Macaroni and Cheese Mix with Prepared Cheese Sauce, Prepared	0.5	CUP	178.96	6.76	25.01	5.57	13.76	3.19
Spaghetti with Tomato Sauce, Meatless	1	CUP	229.41	7.03	41.48	3.65	0.00	0.52
Lasagna with Meat and/or Poultry	1	PIECE	369.89	21.74	37.63	14.67	54.94	7.56
Cheese Pizza, Thick Crust	1	SLICE	202.02	7.49	27.54	6.69	7.29	2.49
SALADS:								
Tuna Salad	0.5	CUP	191.68	16.44	9.65	9.49	13.33	1.58
Potato Salad	0.5	CUP	178.75	3.35	13.96	10.25	85.00	1.79
Coleslaw	0.5	CUP	41.40	0.77	7.45	1.57	4.80	0.23
Chicken Salad	0.5	CUP	208.62	14.75	1.25	15.93	53.01	2.82
Macaroni Salad	0.5	CUP	134.43	2.76	21.32	4.42	3.12	0.65
ENTREES:								
Hot Dog on Bun	1	ITEM	259.57	8.57	19.62	15.99	24.23	5.65
Hamburger, Single Patty with Condiments	1	ITEM	272.42	12.32	34.25	9.77	29.68	3.56
Cheeseburger, Single Patty with Condiments	1	ITEM	294.93	15.96	26.53	14.15	37.29	6.31
Fish Sticks, Frozen, Heated	3	ITEM	228.48	13.15	19.95	10.27	94.08	2.65
Taco, Prepared	1	ITEM	369.36	20.66	26.73	20.55	56.43	11.37
Bean and Cheese Burrito	1	ITEM	188.79	7.53	27.48	5.85	13.95	3.42
SIDES:								
Bread Stuffing, Prepared from Mix	0.5	CUP	178.00	3.20	21.70	8.60	0.00	1.73
Hashed Brown Potatoes	0.5	CUP	163.02	1.89	16.63	10.85	0.00	4.24
Mashed Potatoes with Whole Milk	0.5	CUP	80.85	2.04	18.43	0.62	2.10	0.35
Potato Chips, Salted	1	OUNCE	152.22	1.99	15.02	9.83	0.00	3.11
Potatoes, Scalloped	0.5	CUP	105.35	3.52	13.21	4.51	14.70	2.76
Potato Puffs, Frozen, Heated	0.5	CUP	142.08	2.14	19.51	6.87	0.00	3.26
French Fried Potatoes, Frozen, Heated	10	ITEM	100	1.585	15.595	3.78	0	0.631
Onion Rings, Frozen, Heated	7	ITEM	284.90	3.74	26.71	18.69	0.00	6.01
	3.00	OUNCE	117.57	1.41	14.78	6.15	0.00	0.78

Sodium	Potas	Beta-C	Vit C	Calcium	Iron	Vit E (IU)	Zinc	Diet Fiber	Sugar
695.65	137.02		0.01	218.58	1.76		1.15	1.17	
425.39	171.58		0.3	91.76	1.36		1.17	0	
1207.35	368.8		0.47	374.87	2.4		2.99	0	
934.29	246.97		0.04	219.21	2.25		2.03	1.33	
311.35	87.1		0.19	65	1.08		0.44	1.92	
655.97	381.05		10.59	29.86	1.90		2.06	3.72	
607.96	532.76		11.61	43.91	1.05		0.54	2.12	
695.40	263.52	68.30	66.37	12.20	1.76		0.24	0.49	0.00
775.92	209.84	0.00	0.00	9.76	0.51		0.25	0.00	
792.74	287.60		3.66	23.80	1.12		1.39	0.99	
866.40	336.00		6.96	31.20	2.33		2.64	1.44	2.37
888.54	175.70	75.30	1.26	25.10	1.73		1.00	1.51	
917.50	190.00	20.00	1.75	27.50	1.95		1.71	2.75	3.29
868.46	84.09	0.00	1.13	32.63	0.53		0.59	0.38	
820.98	181.66		3.38	36.40	2.66		1.42	1.28	
1354.15	336.54		21.53	27.54	2.04		1.19	1.55	
392.64	54.27		0.02	58.38	1.25		0.67	1.11	
590.93	454.86		11.46	38.84	2.50		0.80	4.07	
741.32	433.88		13.65	255.39	2.91		3.15	2.60	
423.57	123.54		2.60	117.58	1.79		0.73	1.29	
412.05	182.45		2.26	17.43	1.03		0.57	0.00	
661.25	317.50		12.50	23.75	0.81		0.39	1.63	
13.80	108.60	132.00	19.62	27.00	0.35		0.12	0.90	
145.10	165.30		1.59	19.25	0.79		1.11	0.39	
480.53	58.89		1.12	11.24	0.89		0.33	1.03	
747.32	132.45	0.00	0.00	56.13	1.72		1.12	0.99	
534.24	251.22		2.23	126.14	2.71		2.25	2.33	
615.85	222.61		1.92	110.74	2.43		2.09		
488.88	219.24		0.00	16.80	0.62		0.55	0.00	6.70
801.99	473.67	62.80	2.22	220.59	2.41		3.93		10.50
583.11	248.31	3.16	0.84	106.95	1.14		0.82		
543.00	74.00		0.00	32.00	1.09		0.28	2.90	0.87
18.72	250.38	0.00	4.45	6.24	0.63		0.23	1.56	
318.15	313.95	0.00	7.04	27.30	0.28		0.31	2.10	0.16
168.70	362.10	0.00	8.83	6.82	0.46		0.31	1.28	4.10
410.38	463.05	4.50	12.99	69.83	0.70		0.49	2.33	0.28
477.44	243.20	4.42	4.42	19.20	1.00		0.19	2.05	
15	209	0	5.05	4	0.62		0.2	1.6	0.25
262.50	90.30	0.32	0.98	21.70	1.18		0.29	0.91	
197.29	277.77		8.11	5.51	0.25		0.23	1.42	

359

FATS	Amount	Portion	Kcal	Protein	Carb	Fat	Chol	Sat Fat	Sodium	Potas	
Butter	1	TBSP	107.55	0.13	0.01	12.17	32.84	7.57	123.90	3.90	
Butter, Whipped	1	TBSP	81.72	0.10	0.01	9.25	24.96	5.76	94.22	2.96	
Margarine, with Unspecified Oils	1	TBSP	101.34	0.13	0.13	11.35	0.00	2.23	133.02	5.98	
Whipped Margarine	1	TBSP	64.44	0.07	0.05	7.24	0.00	1.17	97.11	3.42	
Fat Free Margarine-Like Spread, Salted	1	TBSP	4.90	0.20	0.20	0.21	0.00	0.03	90.02	0.00	
Mayonnaise, with Soybean Oil	1	TBSP	98.91	0.15	0.37	10.96	8.14	1.63	78.44	4.69	
Low Calorie Mayonnaise	1	TBSP	37.05	0.04	2.56	3.07	3.84	0.53	79.52	1.60	
Sour Cream Dip	2	TBSP	66.97	1.16	2.47	6.01	12.55	3.69	227.56	56.16	
OILS:											
Corn Oil	1	TBSP	120.22	0.00	0.00	13.60	0.00	1.73	0.00	0.00	
Olive Oil	1	TBSP	119.34	0.00	0.00	13.50	0.00	1.82	0.01	0.00	
Coconut Oil	1	TBSP	117.23	0.00	0.00	13.60	0.00	11.76	0.00	0.00	
Peanut Oil	1.00	TBSP	119.34	0.00	0.00	13.50	0.00	2.28	0.02	0.00	
Soybean Oil, with Soybean and Cottonseed Oil	1.00	TBSP	120.22	0.00	0.00	13.60	0.00	2.45	0.00	0.00	
Sesame Vegetable Oil	1.00	TBSP	120.22	0.00	0.00	13.60	0.00	1.93	0.00	0.00	
Canola Oil	1.00	TBSP	120.22	0.00	0.00	13.60	0.00	0.97	0.00	0.00	
Cottonseed Oil	1.00	TBSP	120.22	0.00	0.00	13.60	0.00	3.52	0.00	0.00	
Grapeseed Oil	1.00	TBSP	120.22	0.00	0.00	13.60	0.00	1.31	0.00	0.00	
Soybean Oil	1.00	TBSP	120.22	0.00	0.00	13.60	0.00	1.96	0.00	0.00	
Flaxseed Oil	1.00	TBSP	114.92	0.00	0.00	13.00	0.00	1.22	0.00	0.00	
DRESSING:											
Blue Cheese Salad Dressing	1	TBSP	77.11	0.73	1.13	8.00	2.60	1.52	167.38	5.66	
French Salad Dressing	1	TBSP	67.03	0.09	2.73	6.40	0.00	1.48	213.72	12.32	
Italian Salad Dressing	1	TBSP	68.69	0.10	1.50	7.10	0.00	1.03	115.69	2.21	
Mayonnaise-Type Salad Dressing	1	TBSP	57.28	0.13	3.51	4.91	3.82	0.72	104.49	1.32	
Thousand Island Salad Dressing	1	TBSP	58.85	0.14	2.37	5.57	4.06	0.94	109.20	17.63	
Low Calorie Thousand Island Salad Dressing	2	TBSP	48.53	0.24	4.96	3.27	4.59	0.49	306.00	34.58	

Beta-C	Vit C	Calcium	Iron	Vit E (IU)	Zinc	Diet Fiber	Sugar
12.42	0.00	3.60	0.02		0.01	0.00	0.00
9.45	0.00	2.68	0.02		0.01	0.00	0.00
12.60	0.02	4.22	0.01		0.00	0.00	0.00
	0.01	2.34	0.00		0.00	0.00	0.00
	0.00	0.00	0.00		0.00	0.00	
	0.00	2.48	0.07		0.02	0.00	0.00
0.00	0.00	0.00	0.00		0.02	0.00	
	0.30	35.94	0.05		0.09	0.25	
0.00	0.00	0.00	0.00		0.00	0.00	0.00
0.00	0.00	0.02	0.05		0.01	0.00	0.00
0.00	0.00	0.00	0.01		0.00	0.00	0.00
0.00	0.00	0.01	0.00		0.00	0.00	0.00
0.00	0.00	0.00	0.00		0.00	0.00	0.00
0.00	0.00	0.00	0.00		0.00	0.00	0.00
0.00	0.00	0.00	0.00		0.00	0.00	0.00
0.00	0.00	0.00	0.00		0.00	0.00	0.00
0.00	0.00	0.00	0.00		0.00	0.00	0.00
0.00	0.00	0.01	0.00		0.00	0.00	0.00
0.00	0.00	0.00	0.00		0.00	0.00	0.00
	0.31	12.39	0.03		0.04	0.00	
	0.00	1.72	0.06		0.01	0.00	2.21
	0.00	1.47	0.03		0.02	0.00	0.37
	0.00	2.06	0.03		0.03	0.00	
	0.00	1.72	0.09		0.02	0.00	
	0.00	3.37	0.18		0.05	0.37	

BEVERAGES JUICE:	Amount	Portion	Kcal	Protein	Carb	Fat	Chol	Sat Fat
Apple Juice, Canned	8	FL OZ	116.56	0.15	28.97	0.27	0.00	0.05
Grapefruit Juice	8	FL OZ	96.33	1.24	22.72	0.25	0.00	0.04
Orange Juice	8	FL OZ	111.60	1.74	25.79	0.50	0.00	0.06
Pineapple Juice, Canned	8	FL OZ	140.00	0.80	34.45	0.20	0.00	0.01
Lemonade, Frozen Concentrate, Prepared with Water	8	FL OZ	99.20	0.25	26.04	0.00	0.00	0.00
Grape Juice, Unsweetened	1	CUP	154.33	1.42	37.85	0.20	0.00	0.06
Cranberry Juice Drink with Vitamin C Added	1	CUP	144.21	0.00	36.43	0.25	0.00	0.02
Fruit Punch Drink Mix, Prepared with Water	8	FL OZ	96.94	0.00	24.89	0.00	0.00	0.00
Tomato Juice, Canned	8	FL OZ	41.48	1.85	10.32	0.15	0.00	0.02
Carrot Juice, Canned	8	FL OZ	98.40	2.34	22.85	0.37	0.00	0.07
Vegetable Juice, Canned ALCOHOL:	8	FL OZ	45.98	1.53	11.01	0.22	0.00	0.03
Beer	12	FL OZ	146.12	1.07	13.19	0.00	0.00	0.00
Light Beer	12	FL OZ	99.12	0.71	4.60	0.00	0.00	0.00
Distilled Alcohol, 80 Proof	1	FL OZ	64.22	0.00	0.00	0.00	0.00	0.00
Distilled Alcohol, 86 Proof	1	FL OZ	69.50	0.00	0.03	0.00	0.00	0.00
Table Wine SOFT DRINKS:	4	FL OZ	82.6	0.236	1.652	0	0	0
Club Soda	12	FL OZ	0.00	0.00	0.00	0.00	0.00	0.00
Cola	12	FL OZ	151.53	0.00	38.43	0.00	0.00	0.00
Low Calorie Cola	12	FL OZ	3.55	0.36	0.36	0.00	0.00	0.00
Ginger Ale	12	FL OZ	124.44	0.00	31.84	0.00	0.00	0.00
Root Beer COFFEE/TEA:	12	FL OZ	151.54	0.00	39.18	0.00	0.00	0.00
Coffee, Brewed	8	FL OZ	4.74	0.24	0.95	0.00	0.00	0.00
Tea, Brewed	8	FL OZ	2.37	0.00	0.71	0.00	0.00	0.00
Herbal Tea, Prepared with Water	8	FL OZ	2.37	0.00	0.47	0.00	0.00	0.00
Coffee, Brewed, Decaffeinated	8	FL OZ	4.74	0.24	0.94	0.00	0.00	0.00
Decaffeinated Tea, Leaf, Unsweetened MISC:	8	FL OZ	2.37	0.00	0.71	0.00	0.00	0.00
Tap Water	8	FL OZ	0.00	0.00	0.00	0.00	0.00	0.00
Soy Milk	8.00	FL OZ	79.20	6.60	4.34	4.58	0.00	0.51

Sodium	Potas	Beta-C	Vit C	Calcium	Iron	Vit E (IU)	Zinc	Diet Fiber	Sugar
7.44	295.12	0.00	2.23	17.36	0.92		0.07	0.25	27.00
2.47	400.14		93.86	22.23	0.49		0.12	0.25	15.50
2.48	496.00		124.00	27.28	0.50		0.12	0.50	25.30
2.50	335.00	0.00	26.75	42.50	0.65		0.28	0.50	31.30
7.44	37.20		9.67	7.44	0.40		0.10	0.25	22.80
7.59	333.96		0.25	22.77	0.61		0.13	0.25	
5.06	45.54	0.00	89.56	7.59	0.38		0.18	0.25	
36.68	2.62	0.00	30.92	41.92	0.13		0.08	0.00	9.51
880.84	536.80	137.00	44.65	21.96	1.42		0.34	0.98	8.00
71.34	718.32	6334.00	20.91	59.04	1.13		0.44	1.97	
653.40	467.06	283.00	67.03	26.62	1.02		0.48	1.94	8.20
17.82	89.10	0.00	0.00	17.82	0.11		0.07	0.71	1.49
10.62	63.72	0.00	0.00	17.70	0.14		0.11	0.00	2.50
0.28	0.56	0.00	0.00	0.00	0.01		0.01	0.00	0.00
0.28	0.56	0.00	0.00	0.00	0.01		0.01	0.00	0.00
9.44	105.02	0	0	9.44	0.484		0.083	0	1.652
74.59	7.10	0.00	0.00	17.76	0.04		0.36	0.00	0.00
14.78	3.69	0.00	0.00	11.08	0.11		0.03	0.00	38.40
21.31	0.00	0.00	0.00	14.21	0.11		0.28	0.00	0.00
25.62	3.66	0.00	0.00	10.98	0.66		0.18	0.00	31.80
48.05	3.70	0.00	0.00	18.48	0.19		0.26	0.00	39.24
4.74	127.98	0.00	0.00	4.74	0.12		0.05	0.00	0.00
7.10	87.62	0.00	0.00	0.00	0.05		0.05	0.00	0.00
2.37	21.31	0.00	0.00	4.74	0.19		0.10	0.00	0.00
4.74	128.00	0.00	0.00	4.74	0.12		0.05	0.00	0.00
7.11	87.69	0.00	0.00	0.00	0.05		0.05	0.00	
7.11	0.00	0.00	0.00	4.74	0.02		0.07	0.00	0.00
28.80	338.40	7.20	0.00	9.60	1.39		0.55	3.12	

SWEETS	Amount	Portion	Kcal	Protein	Carb	Fat	Chol	Sat Fat	Sodium	Potas
CAKES & PIES:										
Devil's Food Cake with Chocolate Frosting, Prepared from Mix	1.00	SLICE	235.00	3.00	40.00	8.00	37.00	3.50	181.00	90.00
Devil's Food Cupcake with Chocolate Frosting	1.00	ITEM	120.00	2.00	20.00	4.00	19.00	1.80	92.00	46.00
White Cake with Frosting	1.00	SLICE	251.92	2.84	38.76	10.23	2.79	2.79	185.92	71.30
Carrot Cake with Cream Cheese Frosting, Prepared	1.00	SLICE	484.00	5.11	52.40	29.30	59.90	5.43	273.00	124.00
Butter Pound Cake, Ready to Eat	1.00	SLICE	116.40	1.65	14.64	5.97	66.30	3.47	119.40	35.70
Yellow Cake, Ready to Eat, with Chocolate Frosting	1.00	SLICE	242.56	2.43	35.46	11.14	35.20	2.98	215.68	113.92
Apple Pie, Prepared	1.00	SLICE	410.75	3.72	57.51	19.38	0.00	4.73	327.05	122.45
Pumpkin Pie, Prepared	1.00	SLICE	316.20	6.98	40.92	14.42	65.10	4.92	348.75	288.30
Chocolate Creme Pie, Ready to Eat	1.00	SLICE	343.52	2.94	37.97	21.92	5.65	5.61	153.68	143.51
BAKED GOODS:										
Fig Bar	2.00	ITEM	111.36	1.18	22.69	2.34	0.00	0.36	112.00	66.24
Cinnamon Bun, Frosted	1.00	ITEM	208.56	2.77	31.12	8.40	29.12	2.09	193.80	50.91
Brownie, Prepared	1.00	ITEM	111.84	1.49	12.05	6.98	17.52	1.76	82.32	42.24
Corn Muffin, Prepared with 2% Lowfat Milk	1.00	ITEM	180.12	4.05	25.19	7.01	23.94	1.32	333.45	82.65
Oat Bran Muffin	1.00	ITEM	153.90	3.99	27.53	4.22	0.00	0.62	224.01	288.99
Plain Cake Doughnut, Glazed	1.00	ITEM	191.70	2.34	22.86	10.31	14.40	2.67	180.90	45.90
COOKIES:										
Vanilla Sandwich Cookie with Creme Filling	3.00	ITEM	144.90	1.35	21.63	6.00	0.00	0.89	104.70	27.30
Chocolate Sandwich Cookie, with Creme Filling	3.00	ITEM	141.60	1.41	21.09	6.18	0.00	1.10	181.20	52.50
Butter Cookie, Ready to Eat	6.00	ITEM	140.10	1.83	20.67	5.64	35.10	3.32	105.30	33.30
Chocolate Chip Cookie, Prepared with Butter	2.00	ITEM	156.16	1.82	18.62	9.09	22.40	4.50	109.12	70.72
Oatmeal Cookie with Raisins, Prepared	2.00	ITEM	130.50	1.95	20.52	4.86	9.90	0.97	161.40	71.70
Peanut Butter Cookie, Ready to Eat	2.00	ITEM	143.10	2.88	17.67	7.08	0.30	1.35	124.50	50.10
Shortbread Cookie, Ready to Eat	3.00	ITEM	120.48	1.46	15.48	5.78	4.80	1.47	109.20	24.00
Granola Bar, with Oats, Sugar, Raisins, Coconut	1.00	ITEM	195.22	4.21	28.68	7.57	0.00	5.46	119.54	140.18
Sugar Cookie, Ready to Eat	2.00	ITEM	143.40	1.53	20.37	6.33	15.30	1.63	107.10	18.90
FROZEN DESSERTS:										
Vanilla Ice Cream, Rich	0.50	CUP	178.34	2.59	16.58	11.99	45.14	7.38	41.44	117.66
Ice Cream with Cone, Flavor Other Than Chocolate	1.00	ITEM	166.41	2.94	20.88	8.40	32.36	5.04	65.21	151.34
Ice Cream Bar, Chocolate Covered	1.00	ITEM	169.33	1.66	14.36	12.51	19.47	9.59	35.55	103.57
Ice Cream Sandwich	1.00	ITEM	143.63	2.62	21.75	5.61	19.78	3.24	36.37	122.39
Ice Pop (Popsicle), Ready to Eat	1.00	ITEM	42.48	0.00	11.15	0.00	0.00	0.00	7.08	2.36
Sherbet, All Flavors	0.50	CUP	133.17	1.06	29.34	1.93	4.83	1.12	44.39	92.64
Frozen Yogurt, Fruit Varieties	0.50	CUP	143.51	3.39	24.41	4.07	14.69	2.63	71.19	176.28
Vanilla Frozen Yogurt, Soft Serve	0.50	CUP	114.48	2.88	17.42	4.03	1.44	2.46	62.64	151.92
CANDIES:										
Gumdrops	10.00	ITEM	138.96	0.00	35.60	0.00	0.00	0.00	15.84	1.80
Hard Candy	2.00	PIECE	47.28	0.00	11.76	0.02	0.00	0.00	4.56	0.60
Marshmallows	4.00	ITEM	91.58	0.52	23.41	0.06	0.00	0.02	13.54	1.44
Taffy	3.00	PIECE	169.20	0.05	41.10	1.49	4.05	0.92	39.90	1.80
Fruit Leather Roll	1.00	ITEM	73.50	0.21	17.70	0.63	0.00	0.14	12.81	61.74
Licorice	1.00	ITEM	69.73	0.00	17.69	0.10	0.00	0.03	4.75	7.03
Chocolate Pudding, Canned	0.50	CUP	173.57	3.52	29.75	5.22	3.92	0.93	168.35	234.90
Milk Chocolate Bar	1.00	ITEM	503.23	6.55	52.73	29.85	20.02		83.72	413.00

Beta-C	Vit C	Calcium	Iron	Vit E (IU)	Zinc	Diet Fiber	Sugar
	0.00	41.00	1.40			1.52	
	0.00	21.00	0.70			0.70	
	0.00	65.07	0.63		0.24	0.78	
	1.22	27.80	1.39		0.54	1.33	
	0.00	10.50	0.41		0.14	0.15	
	0.00	23.68	1.33		0.40	1.15	
	2.64	10.85	1.74		0.29		47.90
	2.64	145.70	1.97		0.71		
0.00	0.00	40.68	1.21		0.26	2.26	
	0.10	20.48	0.93		0.13	1.47	
	0.89	33.12	0.71		0.27	1.06	
	0.07	13.68	0.44		0.23		
	0.17	147.63	1.49		0.35	1.14	
0.00	0.00	35.91	2.39		1.05	2.62	2.11
	0.05	27.00	0.48		0.20	0.68	7.61
0.00	0.00	8.10	0.66		0.12	0.45	
0.00	0.00	7.80	1.16		0.24	0.96	12.30
	0.00	8.70	0.09		0.11	0.24	
	0.06	12.16	0.79		0.30		8.00
	0.15	30.00	0.80		0.26		
	0.00	10.50	0.75		0.16	0.54	
	0.00	8.40	0.66		0.13	0.43	
	0.43	25.80	1.37		0.69	1.33	
	0.03	6.30	0.64		0.13	0.23	
	0.52	86.58	0.04		0.30	0.00	13.02
	0.44	95.25	0.23		0.54	0.13	
	0.27	57.35	0.14		0.35	0.18	
	0.27	60.02	0.28		0.44	0.55	
0.00	0.00	0.00	0.00		0.01	0.00	
	4.15	52.11	0.14		0.46	0.48	
0.00	0.79	113.00	0.52		0.32	0.00	
	0.58	102.96	0.22		0.30	0.00	
0.00	0.00	1.08	0.14		0.00	0.00	23.76
0.00	0.00	0.36	0.04		0.00	0.00	7.55
0.00	0.00	0.86	0.07		0.01	0.03	16.13
	0.00	1.35	0.03		0.02	0.00	30.00
0.21	1.28	6.72	0.21		0.04	0.76	
0.00	0.00	0.57	0.21		0.01	0.00	
	2.35	117.45	0.67		0.55	1.31	
0.00	0.82	195.65	1.09		1.00	1.73	

CONDIMENTS	Amount	Portion	Kcal	Protein	Carb	Fat	Chol	Sat Fat	Sodium	Potas
SAUCE/GRAVY:										
Tomato Sauce, Canned	0.25	CUP	18.37	0.81	4.40	0.10	0.00	0.02	370.56	227.24
Tomato Paste, Canned	2	TBSP	26.90	1.20	6.33	0.18	0.00	0.03	28.86	307.34
Barbecue Sauce	2	TBSP	23.43	0.56	4.00	0.56	0.00	0.08	254.69	54.38
Sweet and Sour Sauce	0.25	CUP	73.75	0.18	18.18	0.02	0.00	0.00	195.00	16.45
Beef Gravy, Canned	0.25	CUP	30.74	2.17	2.79	1.37	1.74	0.67	324.80	46.98
Turkey Gravy, Canned	0.25	CUP	30.60	1.56	3.06	1.26	1.20	0.37	346.20	65.40
Steak Sauce, Tomato-Base	1	TBSP	9.67	0.25	2.45	0.04	0.00	0.01	232.63	64.26
Pepper Sauce (Tabasco)	1	TSP	0.60	0.06	0.04	0.04	0.00	0.01	31.65	6.40
Soy Sauce (Shoyu)	1	TBSP	9.54	0.93	1.53	0.01	0.00	0.00	1028.70	32.40
Spaghetti Sauce with Beef/Meat (not Lamb or Mutton)	0.5	CUP	143.82	8.12	10.60	8.37	23.28	2.26	588.69	549.98
Cocktail Sauce	0.25	CUP	59.47	0.92	15.15	0.44	0.00	0.06	626.85	275.51
Tartar Sauce	1	TBSP	72.07	0.14	1.98	7.25	5.42	1.07	99.75	5.11
Cranberry Sauce, Sweetened with Sugar, Canned	0.25	CUP	104.56	0.13	26.94	0.10	0.00	0.01	20.08	18.01
TOPPINGS/ACCOMPANIMENTS:										
Salsa	2	TBSP	4.48	0.20	1.00	0.04	0.00	0.01	69.44	34.08
Catsup	1	TBSP	15.60	0.22	4.09	0.05	0.00	0.01	177.90	72.15
Yellow Mustard	1	TSP	5.00	0.10	0.10	0.20	0.00	0.00	63.00	7.00
Dill Pickle	1	ITEM	11.70	0.40	2.68	0.12	0.00	0.03	833.30	75.40
Sweet (Gherkin) Pickle, Small	1	ITEM	17.55	0.05	4.77	0.04	0.00	0.01	140.85	4.80
Black Olives, Ripe, Canned	3	ITEM	15.18	0.11	0.83	1.41	0.00	0.19	115.10	1.06
Bacon Bits, Meatless	1	TBSP	31.08	2.24	2.00	1.81	0.00	0.28	123.90	10.15
Honey	1	TSP	21.28	0.02	5.77	0.00	0.00	0.00	0.28	3.64
Jam (Preserves)	1.00	TBSP	48.40	0.14	12.88	0.04	0.00	0.00	8.00	15.40
Jelly	1.00	TBSP	51.49	0.08	13.45	0.02	0.00	0.00	6.84	12.16
Light Corn Syrup	1	TBSP	56.40	0.00	15.32	0.00	0.00	0.00	24.20	0.80
Maple Syrup	0.25	CUP	209.60	0.00	53.76	0.16	0.00	0.03	7.20	163.20
Reduced Calorie Pancake Syrup	0.25	CUP	98.40	0.00	26.58	0.00	0.00	0.00	120.00	1.80
Chocolate Syrup, Thin	2	TBSP	81.75	0.71	22.09	0.34	0.00	0.19	36.00	84.00
Whipped Cream Topping, Pressurized	2	TBSP	19.29	0.24	0.94	1.67	5.70	1.04	9.75	11.05
Non-Dairy Dessert Topping, Semi Solid, Frozen	1	TBSP	38.19	0.15	2.77	3.04	0.00	2.61	3.04	2.18
White Granulated Sugar	1	TSP	15.48	0.00	4.00	0.00	0.00	0.00	0.04	0.08
Brown Sugar	1	TSP	11.28	0.00	2.92	0.00	0.00	0.00	1.17	10.38
Powdered Sugar, Sifted	1	CUP	389.00	0.00	99.50	0.10	0.00	0.02	1.00	2.00

Beta-C	Vit C	Calcium	Iron	Vit E (IU)	Zinc	Diet Fiber	Sugar
	8.02	8.58	0.47		0.15	0.86	2.33
	13.91	11.48	0.64		0.26	1.35	0.79
27.25	2.19	5.94	0.28		0.06	0.38	3.65
0.00	0.00	10.18	0.41		0.02	0.16	
0.00	0.00	3.48	0.41		0.58	0.23	
0.00	0.00	2.40	0.42		0.48	0.24	
	2.58	2.80	0.14		0.06	0.28	
3.05	0.23	0.60	0.06		0.01	0.03	0.00
0.00	0.00	3.06	0.36		0.07	0.14	1.53
	18.72	29.49	1.76		1.72	2.10	
	9.64	17.03	0.41		0.22	1.90	
	0.07	3.12	0.11		0.03	0.03	
	1.39	2.77	0.15		0.04	0.69	
	2.22	4.80	0.16		0.04	0.26	
14.40	2.27	2.85	0.11		0.03	0.20	1.67
0.00	0.00	4.00	0.10			0.06	0.00
6.50	1.24	5.85	0.35		0.09	0.78	
1.35	0.18	0.60	0.09		0.01	0.17	
0.79	0.12	11.62	0.44		0.03	0.42	
0.00	0.13	7.07	0.05		0.13	0.71	
0.00	0.04	0.42	0.03		0.02	0.01	5.73
0.10	1.76	4.00	0.10		0.01	0.22	9.70
0.19	0.17	1.52	0.04		0.01	0.19	7.89
0.00	0.00	0.60	0.01		0.00	0.00	10.20
0.00	0.00	53.60	0.96		3.33	0.00	50.96
0.00	0.00	0.60	0.01		0.01	0.00	23.03
	0.08	5.25	0.79		0.27	0.68	22.01
	0.00	7.58	0.00		0.03	0.00	
	0.00	0.76	0.01		0.00	0.00	
0.00	0.00	0.04	0.00		0.00	0.00	3.88
0.00	0.00	2.55	0.06		0.01	0.00	2.69
0.00	0.00	1.00	0.06		0.03	0.00	93.00

Index

acesulfame K, 24
adequate intake (AI), 67
aerobics, 155–56, 160, 162
aging, herbal support for, 231–32
alcohol
  and iron deficiency, 88
  and pregnancy, 249
allergies. *See* food allergies
allyl sulphides, 198
aloe, 238
amaranath, 22
amino acids
  as ergogenic aid, 187–88
  essential, 27
  megadosing on supplements, 33
anaphylactic shock, 218
anemia, 74
angel-devil smoothie, 127
anorexia nervosa, 314–16
Anorexia Nervosa and Bulimia Association, 320
antibodies, 217, 218
  function of, 24
antioxidants, 76–78, 186, 196–97
aphrodisiac, 231
apples, 108
apricots, 108
arthritis
  alternative remedy for, 235–36
  herbal remedy for, 235
artichokes, 105
artificial sweeteners, 22–24, 250
asparagus, 105
asparagus with dijon sauce, 328

aspartame, 23
avocados, 108
awesome pineapple cake, 126–27

baby formula, 272
baked chicken parmesan, 123–24
Balance Bar, 185
banana-berry frosty, 277
banana-health split, 128
bananas, 108
barley, 22, 112
beans. *See* legumes
beef, leanest choices, 112–13
bee pollen, 188
benign prostatic hyperplasia (BPH), 230
beriberi, 72
beta-carotene, 5, 70, 76, 198
bilberry, 237
bio-electrical impedance, 291
Bio-X, 185
birth defects, neural-tube, 74
black cohosh, 229
blood pressure
  diastolic, 51
  high, 49–51, 229, 232, 233, 238
  systolic, 50–51
blood sugar
  conditions, 19
  regulation of, 18
blueberries, 108
body fat, methods for measuring, 289–91
body mass index (BMI), 288
body weight, healthy, 287–89

bones
  and calcium, 81–82, 246–47
  peak adult mass, 82
boron, 188
boswella, 235
botulism, 274
breads, 111, 175
breakfast
  dining out for, 141
  healthful recipes, 120–21
  importance of, 12–13
breakfast berry crêpes, 276, 324
brewer's yeast, 188
BridgePoint Centre for Eating Disorders, 320
broccoli, 105
brussels sprouts, 105
buckwheat, 112
bulgur, 112
bulimia nervosa, 316–18
butter, 38
butterfat (BF), 6
buttermilk, 110

cabbage, 105
caffeine
  as ergogenic aid, 186
  and pregnancy, 249–50
  sensitivity to, 225
cajun red beans and rice, 211
calcium
  during pregnancy, 245–47
  and healthy bones, 81–82
  intake according to age, 82–83
  nondairy, 207
  sources of, 83–85

calorie-free, defined, 95
calorie-reduced, defined, 95
calories
    deciphering package
        labels, 95
    defined, 7
    and differences in
        nutrition, 8
    "empty," 7
    equivalents in food
        servings, 9
    excess, 21
    general daily
        requirements, 7–8
    in sample menus, 9–10
    "simple," 17
calories, extra requirement
    during pregnancy, 244–45
calorimeter, 7
Canada's Food Guide to
    Healthy Eating, 3–4
Canadian Society of Allergy
    and Clinical Immunology,
    219
cancer and artificial
    sweeteners, 23–24
cancer prevention
    antioxidants and, 77
    fibre and, 59
    foods and, 195
    fruit and vegetables for,
        198–200
    herbs for, 198, 236
    omega-3 fatty acids and,
        196
    vitamins and, 66
    vitamins for, 197–98
candy. *See* sweets
cantaloupes, 108
carbohydrates
    and blood sugar levels,
        18–19
    complex, 16, 18
    composition of, 16

deciphering nutrition
    labels about, 96
    and endurance sports,
        175–76
    high-glycemic index, 21
    personal requirements,
        20–21
    personal requirements for
        sports, 173–74
    sources of, 4, 22
    and weight gain, 21
"carbo-hydrating," 181
carbo-loading, 177–78
Caribbean rice salad, 330
carnitine, 188
carrots, 105
CATA (Canadian Athletic
    Therapists' Association),
    172
cataracts, 77
cauliflower, 105
cereals, 111
chamomile, 233
cheese, part-skim, 110
cherries, 108
chicken and bean salad,
    121–22
chicken teriyaki over
    linguine, 327
children
    after-school snacks,
        275–76
    dietary guidelines for, 274
    and exercise, 280
    foods to avoid, 273–74
    forming healthy eating
        habits in, 275, 279, 280
    iron deficiency in, 86
    recipes to try, 276–78
    recommended intakes of
        protein, 29
    serving vegetables to,
        279–80
    starting solid foods,
        272–73

and sweets, 278
chili, chunky vegetarian,
    213
Chinese food, 133–34
Chinese green tea, 236
cholesterol
    content, of common
        foods, 40–41
    deciphering package
        labels about, 97
    excess, 39
    fats and high-level of,
        41–41
    function of, 39
    lowering, 59
    recommended intake of,
        43
    saturated fat and, 40
    sources of, 39
cholesterol-free, defined, 97
choline, 188
chondroiten, 235–36
chromium picolinate,
    188–89
chunky vegetable lentil
    soup, 126
cinnamon apple phyllo
    rolls, 329
Cliff Bar, 185
clostridium botulinum, 274
cobalamin, 74
coenzyme Q10, 189
colds. *See* respiratory
    ailments
compulsive overeating,
    318–19
constipation, 251
cooking
    cookbook library, 129
    healthful, 117–20
    modifying recipes with
        substitutions, 120
    oils, 116, 118
cooling down, 156–57, 264

corn, 105–6
    treating allergy to, 220
cottage cheese, dry-cured, 110
coumestans, 200
Cox-2 inhibitors, 198
CPTN (Canadian Personal Trainers' Network), 172
cretine phosphate, 187
cross conditioners, 167
cross-country ski machines, 167
CSEP (Canadian Society for Exercise Physiology), 172
cucumber yogurt dip, 214
curried chicken and rice, 326
cyclamate, 23

dementia, 73, 74
depression, 72
    herbal remedies for, 231–32
dermatitis, 73
desserts, healthful recipes, 126–28
diabetes, 22
diabetes mellitus, 19
diarrhea, 73
diastolic pressure, 51
Dietary Reference Intakes, for calcium, 82–83
dietary reference intakes (DRIs), 67
dieting. *See* weight control; weight loss
dining out
    breakfast, 141
    brunch, 141
    Chinese food, 133–34
    fast food, 140–41
    French food, 134–35
    Indian food, 135–36
    Italian food, 136–37

Japanese food, 137
    key questions to ask before ordering, 132
    Mexican food, 138
    North American food, 138–39
    vegetarians, 209
dinner, healthful recipes for, 123–24
diverticulosis, 59
Dr. Atkins Diet, 286
dong quai, 238
double-blind food-challenge test, 220

eating disorders
    anorexia nervosa, 314–16
    bulimia nervosa, 316–18
    compulsive overeating, 318–19
    getting help for, 319–21
    and ideal of beauty, 313
Eating Disorders Clinic (St. Pauls Hospital, Vancouver), 320
Eating Disorder Unit (Douglas Hospital, Montreal), 321
Eating Disorder Unit (Queen Elizabeth II Health Sciences Centre, Nova Scotia), 321
eating habits
    balanced, 12
    and holidays, 143–44
    moderation principle, 11
    overconsumption of salt, 48
    overeating, 131
    personal eating regimen, 12–13
    variety in diet, 11
echinacea, 234–35
edema, 252
eggplant parmigiana, 326

eggplant, 106
eggs
    allergy treatment for, 220
    daily servings during pregnancy, 246
    nutritional value, 114
    preseparated whites of, 114
    yolk, 7
egg substitute, 114
endurance sports, 175–77
Energy Blast, 185
energy, defined, 95
enzymes, function of, 23
ephedra (ma huang), 189, 238
ergogenic aids, 186–91
estimated average requirement (EAR), 67
evening primrose oil, 229–30
exercise
    activities available, 162–63
    aerobics, 155–56, 160, 162
    benefits of, 154
    "carbo-hydrating," 181
    children and, 280
    consistency of regular activity, 154
    deciding on a program, 161–62
    duration, frequency, 156
    equipment, 166–68
    everyday activities as, 163
    and free radicals, 78
    goals and expectations, 154
    intensity of, 156, 157–58
    major muscle groups, 169–71
    myths, 160–61
    personal trainers, 171–72

pre-event meals, 179–81
recovery foods, 181–82
stretching, 157
weight training, 158–60
See also pregnancy,
exercise

fast foods, 140–41
fat-combo foods, 304–5
fat-free
defined, 97
diets, 44–45
fatigue, herbal remedies for,
232
fats
animal, 37
benefits of, 36
deciphering package
labels about, 96–97
detecting foods with high
content of, 101
in foods, 43
and high cholesterol,
40–42
macronutrient, 15
recommended intake of,
43
reducing intake of, 44
types of, 36–38
feverfew, 236
fibre
deciphering nutrition
labels, 96
dietary, 57
foods rich in, 61–62
increasing intakes of,
60–61
insoluable, 58
overloading on, 63
recommended intake of,
60
for reducing cholesterol,
59

and regularity, 59
soluable, 58, 59
fish
and cancer prevention,
196
daily servings during
pregnancy, 246
fattier varieties, 114
leanest choices of, 114
nutrition value of, 113
signs of freshness, 113
fish-oil supplements, 36
Fit for Life diet, 287
flaxseed, 196
flaxseed oil, 196
fluids
daily servings during
pregnancy, 246
during pregnancy, 249
sports drinks, 184
fluoride, 81
flu. *See* respiratory ailments
folacin. *See* Vitamins, folate
folate, 250
folic acid. *See* vitamins,
folate
food additives, 221
food allergies
and anaphylactic shock,
218
diagnosing, 218–20
and food intolerance,
218, 221
immune system and,
217–18
treating, 220–21
food-combining weight-loss
programs, 287
food-elimination diet, 219
food groups
grain products group, 4–5
meat and alternatives
group, 6

milk products group, 5
other foods group, 6–7
vegetables and fruit
group, 5
food intolerance, 218
lactose intolerance,
221–24
Food and Nutrition Board of
the National Academy of
Sciences, 67
food plans
1,200-calorie, 296–97
1,400-calorie, 298–99
1,600-calorie, 300–1
1,800-calorie, 302–3
food poisoning, 218
foods
grain, 22
processed, 52
raw, 249
food sensitivity, 218
caffeine, 225
free radicals, 76, 196–97
free weights, 168
French food, 134–35
fructose, 16, 17
fruit
beta-carotene rich, 248
canned, 107
children, dietary
guidelines for, 274
cooking with, 119
daily servings during
pregnancy, 245
drinks and cocktails, 6
freshness, 104
frozen, 104, 107
guidelines for vegetarian
diet, 204
in high-carb diet, 175
juices, 5, 17, 107–8, 310
nutrients in, 5, 17
puréed, 118

vitamin C-rich, 248

gamma-linolenic acid (GLA), 229
gamma-oryzanol, 189
garden tostada, 325
garlic, 198, 233
Genisoy, 186
ginger, 237
gingko biloba, 231
ginseng, Asian, 232–33
glandular extracts, 189
gliadin, 224
glucosamine sulphate, 235–36
glucose, 16, 18
gluten, 224
gluten-sensitive enteropathy, 224
glycemic index (GI), 19
glycogen, muscle, 176–77
GMP (good manufacturing practices) label, 89
goldenseal, 234
grain products
    children, dietary guidelines for, 274
    daily servings during pregnancy, 245
    nutrients in, 4
    in vegetarian diet, 204
grapefruits, 108
grapes, 108
Greek "village" salad, 324
green tea, Chinese, 236

Harvey's, 141
hawthorn, 233
HDL, 41–42
headaches, migraines, 236
heartburn, 253
heart disease
    antioxidants and, 77

cholesterol and, 39
herbal remedies for, 233–34
and vegetarian diet, 205
vitamins and, 66
heme iron, 87, 207
hemoglobin, 85
    function of, 24
hemorrhaging, 72, 76
herbal teas, 250
herbs
    for female health, 228–30
    for male health, 230–31
    quality of supplements, 227–28
high-calorie nutritional snacks, 311
high-carb diet, 175
high-fat foods, daily servings during pregnancy, 246
high-protein, no-carb weight-loss programs, 286
high source of dietary fibre, meaning of, 96
honey glazed carrots, 125
hormones, function of, 24
hydration, 183–84
hydrogenation, 38
hyperglycemia, 19
hypertension
    condition, 49
    herbal remedies for, 229, 233
    herbs to avoid for, 232, 238
    risk factors, 50
    treating, 51
    and vegetarian diet, 205
hypertrophy, 33, 158, 160
hypoglycemia, 19

ice cream, low-fat, 110
immune system, antioxidants and, 77

Indian food, 135–36
indigestion, 237
infants
    baby formula, 272
    breastfeeding, 271
    convulsions in, 74
    recommended intakes of protein, 29
ingredient lists, 100–1
insomnia, 229, 232
insulin, 22
iron
    absorption, 85, 89

    deficiency, 86, 87–88
    heme, 87, 207, 248
    increasing intake, 86–87
    nonheme, 87, 207, 248
    and red blood cells, 85
    role of, 85–86
    sources of, 87, 207, 248
    supplements, 85, 89
irritable bowel syndrome, 225
isoflavones, 200
isolated soy protein, 206
Italian food, 136–37

jam in popovers, 323
Japanese food, 137

kasha, 112
kava-kava, 232
Kegal exercises, 267
kiwi, 108

labels, package, deciphering, 93–99, 100–1
lactase enzyme pills, 223
lactose intolerance, 221–24
lacto-vegetarians, 205
lamb, leanest choices, 113
LDL, 42

legumes, 114
lemons, 108
lettuce, 106
light, claim, 101
lignans, 200
Lindsay, Anne, 129
"lite," claim, 101
liver, and production of cholesterol, 39
liver disease, herbal remedy for, 234
low-calorie, defined, 95
low in cholesterol, defined, 97
low-fat apple streusel pot pie, 148
low in fat, defined, 97
low in saturated fat, defined, 97
lunch, healthful recipes for, 121–22
lycopene, 198

McDonald's, 141
macronutrients
    ideal proportions in daily diet, 15–16
    See also under specific macronutrient
ma huang. *See* ephedra
mangos, 108
margarine, 38
MCT (medium chain triglycerides), 189–90
meals
    Christmas, 148–49
    Easter, 144
    Hanukkah, 147–48
    Passover, 144–45
    pre-event (sports), 179–81
    summer long weekends, 145–46
    Thanksgiving, 146–47

meat
    beef, 112–13
    children, dietary guidelines for, 274
    cured and smoked, 54
    daily servings during pregnancy, 246
    grading symbols for beef, 112
    lamb, 113
    nutrients in, 6
    pork, 113
    trimming, 118
    veal, 113
menopausal symptoms, herbal remedies for, 230, 238
menstruation symptoms, herbal remedies for, 229–30, 233, 237, 238
MET Rx, 185
Mexican food, 138
Mexican-style egg white omelet, 121
micronutrients, 66
migraines, 236
milk
    1%, 110
    allergy treatment for, 220
    breast, 271
    cow's, 220
    evaporated skim, 110
    skim, 110
milkfat (MF), 6
milk products
    daily servings during pregnancy, 246
    in high-carb diet, 175
    low-fat, 110
milk thistle, 234
millet, 22, 112
minerals, 66, 78–79

Recommended Daily Intakes for, 99
    See also under specific minerals
Mr. Sub, 141
moderate-protein, moderate-carb weight-loss programs, 286
monounsaturated fat, 37
morning sickness, 237, 251–52
MSG (monosodium glutamate), 54, 221, 250
muscle glycogen, 176–77
mushrooms, 106
myoglobin, 85
Myoplex Plux, 185

National Eating Disorder Information Centre, 320
nectarines, 108
nervous disorders, 74
niacin, 73
nitrates, 249
nitrites, 249
nitrosamines, 249
nonheme iron, 87, 207
North American food, 138–39
nutrition label challenge, 99–100
nuts
    allergy treatment for, 220
    daily servings during pregnancy, 246
    toasting, 118

okra, 106
older adults, and iron deficiency, 85, 88
olive oil, extra-virgin, 118
omega-3 fatty acids, 37
onions, 106

oranges, 108
Ornish, Dean, 129
osteoarthritis, 235
oxidation, 76

pain, 160
papaya sorbet, 331
peaches, 108
peanut butter yogurt milkshake, 278
pears, 108
peas, 106, 114
penne with mushroom and spicy tomato sauce, 123
peppermint, 237–38
peppers, sweet, 106
percentages, on nutritional labels, 98
personal trainers, 171–72
pesco-vegetarians, 205
PFLC (Professional Fitness and Lifestyle Consultant), 172
phosphates, 187
phosphorous, 81
phytochemicals, 198, 199
phytoestrogens, 200
phytonutrients, 200
Pickhaven Centre, 320
pineapples, 108
Pizza Hut, 141
PKU, 23
polenta, 112
polyunsaturated fat, 37, 116
and cancer prevention, 196
popcorn, jazzed-up, 277
pork, leanest choices, 113
potato and caramelized onion gratin, 149
potatoes, 18, 106
poultry, leanest choices, 113
Power Bar Harvest, 185

pregnancy
benefits of being physically fit, 261, 263
calcium requirements, 246–47
caloric needs, 244–45
eating plan, 244–45
five-day meal plan, 253–59
foods to avoid, 249
fruit and vegetables for healthy baby, 248
iron, 248
proper hydration, 249
recommended intake of protein during, 30
side effects, 250–53
weight gain, 244–45
————. exercise
conditions precluding, 263
guidelines for, 262–63
intensity of, 264–65
low risks, 261–62
prenatal classes, 266–67
proper warm-up and cooling down, 264
safe forms of, 265–68
types of activity to avoid, 265–66
See also exercise
premenstrual syndrome (PMS), 230
PR Ironman, 185
PromaxBar, 185
prostaglandins, 230
prostate disorders, 230
protein powder, 33
Protein Power Diet, 286
proteins
animal and plant, 27–29
building blocks of, 26

combining complementary, 28–29
complete, 27
composition of, 26
content, in common foods, 30–31
content, in typical meal, 32
deciphering nutritional labels about, 95
deficiency of, 34
excess, 32–33
function of, 25–26
growth and maintenance, 24
incomplete, 27–28
and muscle development, 33, 160
personal requirements, 29–30
requirements for athletes, 178–79
sources of, 6
soy, 206–7
Pure Protein, 185
pygeum africanum, 230
pyridoxine, 74
pyruvate, 190

quinoa, 22

raspberries, 108
RAST (radioallergosorbent test), 219
recommended dietary allowances (RDAs), 67
recommended nutrient intakes (RINs), 66
Recommended Nutrient Intakes (RNIs), 29–30, 98–99
Reisman, Rose, 129
respiratory ailments, herbal remedies for, 234–35

rhubarb, 106
riboflavin, 73
rice
    brown, 112
    instant white, 112
    polished white, 112
    wild, 22
rosemary, 237
rowing machines, 167

St. John's Wort, 232
salad bar, 105
salt
    common foods high in,
        52–53
    composition of, 48
    deciphering nutrition
        labels about, 98
    detecting foods with high
        content of, 101
    and high blood pressure,
        49–50
    recommended intake, 52
    reducing intake of, 53–54
    and thirst, 48
    and water retention, 49
salt-free, defined, 98
saturated fat, 37, 40, 97
sautéed spinach with pine
    nuts, 125
saw palmetto, 230
Scarsdale Diet, 286
Scientific Review Committee
    (Health and Welfare
    Canada), 66
scrambled tofu, 214
scurvy, 76
seasonal affective disorder,
    232
semivegetarians, 205
serving size, on package
    labels, 95
shakes, for weight gain, 311

shellfish, treating allergy to,
    220
shopping
    for breads and cereals,
        111
    for canned soups, 115
    for condiment, 115

    for dairy products, 110
    for dressings, 116
    for eggs, 114
    for fats, 116
    for fish and seafood,
        113–14
    for frozen meals, 115
    for fruits, 107–9
    for grains, 112
    for legumes, 114
    list, 103–4
    for meat, 112–13
    for pasta, 112
    for poultry, 113
    for rice, 112
    for sauces, 115
    snacks, 115
    for spreads, 116
    for vegetables, 104–7
side dishes, recipes for,
    125–26
sit-ups, 268
skillet pork chops with sweet
    potatoes and couscous, 124
skin conditions, 73
skin-fold calipers, 290
skin test, 219
sleep problems, herbal
    remedies for, 231–32
smilax, 190
smoking, and calcium
    deficiency, 88
snacks
    after-schools, 275–76

high-calorie and
    nutritional, 311
    shopping for, 115
    for weight gain, 310
sodium, 48, 97–98
    See also salt
sodium bicarbonate, 187
sodium-free, defined, 98
soft drinks, 17
See also sweets
Somers, Suzanne, 287
Something Fishy Website on
    Eating Disorders, 320
source of dietary fibre,
    meaning of, 96
soy
    beverages, 206
    and cancer prevention,
        200–1
    flour, 206
    milk fortified with
        calcium, 223
    protein, 206–7
    sources of, 201
    treating allergy to, 220
soybeans, vegetable-type,
    206
SoyOne, 186
spicy poached pears, 332
spinach, 106
sports bars, 184–86
sports drinks, 184
Sports-Rx, 185
"spot reducing," myth of,
    159, 161
squash, 107
stairclimbers, 167
starch, 16
stationary bikes, 167
Steel Bar, 185
steroids, 166
Stern, Bonnie, 129
stinging nettle, 230

strawberries, 108
stress, herbal remedies for, 229, 232
stretching, 157, 264
substitutions, low-fat, 120
succinate, 190
sucralose, 23
sugar
    complex, 16, 18
    content, in cereals, 111
    detecting foods with high content of, 101
    simple, 16–17
    See also blood sugar
SugarBusters! diet, 286
sulphites, 221
sweet potatoes, 107
sweet potato stew, 331
sweets, 16–17
Swiss Chalet, 141
systolic pressure, 50–51

"talk" test, 158
tangerines, 108
tartrazine, 221
tea
    black, 198
    green, 198, 236
tempeh, 206–7
texturized vegetable protein (TVP), 206
thiamin, 72–73
tocopherols, 71–72
tofu, 207, 214, 246
tolerable upper limit (UL), 67
tomatoes, 107
    and cancer prevention, 198
tooth decay, 17
total blood cholesterol, 41
trace minerals, 79
traditional tapioca, 328

training heart rate formula, 157–58
trans-fatty acids, 38
treadmills, 167
triglyceride (TG), 36–37, 39
tuna salad cones, 277
tuna salad melt, 122

underwater weighing, 290
underweight, 309–312

upset stomach, 237
urine, and hydration, 184

valerian root (valeriana officinalis), 228–29
vanadyl sulphate, 190
vanilla French toast with fresh fruit, 120
veal, leanest choices, 113
vegans, 205
vegetables
    benefits of, 205
    beta-carotene rich, 248
    and cancer prevention, 198–200
    children, dietary guidelines for, 274
    cooking, 204
    daily servings during pregnancy, 246
    as fat replacements, 119
    freshness, 104
    frozen, 104
    getting children to eat, 279–80
    guidelines for vegetarian diet, 204
    high-calcium, 204
    in high-carb diet, 175
    nutrients in, 5
    prewashed, precut salad, 104

proteins derived from, 27–28
    shopping tips for buying, 104–7
    vitamin C-rich, 248
vegetarian diet
    B-12 deficiency in, 208
    and dining out, 209
    guidelines for, 203–4
    and iron deficiency, 86, 88
    iron needs, 207
    meal plan, 208–9
    meat alternatives, 204
    meatless recipes, 210–15
    milk alternatives, 204
    non-diary calcium for, 207
    protein sources, 205–7
    types of, 205
    zinc needs, 208
vegetarian spinach lasagna, 212
very high source of dietary fibre, meaning of, 96
vitamin A, 70–71
beta-carotene, 5, 76, 198
vitamin B
    B-1, 71–72
    B-2, 73
    B-3, 73
    B-6, 74
    B-12, 74, 190–91, 208
vitamin C, 66, 75–76, 76, 197
vitamin D, 71, 81
vitamin E, 66, 71, 76, 78, 197
vitamin K, 72
vitamins
    fat-soluable, 67
    folate, 66, 74–75, 250
    ingesting prenatal, 252

megadosing on, 65–66
organic compounds, 67
prenatal, 75
Recommended Daily
    Intakes for, 98–99
recommended dietary
    allowances, 68–69
water-soluable, 70, 72–76

walking, as exercise, 265–66
warm-up, 155, 264
water
    loss of, 32
    plain, 184
    retention, 48–49
watermelon, 108
water *See* fluids
weight control
    and artificial sweeteners,
        23
    and excess protein, 32–33
    exercise and, 306
    measures for, 306
    reducing fat intake, 44
    and triglycerides, 39
weight gain
    during pregnancy, 244–45
    and fat intake, 42
    and high-fat foods, 21
    increasing calorie intake,
        310
    sample menu for, 312
weight loss
    1,200-calorie food plan,
        296–97

1,400-calorie, 298–99
1,600-calorie, 300–1
1,800-calorie food plan,
    302–3
charting daily food
    intake, 295–303
determining target calorie
    intake, 291–92
and eating behaviour, 287
exercise and, 306
fad diets, 285–87
fat-combo foods, 304–5
food-combining
    programs, 287
food plans, 292–95
and high-protein diets,
    32–33
high-protein, no-carb
    programs, 286
moderate-protein,
    moderate-carb programs,
    286
personal plan, 292
realistic goals, 305
reasons for failure, 304
weight training
    benefits of, 159
    combining cardio and,
        160
    during pregnancy, 267–68
    exercises, 170–71
    machines, 168
    and muscle bulk, 161
    split routines, 159
    terminology, 165–66
Wendy's, 141

Westwind Eating Disorder
    Recovery Centre, 321
wheat
    allergy treatment, 220,
        224
    cracked, 112
wheat berries, 22, 112
wheat bread, 111
whole-wheat bread, 111
whole-wheat flour, 119
women
    herbal remedies for,
        228–30, 233, 237, 238
    and hormone-related
        cancers, 200
    and iron deficiency, 86,
        88
    and irritable bowel
        syndrome, 225
    morning sickness, 251–52
    postpartum, 266
    realistic body weight, 289
    recommended intakes of
        protein, 30
    See also pregnancy;
        pregnancy, exercise

yogurts, low-fat, 110
yohimbe, 231

The Zone Diet, 286

About the Authors

Leslie Beck, a registered dietitian, is one of Canada's leading nutritionists and operates a successful private practice and corporate practice with many of Canada's leading businesses, international food companies, and sports organizations. For the past 12 years, she has helped over 1,500 individuals achieve their nutrition and health goals. Leslie operates an "integrative nutrition practice," offering clients both dietary advice and science-based recommendations on the use of nutritional and herbal supplements.

The media recognizes Leslie Beck as an authority on nutrition and food issues. Leslie has appeared as guest and host on a variety of nutrition-related television shows and she appears regularly as a nutrition expert on *Canada AM*. She has written for numerous publications and is author of *Managing Menopause with Diet, Vitamins and Herbs: An Essential Guide for the Peri and Post Menopausal Years* and contributing author of Rose Reisman's *Sensationally Light Pasta & Grains*. Born and raised in Vancouver, Leslie now lives in Toronto.

Joy Bauer a registered dietitian, recently named "Best Nutritionist in New York City" by New York magazine, maintains a thriving private practice where she provides counselling to both adults and children dealing with a variety of nutritional concerns, including weight management, eating disorders, cardiac rehabilitation, sports nutrition, food allergies, gastrointestinal disorders, pregnancy, lactation, and menopause.

In addition, Joy serves as the nutrition consultant for Columbia Presbyterian Medical Center in Manhattan, where she designs and supervises the nutritional component of ongoing research in the area of eating disorders. An active speaker in her field, Joy regularly lectures and conducts workshops on nutrition and fitness for corporations, public and private schools, colleges, and universities. Joy lives in New York City with her husband, Ian, her daughter, Jesse, and her son, Cole.